OVER THE COUNTER

PILLS THAT DON'T WORK

OVER THE COUNTER

PILLS THAT DON'T WORK

Joel Kaufman
Linda Rabinowitz-Dagi
Joan Levin
Phyllis McCarthy
Sidney Wolfe, M.D.
Eve Bargmann, M.D.
and the Public Citizen Health
Research Group

Pantheon Books, New York

ACKNOWLEDGMENTS

OTC Pills That Don't Work is the product of the talent, time, labor and dedication of many people. The entire staff of Public Citizen Health Research Group shared in the authorship and production of this book, and others gave generously of advice and support during many months of research and writing.

Four people deserve special thanks:

Allegra Fishel spent long hours producing and editing hundreds of pages of manuscript and making suggestions that resulted in making this a better book.

Michael Coscia, Beth Sharpe, and Richard Anderson of Smith Graphics, Washington, D.C., performed a miracle in producing the final version in recordbreaking time.

Public Citizen Staff:

Cary LaCheen, Health Research Group Science Researcher, assisted with editing, prepared the glossary, helped to compile detailed charts, and made many helpful suggestions resulting in a more understandable book.

Barbara Freese, Health Research Group Science Researcher, prepared footnotes, carried out labeling verification and assisted with text editing and the final compilation of the products chart.

Henry Bergman, Health Research Group Health Care Specialist, assisted with research on drug pricing.

Maggie White, Health Research Group Publications Manager, assisted with countless details of production and provided helpful counsel on design.

Bill Schultz and John Sims, Public Citizen Litigation Group Staff Attorneys, reviewed the manuscript and offered many valuable suggestions.

Alan MacDuffie, Public Citizen's Publication Business Manager, helped with production and gave advice on text design.

Allen Greenberg, Health Research Group Staff Attorney, contributed his proofreading and editing skills and assisted with product labeling verification.

Benjamin Gordon, Health Research Group Staff Economist, contributed to sections on the economics of the pharmaceutical industry.

Others:

Peter Serafino, John Levin, and Lois Frankel provided needed technical advice and assistance.

Medical Consultants:

Many experts representing several medical specialties graciously reviewed drafts of individual chapters, and offered suggestions which have resulted in a book which we believe represents the best in current medical thinking:

John Adriani, M.D., Professor of Pharmacology and Anesthesiology, Louisiana State University Medical Center, Emeritus Professor of Surgery, School of Medicine, Tulane University, Emeritus Director of the Department of Anesthesiology, Charity Hospital, all of New Orleans, Louisiana, and former member of the American Medical Association Council on Drugs, reviewed the section on pain.

James Butt, M.D., Professor of Medicine, University of Missouri School of Medicine, Columbia, Missouri, reviewed the sections on constipation, diarrhea, nausea and vomiting, and hemorrhoids.

Sol Katz, M.D., Professor of Medicine, Georgetown University School of Medicine, Washington, D.C., reviewed the sections on cough, cold, allergy and asthma.

Paul Lavietes, M.D., Professor of Medicine, Yale University School of Medicine, New Haven, Connecticut, reviewed the entire book.

Michael Newman, M.D., a physician in private practice in Washington, D.C., reviewed the entire book.

Ethan Sims, M.D., Professor of Medicine, University of Vermont College of Medicine, reviewed the section on weight loss.

Fredric Solomon, M.D., Director of the Division of Mental Health and Behavioral Medicine of the Institute of Medicine of the National Academy of Sciences, Washington, D.C., and Study Director of the Institute of Medicine study *Sleeping Pills, Insomnia, and Medical Practice* reviewed the section on sleep.

Countless others — at Public Citizen and elsewhere — provided help, counsel and encouragement as needed. To them, our appreciation for assisting in a project which we hope will benefit many. And, finally, we acknowledge with special pride and thanks the thousands of Public Citizen contributors in the United States and abroad, whose steady support provides the foundation for the work of Public Citizen Health Research Group.

TABLE OF CONTENTS

TOP-SELLING OTC (OVER THE COUNTER) DRUGS WITH INGREDIENTS LACKING EVIDENCE OF SAFETY OR EFFECTIVENESS (ALL IN TOP 40 DRUGS FOR 1981)[1]

DRUG	1981 RETAIL SALES[2] (MILLIONS)
ANACIN (TABS, CAPS, & EXTRA-STRENGTHS)	$112
LISTERINE MOUTHWASH	$87
NYQUIL	$63.1
PREPARATION H	$61.4
EXCEDRIN	$55.7
DRISTAN TABLETS	$50
SCOPE MOUTHWASH	$41
ROBITUSSIN COUGH SYRUP[3]	$28.5
SINUTAB	$25.5
TOTAL	**$524.2 MILLION**

[1] Top 40 ranking, based on drug product sales in chain drug stores (*Chain Drug Reviews*, February 15, 1982).
[2] 1981 retail sales from a leading drug industry marketing consultant.
[3] Guaifenesin, the only active ingredient in ROBITUSSIN Cough Syrup, was found lacking in evidence of effectiveness by the FDA OTC Review panel and all prescription drugs with this ingredient also lack evidence of effectiveness. FDA has, however, recently begun the process of re-classifying guaifenesin as effective based on a poor-quality study.

INTRODUCTION

What top selling brew costs $10.60 a fifth, is 50 proof and is usually taken straight in a shot glass? Jim Beam? Jack Daniels? No, guess again. This best-selling product is found not in liquor stores but in drug stores. You probably know it best as "the nighttime-sniffling-sneezing-coughing-aching-stuffy-head-fever-so you-can-rest medicine" called NYQUIL. It even comes with its *own* shot glass.

Although the former director of Clinical Research at Vick's Laboratories (now Richardson-Vick) has called NYQUIL, Vick's product, "a witch's brew because it contains everything under the sun,"[1] Americans have spent hundreds of millions of dollars for this heavily advertised product. Like many other best-selling drugs in this book, NYQUIL contains an ingredient which the Food and Drug Administration (FDA) found to lack evidence of effectiveness. NYQUIL, with its four active ingredients, is also an irrational combination — that is, a drug which takes an illogical "shotgun" approach to illness. Clearly, it is less expensive, more effective and safer to treat the particular symptom which bothers you with a single-ingredient drug (if any drug is needed) than to go for the shotgun approach taken by NYQUIL (and many other products). With hundreds of products like NYQUIL, the "uniqueness" they promote is in treating multiple symptoms (which are rarely all present at the same time) with expensive multiple ingredients, which are rarely all safe and effective.

Another kind of hustle involves a "unique" symptom such as an "Excedrin headache" or a seemingly unique ingredient such as "the pain reliever doctors recommend most." Just as NYQUIL represents a classic example of the 3-way, 4-way, or 5-way product approach, over the counter (OTC) pain relievers, with annual sales of well over one billion dollars, are the best example of expensive and contrived variations on a profitable theme.

QUESTION: WHAT IS THE ONLY SAFE AND EFFECTIVE INGREDIENT FOR TREATING PAIN CONTAINED IN THE FOLLOWING PRODUCTS?
ALKA SELTZER PAIN RELIEVER AND ANTACID, ANACIN, MAXIMUM STRENGTH ANACIN, BAYER ASPIRIN, BAYER TIMED-RELEASE ASPIRIN, BUFFERIN, ARTHRITIS STRENGTH BUFFERIN, and COPE.

ANSWER: Aspirin. Any additional ingredients in these products lack evidence of safety or effectiveness for treating pain. The ANACINs and COPE have, for example, caffeine, which lacks evidence of effectiveness. BAYER timed-release dosage form also lacks evidence of effectiveness. If you bought enough of each of these products to be equivalent (in aspirin content) to a bottle of 100 plain 325 mg. aspirin tablets (which you can purchase in a generic or house brand for about $0.99), it would cost you as "little" as $1.99 for BAYER ASPIRIN and as much as $5.50 for ALKA SELTZER. In other words, you pay from 2 to 5½ times as much for aspirin if you buy these heavily advertised brand names than you do if you buy the equally effective generic or store brand aspirin.

QUESTION: WHAT ABOUT ANACIN−3, MAXIMUM STRENGTH ANACIN 3, DATRIL, DATRIL 500, EXCEDRIN PM, PERCOGESIC, TYLENOL, AND EXTRA-STRENGTH TYLENOL?

ANSWER: The only safe and effective pain-killer in any of these is acetaminophen. EXCEDRIN PM and PERCOGESIC both contain antihistamines, which lack evidence of effectiveness for treating pain. If you buy 100 regular acetaminophen tablets generically, it will cost you about $1.79. If you buy enough of the above brand name products to contain an amount of acetaminophen equivalent to 100 regular 325 mg. pills, it will cost from about $3.15 for ANACIN-3 to as much as $7.70 for PERCOGESIC. (66 EXTRA-STRENGTH TYLENOL equals 100 regular acetaminophen.) Once again, if you make the mistake of buying brand name acetaminophen it will cost you from 1.8 times to 4.3 times as much as generic or house brand acetaminophen, with no gain — except to those selling the products.

Every day, on television, on the radio, in newspapers, in magazines, drug companies spend millions of your dollars to tell you about the wonders of their special and "unique" over the counter (OTC) remedies for all that ails you.

You listen, you buy. If you are an average American, you spend over $40.00 a year on over the counter drugs — well over $100 a year for a family of four. Many of you spend much more, particularly older people and anyone living alone. You are buying some of an estimated 300,000 "different" over the counter drug products which are concocted **OUT OF A MERE 1000 OR SO DIFFERENT INGREDIENTS.** But listen: it turns out that **FEWER THAN 1/3 OF THESE OVER THE COUNTER DRUG INGREDIENTS HAVE BEEN SHOWN TO BE SAFE AND EFFECTIVE FOR THEIR INTENDED USES.**

In other words, many OTC drug products which you purchase contain one or more ingredients which do not meet the Federal drug law standards for safety, effectiveness or both. Examples include ANACIN, DRISTAN TABLETS, EXCEDRIN, NYQUIL, PERCOGISIC, PREPARATION H and many more. Of the more than 10 billion dollars Americans spend each year on OTC drugs, at least 3 or 4 billion dollars are wasted on grossly overpriced products or products with ingredients lacking evidence of safety or effectiveness.

Since all drug ingredients have risks, extra ingredients which aren't effective or which lack evidence of effectiveness subject you to extra risks without providing compensating benefits. So you are not only wasting your money when you buy products with such ingredients, but you are also risking your health and that of your family. By now, you must have some questions:

QUESTION: WHO SAYS THESE OVER THE COUNTER DRUG INGREDIENTS LACK EVIDENCE OF SAFETY OR EFFECTIVENESS?

ANSWER: Starting 10 years ago, the U.S. Food and Drug Administration (FDA) established a large number of over the counter drug advisory panels — including physicians, pharmacists and other technically qualified people. They reviewed, by therapeutic category (such as cough and cold, or nighttime sleep-aids), the ingredients contained in approximately 300,000 brands of over the counter (OTC) drugs to determine if these ingredients were safe and effective.

As mentioned above, and according to the FDA's Director of OTC Drug Evaluation, Dr. William Gilbertson, only "about ⅓ of the ingredients reviewed by the panels have been shown to be safe and effective for their intended uses."

In addition to ingredients or combinations of ingredients not found safe and effective by the FDA panels, in a number of instances other ingredients such as PPA (phenylpropanolamine, the main ingredient in most OTC diet pills) have been judged by the Public Citizen Health Research Group and its consultants (based on published medical studies) to lack evidence of safety or effectiveness. As seen in the BRAND NAME INDEX in Part II, when HRG disagrees with the FDA panel finding (FDA, YES; HRG, NO), the reason is stated.

QUESTION: BUT I'VE USED MANY OF THE PRODUCTS WITH INGREDIENTS YOU SAY DON'T WORK. THEY SEEMED TO WORK FOR ME.

ANSWER: There are two main reasons why people seem to get better, and often do get better, when taking OTC drugs. First, most of the diseases for which self-medication is appropriate are so-called self-limiting diseases, like the cold, which get better no matter what you do. Second, many of the products with ingredients lacking evidence of effectiveness have at least one effective ingredient. So if your symptoms respond quickly, even sooner than if the problem ran its natural course, it is probably due to that ingredient, such as aspirin or acetaminophen in a multiple ingredient pain-relief product. The other, ineffective ingredients are not only costing you additional money but are also exposing you to the unneeded risks of ingredients which don't work. (See later part of INTRODUCTION, in which Combination Drug Products are discussed.)

QUESTION: IF FDA EXPERT PANELS HAVE FOUND ONLY ⅓ OF THE INGREDIENTS THEY REVIEWED TO BE SAFE AND EFFECTIVE FOR THEIR INTENDED USES, WHY ARE PRODUCTS CONTAINING UNPROVEN INGREDIENTS STILL BEING SOLD?

ANSWER: This question has a practical answer and a legal answer. The practical answer is that too many companies are making too much money from these products to do otherwise. If they reformulated, omitting all ingredients which are not safe and effective, there would be far fewer "different" products on the market. This would be simpler and less expensive for consumers, but less profitable for the drug industry.

The legal answer is that the FDA is violating the drug laws by allowing these ingredients, which do not meet the legal standards for safety and effectiveness, to remain on the market. Even though the expert FDA panels made decisions on many of these ingredients as long as several years ago, FDA officials, under pressure from the OTC drug companies, have not implemented the findings of the panels. The Public Citizen Litigation Group, on behalf of several consumers, has sued the FDA in federal court to speed up the process of removing these products from the market. These lawsuits continue.

QUESTION: ARE YOU AGAINST SELF-MEDICATION? WOULD YOU RATHER HAVE PEOPLE GO TO THE DOCTOR EVERY TIME THEY ARE SICK, WHICH WILL NOT ONLY COST MORE BUT USUALLY RESULT IN A PRESCRIPTION DRUG WHICH MAY BE MORE DANGEROUS THAN MOST OTC DRUGS?

ANSWER: No. Quite the opposite. Aside from listing many widely-sold OTC drugs containing ingredients which are not safe and effective, the other main purpose of this book is to be a guide to appropriate self-treatment for a variety of problems. Self-treatment, although it includes self-medication, also includes many non-drug approaches to problems such as sleeping difficulties, losing weight, coughs and colds, constipation and other ailments. Another purpose of this book is to discuss those warning signals of serious illness which should prompt a trip to the doctor or other health care professional.

QUESTION: WHAT IS A HEALTH CARE PROFESSIONAL?

ANSWER: When used in this book, the term refers to someone who is trained to diagnose disease and determine whether there is a need for medical treatment. Examples include physicians, physicians' assistants, and nurse practitioners.

You still have questions?

QUESTION: Are there some people who should be particularly careful about taking drugs, especially often questionable over the counter drugs?

ANSWER: Certainly. Pregnant or nursing women, because they pass the drug on to the fetus or infant; and the elderly. Older people often do not metabolize or clean drugs out of their bodies as easily as younger people.

QUESTION: Is there *ever* any advantage to brand name OTC products when a less expensive alternative is available?

ANSWER: No, unless you enjoy subsidizing TV ads at your own expense. The main difference is that "created" by advertising geniuses.

OTC DRUG ADVERTISING: IT WORKS

ADS FOR CONSUMERS

The story of why 10 billion dollars worth of OTC drugs are bought every year is mainly a story of successful and expensive advertising. Listen to Harvard Medical School Professor Dr. Franz Ingelfinger, the former editor of the *New England Journal of Medicine*:

The promoter, in coaxing or authoritarian tones, advises you to put your faith in the health or comfort-promoting effects of a "special ingredient," a product with "extra strength" or an agent "most recommended by doctors," but the nature of the potent miracle drug is not revealed. It might be snake oil, sassafras, or Dr. Pangloss' magic powder. Such ads are designed to outsmart too trusting or unwary prospects. . .

Drugs affect health, the most precious of human possessions. Yet OTC products are marketed on TV by methods similar to those used to promote underwear, house paint, and laundry soap. Indeed, as described by one TV ad creator, TV commercials observe a basic routine: "Thirty times a night you'll see it. Seven seconds of the problem, fourteen seconds of solution when somebody tells the poor slob with the problem how the product can solve it, seven seconds of reward and a closing two second shot of the package."[3]

The highly competitive pain-killer (internal analgesic) market shows what advertising dollars can buy. In 1981, the 5 leading product lines (the TYLENOLs, ANACINs, BAYERs, BUFFERINs, and EXCEDRINs) spent approximately 150 million dollars in advertising.[4] The largest ad budget for any of these products (possibly the largest for any OTC product) was for ANACIN, tablets and capsules, with 27.5 million dollars spent (45 million for all ANACIN products).

With their massive advertising efforts, these products alone captured over 800 million dollars in sales, or ⅔ of the amount spent on OTC pain-killers. All of these products contain aspirin or acetaminophen (or a combination, as in EXCEDRIN) as their only safe and effective ingredient for killing pain. In other words, by spending 150 million dollars on advertising, their makers convinced people to pay 800 million dollars for aspirin and acetaminophen which should cost 200 or 300 million dollars. A federal court of appeals upheld an FTC (Federal Trade Commission) ruling that ANACIN ads claiming that the product contains "the pain reliever doctors recommend most" was misleading. The ads did not disclose that the pain reliever being referred to was aspirin, while at the same time attempting to convince consumers that ANACIN relieved pain more effectively than aspirin![5]

ADS FOR PHARMACISTS

For good reasons, pharmacists are an important source of information about minor illness, drugs, drug interactions, and health issues in general.

When a pharmacist recommends a non-prescription product, 95% of the time it is purchased.[6] Many excellent pharmacists will, despite the loss of a sale, advise patients to use non-drug self-treatment for many of the illnesses described in the book. But many do not.

Another kind of advertising promotion by the drug industry involves convincing pharmacists to recommend one product over another by ads in pharmacists' journals. A recent ad for MYLANTA headlines "YOUR MYLANTA WINDFALL OF PROFITS," offering free goods (MYLANTA), advertising allowance and promotional display allowance.[7]

Another ad promotes ACTIFED over the counter for colds even though the FDA says it lacks evidence of effectiveness for colds as a prescription drug because of the antihistamine in this drug. The copy reads, "57 tablets have been taken by American astronauts in space."[8] There is evidence that the antihistamine in ACTIFED makes you drowsy when treating your cold (something that astronauts might find risky), a fact recognized even by Burroughs Wellcome, maker of ACTIFED and SUDAFED. SUDAFED ads (SUDAFED is the same as ACTIFED, without the antihistamine) for colds say "potent relief without drowsiness."[9] Nose spray is the treatment we recommend for a stuffy nose.(See Cough and Cold Section.)

Another ad pushes NEOSPORIN ointment, a triple-header antibiotic ointment (originally found lacking evidence of safety and effectiveness but recently upgraded to safe and effective by FDA) saying "FIRST AID FOR PROFITS" with the accompanying irresponsible slogan "If it needs a bandage, it needs Neosporin."[10]

Like the TV ads directed at consumers, these ads pointed at pharmacists also work. In a recent issue of *American Druggist* (September 1982) the brands pharmacists most often recommended to consumers for all categories of OTC drugs were listed. Again, the most heavily advertised products were most often recommended despite the fact that most of them are more expensive (or because of the fact that they are more profitable to the pharmacist as well as the manufacturer) than equally safe and effective alternatives. Many of them, such as PREPARATION H, PERCOGESIC, and KAOPECTATE, also contain ingredients which are not effective.

In addition to bombarding consumers and pharmacists, drug companies are spending heavily on ads in medical journals to influence doctors' recommendations, thus accounting for some doctor-recommended products which may not be in the best financial or health interest of patients.

COMBINATION DRUG PRODUCTS

Most of the drug products in this book are fixed-ratio combinations. This means that these products combine two or more ingredients so that questions relating to their safety and efficacy depend not only on the safety and effectiveness of the individual drugs for specific symptoms, but also on the safety and efficacy of the drugs taken together. Some of the cough and cold preparations found in this guide, for example, contain as many as five different drugs. Although the likelihood of unwanted side effects clearly increases proportionally with the number of drugs a person consumes, increasing the number of different ingredients in a product will rarely make that product better or more effective.

Some of the fixed-ratio combination drugs in this book contain one or more ingredients that are effective when taken alone, but the drugs are not rated effective because they include unproven or ineffective ingredients, thus making the combination more potentially dangerous and at best no more effective than the single drug.

As former FDA Commissioner Donald Kennedy has stated, "the use of an irrational combination product (even though one ingredient may be effective) needlessly exposes the patient to the risks of these ineffective components." Many combination drugs have been explicitly cited as "irrational mixtures" by the *AMA Drug Evaluations* (first edition), a publication of the American Medical Association Council on Drugs.

The Final Report of the National Academy of Sciences (NAS) Drug Efficacy Study (1969), which included a review of 510 OTC drug products, flatly opposed combination drugs:

> It is a basic principle of medical practice that more than one drug should be administered for the treatment of a given condition only if the physician is persuaded that there is substantial reason to believe that each drug will make a positive contribution to the effect he seeks. Risks of adverse drug reactions should not be multiplied *unless there be overriding benefit* (emphasis added). Moreover, each drug should be given at the dose level that may be expected to make its optimal contribution to the total effect, taking into account the status of the individual patient and any synergistic or antagonistic effects that one drug may be known to have on the safety or efficacy of the other.

WHY AND HOW TO USE THIS BOOK

As mentioned above, we believe that appropriate self-treatment for a variety of common ailments not only saves money, but also avoids expensive visits to the doctor.

PART I. COMMON PROBLEMS AND THEIR TREATMENT

This section begins with a SYMPTOMS INDEX which allows you to see where in the book the problems with these symptoms are discussed.

The eight groups of problems are:

Pain, Fever and Inflammation
Cough, Cold, Allergy and Asthma
Weight Loss
Constipation
Excess Acid and Gas
Nausea, Vomiting and Diarrhea
Hemorrhoids
Sleeping Problems

For each of the eight problems discussed in detail in this part, the following pattern is used:

WHAT IS THE DISEASE/PROBLEM?

HOW TO TREAT WITHOUT DRUGS, IF POSSIBLE

WHICH OTC DRUGS TO USE THAT ARE SAFE AND EFFECTIVE

EXAMPLES OF OTC PRODUCTS NOT TO USE BECAUSE OF LACK OF SAFETY, EFFECTIVENESS, OR BOTH, OR BECAUSE THE PRODUCT IS NOT A GOOD BUY

WHEN TO CONSULT A HEALTH PROFESSIONAL, OR WHEN THE PROBLEM REQUIRES MORE THAN SELF-TREATMENT

By learning more about the origin of these problems, you are empowering yourself to take more control over your body. By educating yourself to participate in self-care and self-treatment, you need not always be dependent on a doctor.

PART II. INGREDIENTS INDEX/BRAND NAME INDEX/GLOSSARY

INGREDIENTS INDEX

This book is not an exhaustive list of all brand name OTC drugs. If the drug you are trying to find out about is not listed among those listed in the BRAND NAME INDEX, look at the ingredient chart to see if each active ingredient you see listed on the box or bottle has been shown to be safe and effective. This section lists 1,800 uses for the various ingredients in OTC drugs. If FDA panels or published updates of FDA panel reports have found the ingredient to be safe and effective for a particular use, the chart will say "YES." Otherwise, it will say "NO" under the column "SAFE AND EFFECTIVE."

WATCH OUT! Drug companies often change ingredients in products without changing the brand name. ALWAYS CHECK INGREDIENTS. Bring this book with you to look up ingredients in the INGREDIENTS INDEX.

BRAND NAME INDEX

For each of the drug products listed in the BRAND NAME INDEX in PART II, the following information is given: brand name, use, ingredients evaluation by Food and Drug Administration (FDA) and Health Research Group (HRG), reason for evaluation, and other problems with the drug, such as cost ($), alternative treatments and, finally, page references to more information in the text of this book. For example, ANACIN, a pain-killer, contains aspirin and caffeine. Both FDA and HRG evaluate this product as lacking evidence of effectiveness because there is no evidence that caffeine is effective for pain. In addition, a "$" signifies that HRG believes ANACIN is not a good buy. On pages 7 and 29 more information about proper treatment of pain can be found.

GLOSSARY

For those words used in the book which you may not understand, a glossary is included in PART II.

CONCLUSION

When you read the following section, **COMMON PROBLEMS AND THEIR TREATMENT (PART I),** you will better understand how your body works, what can go wrong, how you can help to heal yourself and when to call for help. You will also understand that you rarely need any of the drugs discussed in this book, and, by looking at the BRAND NAME INDEX in PART II, you will avoid *Over the Counter Pills That Don't Work,* or are unsafe. By avoiding these drugs, you will save much money and protect yourself and your family.

PART I:
COMMON PROBLEMS
AND THEIR TREATMENT

SYMPTOMS INDEX

4

5

PAIN, FEVER AND INFLAMMATION

WHAT ARE ANALGESICS?

Analgesics are drugs taken to relieve pain.

WHAT ARE ANTIPYRETICS?

Antipyretics are drugs taken to reduce fever.

WHAT ARE ANTI-INFLAMMATORY DRUGS?

Anti-inflammatory drugs are taken to reduce inflammation. Inflammation is a body response characterized by pain, heat, redness and swelling.

WHICH OTC DRUGS TO USE FOR PAIN, FEVER AND INFLAMMATION

Use plain single-ingredient aspirin (as an analgesic, antipyretic, or anti-inflammatory agent) or acetaminophen (as an analgesic or anti-pyretic) in 325 mg (5 grain) tablets, or non-alcoholic liquid acetaminophen. One brand of acetaminophen is TYLENOL, but for either aspirin or acetaminophen, purchase a generic or house brand, if available. Adults should not take more than 12 tablets of aspirin or 8 tablets of acetaminophen per day without medical supervision. Children's doses are discussed on p. 20.

EXAMPLES OF OTC DRUGS NOT TO USE

The following products are formulated with ingredients or in dosage forms which lack evidence of safety or effectiveness as analgesics according to FDA panels:

ANACIN, MAXIMUM STRENGTH ANACIN, A.S.A. COMPOUND, A.S.A. ENSEALS, ASPIRIN SUPPOSITORIES, BAYER TIMED-RELEASE ASPIRIN (and other timed-release analgesics), BC POWDER, CYSTEX, ECOTRIN (and all other enteric-coated tablets), EXCEDRIN, EXCEDRIN P.M., EXTRA STRENGTH EXCEDRIN, GOODY'S HEADACHE POWDERS, MOMENTUM MUSCULAR BACKACHE FORMULA, PERCOGESIC, STANBACK TABLETS and POWDER, and VANQUISH.

Although the FDA has tentatively approved the use of the following products, we do not recommend them, largely because they are unnecessarily expensive (usually 2, 3 or more times the price of plain generic aspirin or acetaminophen) without increased effectiveness:

All non-standard dosage forms (pills containing other than 325 mg or 5 grains), including "Extra Strength," "Maximum Strength" and "Arthritis Strength" products, such as ASPIRIN-FREE ARTHRITIS PAIN FORMULA, DATRIL 500, EXTRA STRENGTH TYLENOL, ASCRIPTIN, and ASCRIPTIN A/D;

9

all analgesics sold in CAPSULE form, and aspirin chewing gum, such as ASPERGUM.

WHEN TO SEEK HELP FROM A HEALTH CARE PROFESSIONAL

When pain, fever or inflammation is accompanied by:
- Symptoms which do not respond to the simple self-treatment steps described in this chapter.
- A fever which is greater than 103° F (39.5° C) or lasts for more than three days.

IMMEDIATE MEDICAL ATTENTION FOR A HEADACHE SHOULD BE SOUGHT WHEN

- Any headache is accompanied by marked weakness, paralysis, loss of sensation in any portion of the body, visual disturbance, confusion and giddiness, or personality changes.
- There is any excruciating or incapacitating pain, with or without loss of consciousness, nausea or vomiting.
- A mild to severe headache is associated with a stiff neck *and* a fever.

IMMEDIATE MEDICAL ATTENTION FOR PAIN IN A JOINT SHOULD BE SOUGHT WHEN

- Pain or swelling is very intense and sudden.
- Pain follows an injury.
- Joint problems are accompanied by a fever over 100° F (or 38° C).
- You cannot use a joint.
- There is numbness or a tingling sensation associated with the pain.

ASPIRIN OR OTHER SALICYLATE -CONTAINING PRODUCTS SHOULD NOT BE USED IN (details on pp. 20, 22-24)

- Children 18 years or younger for treatment of chicken pox or during the flu season. The peak months for flu are October or November thru March or April, but scattered cases occur throughout the year. (Aspirin use in children with chicken pox and flu has been associated with Reye's Syndrome, a serious disease.)
- People who are allergic to aspirin.
- People who have any kind of stomach ailment or discomfort.
- Women who are pregnant.
- People who are taking drugs which can interact with aspirin,

such as Coumadin, Orinase, Diabinese, Anturane, Benemid, Probalon, and others (see list on p. 24).

WHAT IS MENSTRUAL PAIN (DYSMENORRHEA)

Dysmenorrea, or painful periods, is a set of symptoms which occurs during menstrual periods. It is often characterized by cramps, backaches, fatigue and tension.

WHAT IS PREMENSTRUAL SYNDROME

Premenstrual syndrome is a set of symptoms which occur the week preceding a menstrual period; it may be marked by tiredness, irritability, depression, breast tenderness, and bloating.

HOW TO TREAT PAINFUL PERIODS AND AVOID PREMENSTRUAL SYNDROME WITHOUT DRUGS

- Hot baths, hot compresses and massage can help to reduce the discomforts of menstrual cramps.
- To reduce premenstrual bloating, reduce the amount of salt you consume for a week before your menstrual period.

WHICH OTC DRUGS TO USE FOR PREMENSTRUAL AND MENSTRUAL SYMPTOMS

Plain 325 mg (5 grain) tablets of aspirin or acetaminophen (if you can't take aspirin) to treat painful periods.

EXAMPLES OF OTC MENSTRUAL PRODUCTS NOT TO USE

The following products contain ingredients which lack evidence of safety, effectiveness or both according to the FDA Panel:
MIDOL, DIUREX, FLUIDEX, LYDIA E. PINKHAM TABLETS and LIQUID, and ODRINIL.

Although the FDA panel has proposed that the ingredients in the following products be approved, we do not recommend their use:
AQUA-BAN, PAMPRIN, SUNRIL, TRENDAR.

WHEN TO SEEK HELP FROM A HEALTH CARE PROFESSIONAL

When premenstrual or menstrual symptoms do not respond to the simple self-treatment steps described in this chapter and you need further evaluation or alternative therapy.

INTRODUCTION

More people purchase over the counter remedies for headache, fever, sore muscles and other kinds of pain than for any other reason, boosting sales of internal analgesics (pain remedies taken internally) to more than $1.3 billion in the U.S. in 1981.[1] Although there are safe and effective products available for these complaints, a large proportion of the 1.3 billion dollars was wasted on products containing ingredients lacking evidence of safety and/or effectiveness, or on products that are a poor value, because their *only* distinguishing feature is a heavily advertised and well-known brand name.

An *analgesic* is a drug taken to relieve pain. An *antipyretic* is a drug taken to reduce fever. *Anti-inflammatory drugs* work to reduce heat, redness and swelling. All effective OTC internal analgesics have antipyretic properties as well; however, not all of them have anti-inflammatory properties. This chapter will discuss pain, fever and inflammation, self-treatment, what kinds of over the counter ingredients and products are available, and how you should buy them.

PAIN, FEVER AND INFLAMMATION
Headache

Headache is one of the most common kinds of pain. Most headaches will resolve without treatment or may be treated safely and effectively with over the counter products. However, certain headaches require medical attention.

Headaches which can be treated without medical supervision include *Tension Headaches* and *Caffeine Withdrawal Headaches*. Other headaches, including fever headaches, usually respond to self-treatment, though medical advice is sometimes required.

"**Sinus Headaches**" often accompany a head cold, and are noted by pain occurring in a small area above or beneath the eyes. They usually respond to self-treatment. If skin is red or tender to the touch in the above-mentioned areas, if fever or draining of pus from the nose occurs, or if such headaches occur often, medical attention should be sought.

Migraine and so-called cluster headaches result from constriction followed by expansion of blood vessels in the head. They are extremely painful, usually throbbing, and usually only on one side of the head. OTC analgesics will do little, if anything, to relieve the pain. Prescription medications are required to treat this type of headache, which tends to recur.

Immediate medical attention is required for certain types of headaches, such as those caused by a brain tumor, narrow angle glaucoma or meningitis. While it is unlikely that your headache is the result of any of these problems, you should CALL YOUR

13

DOCTOR OR GO TO A HOSPITAL EMERGENCY ROOM
WHEN:
- Any headache is accompanied by marked weakness, paralysis, loss of sensation in any portion of the body, visual disturbances, confusion, giddiness, inability to speak or inappropriate speech or personality changes.
- The headache is excruciating or incapacitating, with or without loss or reduction of consciousness, nausea or vomiting.
- Meningitis may be present. Meningitis is characterized by a mild to severe headache, associated with a very stiff neck and a fever, getting worse through the course of a day.

With these symptoms you should seek medical attention immediately; prompt action may prevent severe mental or physical deterioration or even death.

Muscle Aches and Pain

The most common type of localized muscle pain results from overexertion, tension, or minor trauma (wound or injury). For example, the physical stress caused by moving heavy furniture or standing in high-heeled shoes often results in a spasm (an involuntary contraction, which is sometimes prolonged) of the muscles in the back. Pain caused by this type of muscle spasm can usually be safely treated at home. The treatment will be discussed further on in the chapter. Muscle spasms frequently occur in the back, neck, arms and legs.

More diffuse, widespread aches often are part of a variety of viral infections, including flu and "flu-like" diseases. Other symptoms of these infections may include fever, rash, and sore throat; typically they only last a few days, and they rarely require professional attention. Treatment of this type of "achiness" is discussed in greater detail in the chapter on cough and cold products.

If pain is excruciating, persistent or recurring, or if pain is accompanied by weight loss, fatigue, weakness, blood in the urine, or any other unusual symptoms, consult a health care professional. Occasionally, serious medical problems, including kidney and thyroid disorders, can cause back or muscle pain, and professional medical attention should be sought quickly for appropriate diagnosis and treatment of the underlying disorder.

Fever

The temperature of your body, like the temperature of your home, is set by a thermostat. Various factors such as illness, environmental conditions, and certain drugs can act to reset this thermostat at a lever higher than normal. This is fever.

Mild fever is appropriately treated at home. When and how to treat fever is discussed on p. 18. If the cause of the fever is not

14

known, or if the fever is 103° F (39.5° C) or above, if it persists longer than three days or if it recurs, you should consult a health care professional.

Arthritis and Inflammation

Inflammation is a body response marked by pain, heat, redness and swelling. Arthritis simply means an inflammation of a joint (although inflammation is not always present) and it is usually characterized by pain when moving the joint or when bearing weight on the joint. It is a blanket term for a number of ailments with different causes and symptoms, and of different significance.

Pain, stiffness, swelling, or tenderness in any joint, or in the neck or lower back, which lasts longer than six weeks warrants a trip to a doctor to determine the cause of the problem. A long delay in seeking help may result in irreversible damage to joints.

You should seek medical attention for pain in a joint immediately if:

- Joint pain or swelling is very sudden and intense;
- Joint pain follows an injury (you may have a fracture near the joint);
- Joint problems are accompanied by a fever over 100°F. or 38 °C (you may have an infection of the joint);
- You can't use the affected joint; or
- There is numbness or a tingling sensation associated with the pain (you may have nerve damage).

At least 31.6 million Americans suffer from some form of arthritis. The three most common forms of arthritis are osteoarthritis, rheumatoid arthritis, and gout. Each has a different cause, treatment, and probable outcome.

Osteoarthritis is the most common type of arthritis, and is usually related to the aging of the joint. Most of the time it is not crippling and it often can be treated without medical supervision, as is discussed on p. 18.

The most severe form of osteoarthritis is the type which affects joints that bear the body's weight, such as the hips and the knees. This sort of arthritis can cause a great deal of pain, and it occasionally progresses to a point where walking is difficult. It is worsened by obesity and lack of exercise.

Osteoarthritis also frequently strikes the finger joints, where it causes knobby bumps, and the spine, where it causes bone-like growths. These do not commonly cause serious problems.

OTC analgesics, such as aspirin and acetaminophen, are sometimes used to treat the pain of osteoarthritis. Under medical supervision, severe osteoarthritis is sometimes treated with physical therapy, orthopedic devices and, in extreme cases, surgery.

Rheumatoid arthritis is an inflammation of the joints caused by

15

disturbances in the immune system. Rheumatoid arthritis can occur at any age; its victims include infants, teenagers, the middle aged, and the elderly. Although it is more common in women, men also suffer from the disease. It is often characterized by morning stiffness, along with pain and swelling, characteristically in the joints of fingers, ankles, knees, wrists and elbows.

The distribution of affected joints is usually "bilaterally symmetrical;" that is, if your right wrist is afflicted, your left wrist will probably be afflicted as well.

There is no cure for rheumatoid arthritis, but the inflammation may be controlled, under medical supervision, with an over the counter medication such as aspirin (discussed later in the chapter) or with other treatment, including prescription drugs, exercise, and physical therapy.

Gout is related to the formation of uric acid crystals in the joints which causes the release of injurious chemicals. The big toe is a common location of gouty pain. Treatment by a professional is required, and is usually sought, as the pain typically comes on suddenly and is often severe.

The use of OTC formulations which contain aspirin causes retention of uric acid, and may result in a worsening of gouty arthritis. Aspirin also works against the effect of several anti-gout medications. *People who have gout should avoid aspirin and other salicylates.*

Infectious arthritis occurs when a joint is invaded by bacteria, causing it to become red, hot and swollen. It may be difficult to distinguish this type of arthritis from other forms of arthritis, particularly since it frequently occurs in patients with other kinds of arthritis. This type of infection is almost always accompanied by fever and requires antibiotic therapy, as directed by a physician, as soon as possible; otherwise the joint may be destroyed. No over the counter preparations are appropriate as the sole treatment.

Premenstrual Syndrome and Menstrual Pain

While a monthly menstrual period is a normal part of the lives of most premenopausal women, many women experience symptoms before and during menstruation which are uncomfortable, painful, and sometimes incapacitating.

Many women experience cramps, backaches, fatigue, and tension before or during their monthly periods. The week or two preceding the period may be marked by weight gain, skin disorders, painful breasts, swelling, irritability, mood swings, and depression.[2]

The reasons for this menstrual distress are not entirely clear, and scientists continue to seek to explain the processes at work.

Bloating and breast tenderness which occur just before the menstrual period are similarly caused by salt and water retention in bodily tissues. The best way to reduce the severity of these problems is to avoid eating extra salt or sodium in other forms. Your body will not retain as much extra water if there is no extra salt to "hold" it there.

HOW TO TREAT SIMPLE PAIN, FEVER OR INFLAMMATION

If you do not have any of the warning signs discussed on the preceding pages (and listed at the beginning of this chapter), then your discomfort is appropriate for self-treatment. Some pain, fever or inflammation is self-limited and will respond to rest and relaxation or to the passage of a day or two, and in many instances, discomfort will respond to simple over the counter remedies.

Treating Headaches

Tension headaches are best treated by relaxation techniques which attempt to remove some of the tension. Resting in a comfortable position in a quiet place may bring relief. OTC analgesics offer relief when relaxation is unavailable or insufficient. Frequent tension headaches should prompt an analysis of your personal lifestyle to find and eliminate sources of stress, or to develop satisfactory methods of coping with daily pressures.

Caffeine withdrawal headaches will improve without treatment, but OTC analgesics will hasten this process. Be sure not to use a product containing caffeine such as ANACIN, EXCEDRIN, or MIDOL. If you are already a heavy user of products containing caffeine and would like to cut down your use of caffeine, do it gradually; tapering off over several days or weeks will probably help you to achieve this worthwhile health goal without suffering withdrawal headaches.

"Sinus headaches" (described on p. 13) occasionally accompany the congestion of a cold or nasal allergy. The best approach to these headaches is to relieve the underlying congestion, although an OTC analgesic will relieve discomfort. (See the chapter on cough and cold products for a complete discussion of treatment of nasal decongestion during colds.)

Treating Minor Muscle Aches

Muscle aches resulting from overexertion, tension, and trauma are treated safely and effectively at home with the use of non-drug methods, with the addition of OTC internal analgesics if necessary.

The most important part of treating muscle pain of this sort is to rest the injured area for several days in order to allow healing, and to slowly resume full activity. To relieve aching, apply warm, moist heat to the injured area; wrapping the sore area in hot towels or taking a warm bath, shower, or sauna, for example, may be quite helpful. Massage may also relieve some of the pain.

If pain does not respond to these non-drug techniques, the use of aspirin or acetaminophen may be considered. These OTC internal analgesics are effective in the treatment of muscle pain. If pain does not respond, or is excruciating, persistent or recurrent, consult a health care professional.

OTC *external* analgesics (those applied to the skin) marketed for muscle pain are not discussed in detail in this book. Many (including ABSORBINE JR., ASPERCREME, HEET, MYOFLEX, SLOAN'S LINIMENT and VICKS VAPORUB) contain ingredients which lack evidence of safety or effectiveness according to an FDA panel. (See the table of brand names for more examples.)

We do not recommend any of the OTC external analgesics for muscle pain. Not only do many lack evidence of safety or effectiveness, but in our opinion (and the opinion of our consultants), it is probably safer *and* more effective to use the treatment plan just described.

These so-called external analgesics (BEN-GAY is the best-selling example and more are mentioned above) are counter-irritants, which means that they are supposed to create a sensation to distract you from your pain. They are generally not used by the medical profession to treat muscle pain. They need not be used by you either.

Treating Fever: Without Drugs if Possible

Mild fever (less than 103°F or 39.5°C) which lasts for fewer than three days can be treated at home. In most cases fever does not require drug treatment.

Moderate or low fever (below 101 °F or 38.3 °C) usually does not require any drug treatment at all. If a fever makes you uncomfortable, non-drug approaches should be tried, whenever possible. Drinking lots of cool liquids, for example, can make you more comfortable. Sponge baths and light clothing can also help.

OTC analgesics (aspirin and acetaminophen) are also effective antipyretics, and will usually reduce fever when used in recommended doses.

See p. 20 before considering using aspirin to treat fever in a child.

Treating Arthritis and Inflammation

Arthritis or joint stiffness which does not require medical treatment (as discussed on p. 15) can be safely treated at home. Osteoarthritis, for example, is best treated with exercise and weight loss if necessary. (See chapter on losing weight for more details.) OTC analgesics can be used to relieve pain, but should not be used to control inflammation except under the supervision of a health care professional.

When exercise is used to care for osteoarthritis, it should put an affected joint through its full range of motion. Swimming and walking are particularly good for this, and are a good choice because you can start immediately, and gradually improve your strength and flexibility.

For osteoarthritis, plain aspirin (two 325 mg tablets four times a day for adults) is best to relieve the pain of the disorder. Other pain relievers, including acetaminophen, are recommended for the person who can't take aspirin (discussed on pp. 22-24).

Treatment of other forms of joint disorders, including rheumatoid arthritis, gout, and acute problems, should be planned in cooperation with a health care professional.

For rheumatoid arthritis, aspirin is the pain reliever that "doctors prescribe most." The amount of aspirin required for reducing the inflammation of arthritis, however, approaches levels at which some patients may experience a variety of undesirable side effects (see salicylate overdose, p. 23). These dosage levels should never be taken without medical supervision to assess the correct dose and to get the most therapeutic effect with the least side effects. A physician should also be involved in the coordination of your total treatment, including physical therapy and other medications if necessary. You should be aware that all prescription medicines for rheumatoid arthritis are much more expensive than aspirin and have significant side effects. Most are no more effective than aspirin.

While acetaminophen may relieve the *pain* of rheumatoid arthritis, it is not effective in reducing *inflammation*. Therefore, we do not recommend the use of acetaminiphen for the treatment of arthritis unless it is clear that you have osteoarthritis.

Topical preparations marketed for treating arthritis, including external salicylate-containing analgesics to be applied to the skin such as ASPERCREME and MYOFLEX, have no place in arthritis treatment. Salicylates (including aspirin) exert their effect on joints by absorption into the bloodstream, and this is best done by swallowing tablets, not using cream. If arthritis presently bothers you, consult a health care professional and begin an *effective* treatment plan.

Treating Pain, Fever or Inflammation in Children

The FDA Panel reviewed analgesics for children and recommended aspirin or acetaminophen in the dosages listed in the table:

PEDIATRIC DOSE OF INTERNAL (ORAL) ANALGESICS

AGE	Equivalent # Of Tablets Adult Regular Strength 325 mg (5 grains)	Single Dose In Pediatric Aspirin Or Acetaminophen 80 mg (1¼ grains)
Less Than 2 Years	CONSULT YOUR PEDIATRICIAN BEFORE USING ANY DRUG	
2-4 Years	½	2
4-6 Years	¾	3
6-9 Years	1	4
9-11 Years	1¼	5
11-12 Years	1½	6

Aspirin Warning for Children

You should be aware that the use of aspirin in children with influenza (flu) or chicken pox is strongly linked with the subsequent occurrence of Reye's Syndrome, an often fatal disease. Avoid using aspirin or salicylate-containing medicine in children 18 years old or younger for treatment of chicken pox or during the flu season. The peak months for flu are October or November through March or April, but scattered cases occur throughout the year.

Accidental Overdose

Another risk to children from analgesic products is accidental overdose. In 1979, approximately 30,000 children in the United States under the age of 5 years old accidentally ingested aspirin or acetaminophen; some of these overdoses were fatal. Even small overdoses can be life-threatening to young children.

Like all other medication, analgesics should be kept out of the reach of children. Even if you do not have children you should take the additional precaution of making sure that all medication is in child-proof packages in case children should come in to your home. The incidence of accidental poisoning has dropped dramatically since the advent of these safety closures.

By far, most accidental ingestion of internal analgesics occurs with sweetened children's aspirin, as children enjoy its flavor. Because such products are so tempting to children, it is safer (and less expensive) to purchase regular aspirin tablets, break them into the appropriate children's dose, and crush the prescribed amount into apple sauce or fruit juice, rather than keep sweetened children's aspirin or acetaminophen products around the house. (See chart on p. 20 for equivalent doses.)

As with adults, the best choices for children are generic or store brand aspirin tablets, or acetaminophen in either tablet or liquid form. Name brand versions of children's analgesic tablets, such as ST. JOSEPH'S, BAYER CHILDREN'S (both are aspirin) and CHILDREN'S TYLENOL (acetaminophen), are much more expensive.

Liquid analgesics are very popular for the youngest age group. Although aspirin is not available as a liquid, liquid acetaminophen is available as CHILDREN'S TYLENOL Elixir or Infant Drops, TEMPRA ACETAMINOPHEN Drops or Syrup, and LIQUIPRIN. TYLENOL and TEMPRA products contain the alcohol equivalent of 14 proof and 20 proof, respectively. This may result in drowsiness, particularly when the syrup or elixir is given to a small child. LIQUIPRIN (although not as widely available) is preferable to these other forms of liquid acetaminophen because it is alcohol-free.

All of the drawbacks of aspirin for adults (which are discussed on pp. 22-24) also apply to children. There is also the danger of Reye's Syndrome, so special caution should be exercised (see p. 20). If a child is not sensitive or allergic to aspirin (p. 22), *and* is taking no medication which could interact with aspirin (p. 24) *and* doesn't have an upset stomach *and* doesn't have the flu or chicken pox, *and* it isn't flu season, then, and only then, may aspirin be appropriate (in the dosages shown on p. 20).

Remember, most moderate or low fevers do not require any treatment. If the child is uncomfortable, non-drug treatments such as lukewarm sponge baths, drinking cool liquids, and wearing light clothing should be tried first. Prolonged or high fever requires consultation with a health care professional.

Treating Menstrual Pain and Premenstrual Syndrome

If hot compresses, exercise and massage do not relieve the cramps associated with menstruation, then over the counter medication may help.

Aspirin and acetaminophen are good pain relievers which are worth trying for the treatment of cramps. One or the other should be taken in a single-ingredient preparation only. If pain does not respond to either, a health care professional should be consulted.

No over the counter medication is recommended for the treatment of bloating, or "water weight," before or during your menstrual period. If avoiding salt during the week preceding your menstrual period is not enough to reduce the discomfort of bloating, and if discomfort from premenstrual tension is severe, consult a health care professional.

Treating Hangover

Acetaminophen in regular doses (one or two 325 mg tablets) may be helpful in relieving the headache and pain of an alcoholic hangover. Aspirin is not recommended because it can further exacerbate an irritated stomach, which is often part of the hangover. (This is discussed further in the section on overindulgence, pp 107-111.)

OTC PRODUCTS FOR PAIN, FEVER AND INFLAMMATION

According to the FDA Panel on Internal Analgesics, only aspirin, calcium carbaspirin, choline salicylate, magnesium salicylate, sodium salicylate, and acetaminophen are safe and effective analgesics and antipyretics.* All of these except acetaminophen are in a category of drugs called salicylates. All salicylates are denoted as aspirin through the rest of this chapter, since they have basically the same effects. None of the other salicylates are any more effective than aspirin, but they are generally more expensive when available.

All of the following ingredients lack evidence of safety or effectiveness, either as analgesics or as adjuvants (substances added to medication to increase the effect of the primary active ingredient). They have no place in over the counter analgesics: acetanilid, aluminum aspirin, aminobenzoic acid, antipyrine, buchu, caffeine, codeine,** iodoantipyrine, methapyriline fumarate, phenacetin,*** pheniramine maleate, phenyltoloxamine, potassium nitrate, quinine, salicylamide, salsalate, sodium para-amino benzoate (PABA) and uva ursi. Unfortunately, many of these can still be found in products on drugstore shelves. Specific brands containing one or more of these will be discussed later in this section.

ASPIRIN-CONTAINING PRODUCTS

Aspirin is the common name for a chemical called acetylsalicylic acid, or A.S.A. (as it is still known in Canada and some other countries). Aspirin, used as directed, is perhaps the most effective non-narcotic remedy, prescription or nonprescription, for pain, fever and inflammation. Unfortunately, certain people should not use aspirin.

Aspirin Allergies

Some people are allergic to aspirin. These people may experience

---

*These salicylate derivatives are *not* the same as simple "calcium," "choline" and "magnesium" (without the salicylate) available as dietary supplements.

**Codeine is an effective narcotic analgesic, but only effective at doses which are not safe for OTC sales. Codeine is often abused and has a high potential for dependence.

***Phenacetin is a pain-reliever formerly found in many OTC and prescription analgesics, but has been banned following evidence that it causes kidney damage and blood disorders.

a wide variety of reactions to aspirin, including hives, rash, swollen lymph nodes, generalized swelling, severe breathing difficulties or a drop in blood pressure. Simple stomach discomfort following the use of aspirin or any other medication, however, does not indicate that you have an allergy.

Asthmatics seem to be particularly prone to allergies to aspirin, as well as allergies to calcium carbaspirin, another member of the salicylate family.

If you have ever had an allergic reaction to aspirin or any other drug, be sure to tell your physician. This kind of reaction can also occur in response to other, related medications, which include prescription drugs containing salicylates or similar ingredients.

Aspirin and the Stomach

Aspirin is a locally irritating, corrosive substance. Therefore, long-term use of aspirin or use in high doses can increase the likelihood of developing peptic ulcers.[3] If you have ulcers, gastritis, or any form of stomach discomfort, you should not be taking even small quantities of aspirin, in any form.

Aspirin and Bleeding

Aspirin causes bleeding in the stomach; over time, it can weaken the ability to slow and contain bleeding throughout the body. Taking aspirin for a few days can increase the amount of bleeding during childbirth, after tooth extraction, during surgery, and in many other circumstances. Aspirin should not be taken for at least 5 days before surgery, even in small doses. Persons with serious liver disease, Vitamin K deficiency or blood clotting disorders, or persons already taking blood thinners or anticoagulants (as listed on p. 24) should not take aspirin without strict supervision of a health care professional.

Aspirin should not be taken in very large doses (more than 12 regular-strength 325 mg or 5 grain tablets per day) or for more than a few days without the supervision of a physician. Even small doses used over a long period of time may leave certain predisposed individuals at an increased risk of serious bleeding after wounds or cuts.

Aspirin and Pregnancy

Like all medication, aspirin should not be taken during pregnancy except when absolutely necessary and under competent medical advice. It can cause excessive bleeding in the mother and child in the first few days after birth, increase duration of pregnancy, and cause a slight decrease in birth weight.

Aspirin and Salicylate Overdose

Repeated high doses of aspirin and other salicylates or accidental poisoning with salicylates can lead to salicylate overdose. Symptoms of mild overdose include dizziness, continuous ringing in the ears, difficulty in hearing, nausea, vomiting, diarrhea and mental confusion. More severe overdose can also cause hyperventilation, dimness of vision, delirium, hallucinations, convulsions and coma.

In order to avoid overdose, do not take more than the recommended or prescribed amount of aspirin. Also, care should be used if you are taking any other medication containing salicylates. DRISTAN capsules and PEPTO-BISMOL are but two examples of a large number of nonprescription products which contain a salicylate ingredient. Consult a health care professional if any signs of salicylate overdose occur.

Aspirin and Other Drugs

Aspirin and other salicylates should not be used without a physician's direction by people who are taking certain other medications. These medications include:

- anticoagulant "blood thinners" such as warfarin (Coumadin), dicumarol, heparin, and others;
- any oral diabetes medication including tolbutamide (Orinase) or chlorpropamide (Diabinese);
- any medication for gout (discussed earlier in the section on arthritis) including sulfinpyrazone (Anturane) and probenecid (Benemid and Probalan);
- corticosteroids such as cortisol and prednisone;
- methotrexate (Mexate), used in psoriasis and cancer therapy; and
- spironolactone (Aldactone).[4]

If in doubt, consult your physician.

Forms of Aspirin

Aspirin comes in many forms — plain, buffered, chewable, gum, coated, timed-release, capsule, and suppository. If you can take aspirin, plain tablets are generally all that is necessary.

Buffered aspirin is plain aspirin combined with antacids or "buffers." Regularly buffered aspirin (such as the entire BUFFERIN line, ASCRIPTIN, ASCRIPTIN A/D, and ARTHRITIS PAIN FORMULA) all contain relatively small amounts of antacids. Highly buffered aspirin products (such as ALKA-SELTZER EFFERVESCING PAIN RELIEVER AND ANTACID) contain large amounts of antacids, but should still be avoided by people with ulcers or other stomach disorders because they contain aspirin.

Highly buffered aspirin, which must be dissolved in water before use, can actually decrease the acidity of the stomach and reduce much of the bleeding and irritation in the process. Unfortunately, it does so at the cost of high sodium content, which makes it unwise for long-term use; persons on a salt-or sodium-restricted diet should avoid any use of these products. Products like ALKA SELTZER EFFERVESCING PAIN RELIEVER AND ANTACID are also *much* more expensive than plain aspirin (5½ times more expensive at one major Washington, D.C. area drug chain). In our opinion, they are not worth the expense and we do not recommend them for use in relief of simple pain.

Numerous studies sponsored by drug manufacturers have failed to prove conclusively that regularly buffered aspirin is any "gentler" to the stomach than plain aspirin.[5] In order to minimize stomach irritation, we recommend that you always take aspirin with a full glass (8 oz.) of fluid (like water or milk), or immediately following a meal.

Although buffered aspirin may be absorbed more quickly than plain aspirin, buffered aspirin does not provide significantly faster pain relief than plain aspirin tablets.[6]

Aspirin chewing gums, such as ASPERGUM, are marketed as general analgesics as well as for relief of sore throat pain. They offer no advantage over tablets for use in headaches or other types of pain. Also, aspirin chewing gum is not even an appropriate choice for sore throat pain, as it can further irritate the throat surface (see the chapter on cough and cold for *appropriate* therapy). Aspirin chewing gum, in our opinion, should not be used.

Aspirin chewing gum products typically provide a smaller dose of aspirin than standard 5 grain tablets. ASPERGUM, for example, contains only 3½ grains of aspirin.

Aspirin does not exert an anesthetic (sensation-deadening) effect when applied to or placed in direct contact with a painful surface. The chief effect which aspirin has in reducing pain takes place after the drug is absorbed into the bloodstream from the intestine. Aspirin's chief effect on the surface of mucous membrane, including the lining of the mouth and throat, is to cause irritation and burning sensations.[7]

Since there are other products that are safer and more effective for use as analgesics (like swallowed aspirin or acetaminophen tablets) and for relief of sore throat pain (see p. 54), use of aspirin chewing gum like ASPERGUM is not recommended.

Chewable aspirin tablets are usually intended for those who have difficulty swallowing whole tablets. Children's aspirin tablets are typically in this form. Because of the irritating potential of aspirin, each dose should be followed by drinking plenty of water. In addition, chewable aspirin should not be taken less than a week after a tonsillectomy or oral surgery because of the risk of irritation and bleeding.

Parents should know that children often confuse these flavored chewable tablets with candy. (See section on accidental overdose, earlier in this chapter.)

Capsules are a form of medication in which the active ingredient or ingredients are enclosed in a shell, which then dissolves in the digestive tract. They are similar in all ways (absorption and effectiveness, for example) to tablets, although some people find them easier to swallow. Capsules are generally far more expensive than tablets, and, as we discovered tragically in the Tylenol tampering case and the incidents that followed, capsules are much easier to open and tamper with than tablets. *Because capsules pose an unnecessary expense they should be avoided in OTC products.*

Non-standard dosages, with names such as "Extra-Strength," "Maximum-Strength," and "Arthritis Strength," offer no advantage over regular strength products, and are generally much more expensive to use. In addition, the FDA Advisory Panel on Internal Analgesics *recommended* that aspirin and acetaminophen products contain only 325 mg (5 grains) per dosage unit,[8] but allowed for the likelihood that the FDA would allow extra-strength dosages.

These higher ("stronger") dosages typically contain about 500 mg of analgesic, roughly equivalent to 1½ times the regular dose. This higher amount is unnecessary, since the appropriate dosage for self-medication with aspirin or acetaminophen for pain, fever and inflammation, is only 325 to 650 mg (one or two regular-strength tablets) every four hours.

Any higher dose of aspirin which might be recommended by a physician for rheumatoid arthritis can be met with an appropriate number of much less expensive regular-strength tablets. A higher dose lessens the safety and doesn't necessarily increase the effectiveness. (3 regular aspirin or acetaminophen equal 2 extra-strength.)

Enteric coated aspirin, such as ECOTRIN, is aspirin coated with a substance intended to prevent the pill from dissolving in the stomach. The aspirin is intended to dissolve, instead, in the small intestine. The advantage is a decrease in the amount of stomach irritation. The significant drawbacks are that the onset of action is delayed (there's no "fast relief" with these) and the quantity of aspirin absorbed into the blood is unpredictable and variable. Some people do not absorb enough aspirin to have the desired effect. In addition, these products have the same effect on bleeding as other aspirin products. For this reason, an FDA panel of experts classified these products as lacking evidence of effectiveness for use as analgesics. We agree, and recommend against their use.

Timed-release aspirin, such as BAYER TIMED-RELEASE ASPIRIN, suffer from an unpredictably varied rate of absorption. The result is that you may have too little or too much in your blood at one time. The FDA panel concluded that this dosage form lacks evidence of safety and effectiveness.

Aspirin rectal suppositories offer relief from stomach irritation, but may cause rectal irritation instead. This form may be useful for someone who is vomiting; however, the risks and benefits are unclear, and therefore, we cannot recommend its use. Because of the great variability in the amount of aspirin absorbed from these products, the FDA panel found that aspirin suppositories lack evidence of safety and effectiveness.

Powdered aspirin dissolves somewhat more rapidly than aspirin in tablet form. Although you might expect a more rapid therapeutic effect from this form, no significant advantage has been demonstrated.

Magnesium salicylate (in DOAN'S PILLS for example) is equivalent to aspirin in pain relief but not in price. Although DOAN'S PILLS are marketed specifically for muscular backache, magnesium salicylate offers no advantage over plain aspirin in the treatment of this complaint, and the brand name is 10 to 20 times as expensive.

Liquid analgesics are sometimes preferred by people who have difficulty swallowing and are often used in children. Because of its chemical nature, aspirin is not available in liquid form. Choline salicylate, a related effective analgesic, is the usual liquid form of salicylate, but is not widely available. Acetaminophen is more often available in liquid form. (For a discussion of liquid analgesics refer to the section on analgesics for children, p. 21.)

ACETAMINOPHEN-CONTAINING PRODUCTS

Acetaminophen is the active ingredient in non-aspirin analgesics, including TYLENOL, DATRIL, ANACIN-3*, and PER-COGESIC. Like aspirin, acetaminophen reduces fever and pain, but unlike aspirin, it lacks the anti-inflammatory effect which makes aspirin useful for diseases such as rheumatoid arthritis. Fortunately, it does not cause significant irritation to the stomach lining, thus making it the appropriate analgesic choice for a person who experiences stomach discomfort with aspirin. (If you have severe or repeated stomach discomfort, refer to the chapter on indigestion and consult a physician, if necessary.) Further, acetaminophen does not predispose the user to bleeding problems.

There is one serious adverse effect of acetaminophen: overdosage. Taking much more of this medication than the recommended dosage (at one time or over a long period of time) can result in serious and sometimes fatal liver damage, a common occurrence in acetaminophen overdose. The recommended dose of acetaminophen is one or two 325 mg (5 grain) tablets every 4 hours, not to exceed 12 tablets per day. ACETAMINOPHEN OVERDOSE

---

*Non-aspirin ANACIN-3, available over the counter and containing only acetaminophen, should not be confused with ANACIN-3 with Codeine, which is a prescription drug. This labeling is quite confusing, and is complicated by the long identification of Tylenol #3(a prescription pain-killer) as containing acetaminophen with codeine. OTC ANACIN-3 and TYLENOL both contain acetaminophen only, at a price considerably higher than that of widely available identically formulated generic or store brands.

MUST BE TREATED PROMPTLY TO PREVENT PERMA-
NENT LIVER INJURY OR EVEN DEATH. IN CASE OF
OVERDOSE SEEK MEDICAL ASSISTANCE IMMEDIATELY.

As in the case of aspirin, you can save a great deal of money by
purchasing acetaminophen in the generic or store brand form. The
same considerations apply to non-standard dosage forms and capsule forms of acetaminophen as of aspirin (see p. 26).

Although the brand name TYLENOL has, for many people,
become synonymous with acetaminophen, generic or house brand
acetaminophen is the same ingredient at a much lower price. At a
large Washington, D.C.-area drugstore chain, 100 tablets of
TYLENOL Regular-Strength Tablets sell for $3.59. A generic
brand with the identical formula is $1.79 per 100, half as much.

A new acetaminophen product, PANADOL, will be marketed in
the U.S. in the near future. It is no different or better than any of
the others, and your best buy in acetaminophen analgesic products
remains the generic or store brand.

For a discussion of liquid acetaminophen, see the discussion
under treating children p. 21.

PHENACETIN-CONTAINING PRODUCTS

Phenacetin has been classified as unsafe by the FDA. Phenacetin
should not be taken because it is likely to cause kidney damage and
blood disorders following long-term use, because it is a carcinogen
(cancer-causing chemical) and because it has a history of abuse. On
August 10, 1982, the FDA announced plans to remove all
phenacetin-containing products from the market in one year but
will, unfortunately, allow existing stocks to be sold.[9]

Phenacetin is marketed extensively abroad. In the United States,
it has been available most commonly in a combination product
with aspirin and caffeine called APC. Phenacetin-containing products include A.S.A. COMPOUND, CAPRON, DURADYNE
PAC, OS-CAL-GESIC, SAL-FAYNE, and S.P.C. These products
which contain phenacetin are unsafe and should no longer be
available.

SALICYLAMIDE-CONTAINING PRODUCTS

Salicylamide was found by the FDA panel to lack evidence of
safety and effectiveness as an analgesic, antipyretic, and anti-
inflammatory ingredient. It is ineffective at low doses, and has
significant safety problems at higher doses. It commonly causes
dizziness, drowsiness and stomach irritation; long-term use has
resulted in liver problems and damage to blood formation, among
other reactions.

Salicylamide has been available in combination products such as
ARTHRALGEN, BC Powder, BANESIN, CYSTEX, DEWITT
PILLS, and STANBACK Tablets and Powder. Products contain-

ing this ingredient should not be used.

PRODUCTS CONTAINING SEVERAL INGREDIENTS
Combinations of 2 or More Analgesic Ingredients

Some products contain combinations of 2 or more analgesic ingredients. EXCEDRIN, EXTRA-STRENGTH EXCEDRIN, GEMNISYN, GOODY'S HEADACHE POWDER, and VANQUISH, for example, all contain both aspirin and acetaminophen. This combination is irrational and we believe that these products should not be used. Aspirin and acetaminophen together are no more effective than either single ingredient by itself.[10] Further, by taking both of these ingredients, you risk the side effects of both.

Combinations of Analgesics with Non-Analgesic Ingredients

Some products, including a number of widely sold and heavily advertised items, contain aspirin or acetaminophen along with non-analgesic ingredients. These other ingredients usually include caffeine or antihistamines, which lack evidence of safety and effectiveness as analgesic adjuvants (substances added to medication to increase the effect of the primary active ingredient).

Caffeine is added to aspirin and/or acetaminophen in products such as ANACIN, MAXIMUM STRENGTH ANACIN, COPE, EXCEDRIN, EXTRA-STRENGTH EXCEDRIN, GOODY'S HEADACHE POWDER, and VANQUISH. This combination lacks conclusive evidence of being more effective than plain aspirin for reducing pain, fever or inflammation. Caffeine, the stimulant in coffee, may cause side effects such as anxiety, increased blood pressure, and possible withdrawal headaches. It is unnecessary, less desirable, and more expensive to use aspirin or acetaminophen in combination with caffeine.

Products containing aspirin in combination with antihistamines are marketed as analgesics, sleep-aids and cough/cold remedies. In general, we discourage the use of these combination products. Aspirin in sleep-aids and cough/cold remedies is discussed further in the appropriate chapters. In addition, antihistamines have other side effects discussed at length in both chapters.

The antihistamines phenyltoloxamine citrate and pyrilamine maleate are found in PERCOGESIC and EXCEDRIN P.M., respectively. These antihistamines lack evidence of effectiveness as analgesic adjuvants, so combinations like PERCOGESIC and EXCEDRIN P.M. are unnecessary and should not be used.

MOMENTUM MUSCULAR BACKACHE FORMULA contains not only the antihistamine phenyltoloxamine citrate, which lacks evidence of effectiveness as an analgesic adjuvant, but also the ineffective analgesic salsalate. It also contains an ineffective dose of aspirin. This product should be avoided.

PRODUCTS FOR PREMENSTRUAL AND MENSTRUAL SYMPTOMS

The only ingredients available in OTC products which we recommend for premenstrual and menstrual symptoms are aspirin and acetaminophen. (Other salicylates, such as calcium carbaspirin, choline salicylate, magnesium salicylate, and sodium salicylate are also good, but no better than aspirin.) They are the only proven, effective, over the counter medications to treat cramps, backache or headache associated with menstruation. Other ingredients sold in products for premenstrual and menstrual symptoms include antihistamines, smooth muscle relaxants and diuretics.

Antihistamines

An FDA advisory panel found pyrilamine maleate (an ingredient in PAMPRIN and SUNRIL) to be safe and effective for the treatment of emotional changes in the premenstrual period, such as anxiety, irritability and tension in combination with other ingredients only. However, the FDA has suggested it may reverse the approval of pyrilamine maleate since there may not be sufficient evidence of effectiveness for the treatment of Premenstrual Syndrome.[11]

Like other antihistamines, whose side effects are discussed at length with sleep-aids (see pp. 160-161) and cough and cold remedies (see pp. 46-47), pyrilamine maleate can cause drowsiness. The FDA Panel on OTC Sedative, Sleep-Aid, and Tranquilizer Drug Products found that antihistamines cause drowsiness but do not relieve anxiety, irritability, and tension.[12] We therefore do not recommend the use of products with pyrilamine maleate for treating these symptoms during Premenstrual Syndrome.

Smooth Muscle Relaxants

Although muscle relaxants are presumably of value in relaxing muscles to relieve menstrual cramps, no ingredients in OTC products were found to be effective as smooth muscle relaxants. (Smooth muscle is the kind of muscle in the uterus.) According to the FDA panel, cinnamedrine hydrochloride (in MIDOL) lacks evidence of effectiveness in treating menstrual symptoms.

Diuretics

These agents are designed to eliminate excess water accumulation in body tissue during the week prior to the onset of the menstrual flow. The FDA panel rated ammonium chloride (in AQUA-BAN), caffeine (in AQUA-BAN and MIDOL), and pamabrom (in PAMPRIN and TRENDAR) as safe and effective diuretics. (Caffeine was also found safe and effective for treatment of fatigue.) However, we do not recommend the use of the OTC diuretics for self-medication of premenstrual water accumulation. Mineral and chemical imbalances can occur as a result of the use of these ingredients, and this may well outweigh any benefit that they may have.[13] Bloating is best treated by limiting consumption of salt, especially for the week before the onset of symptoms.

Other Unproven Ingredients

A number of assorted herbal ingredients which are not recognized as safe and effective by the FDA are found in menstrual products. They should be avoided. These include: uva ursi, buchu, couch grass, corn silk, Jamaica dogwood, and pleurisy root, among others. Products containing some of these include DIUREX, FLUIDEX, LYDIA E. PINKHAM Tablets and Liquids, and ODRINOL.

VALUE AND ANALGESICS

A vigorous pharmaceutical industry advertising campaign supported by your drugstore dollars is working to keep you from getting the best value for your money. You may be unwittingly footing the bill for this effort.

There is no reason to pay extra for any of the following types of analgesic products:

1) **Brand name products when a generic or store brand version is available.** There is no evidence that BAYER ASPIRIN, for example, is any better than any other aspirin tablet approved by the FDA. When you buy BAYER ASPIRIN at 2-3 times the price of the generic or house brand equivalent, you are helping to pay for the $22.4 million (1981) advertising campaign of Sterling Drug's BAYER ASPIRIN products.[14] The same goes for TYLENOL, and the $42.9 million spent in 1981 on the TYLENOL line of products.[15] At one large Washington, D.C. area drugstore chain,* 100 BAYER Aspirin tablets are $1.99, while an equivalent store brand (with identical ingredients) is $0.99. 100 tablets of TYLENOL are $3.59, while an equivalent store brand (with identical ingredients) is $1.79 for 100 tablets.

2) **Extra ingredients.** No ingredients or combinations of ingredients available OTC are more effective than plain aspirin or acetaminophen. ANACIN, for example, contains caffeine (the amount in about half a cup of coffee) in addition to aspirin. In addition to paying for this ineffective ingredient, you support the $27.5 million in advertising spent on ANACIN.[16] 100 tablets of ANACIN are $2.99, of EXCEDRIN $3.09 and of BUFFERIN $3.29, while 100 tablets of the store brand aspirin, providing the pain relief we recommend, are $0.99.

3) **Capsules rather than tablets.** Capsules are no more effective or faster-acting than tablets. They may be easier to swallow for some, but so are tablets if they are ground up and put in food or drink. Tablets are relatively tamper-proof as well. 100 *capsules* of

31

EXTRA-STRENGTH TYLENOL are $6.57, while 100 EXTRA-STRENGTH TYLENOL *tablets* with the identical ingredients and action are $5.37. (The same amount of generic acetaminophen costs $2.75.)

4) "Extra-Strength," "Arthritis-Strength," or "Maximum-Strength" products. For discomfort that is appropriate for self-treatment, one or two regular-strength generic tablets are appropriate, and *no more* is necessary. For higher doses, as directed by a physician, and for the treatment of arthritis, you should be able to get whatever strength is required with the correct number of inexpensive regular-strength tablets. There is no reason to pay 1½ times the price for the same amount of relief. 100 tablets of EXTRA-STRENGTH TYLENOL are $4.95, while 100 tablets of regular-strength TYLENOL, which provide adequate pain relief and safer dosage, are $3.59.(Note that your best value would be in the store brand acetaminophen, with identical ingredients, for $1.79 per 100 tablets.)

5) "Timed-release" formulations. These lack evidence of safety and effectiveness, according to the FDA panel. 72 tablets of BAYER TIMED-RELEASE ASPIRIN are $4.39 ($6.10 per 100) while an equivalent amount of regular store brand aspirin, which can be taken with a greater assurance of effectiveness, although it must be taken twice as often, is $1.50 ($1.88 buys 250 generic aspirin).

6) Enteric-coated tablets. These lack evidence of effectiveness, according to the FDA Panel. 100 tablets of ECOTRIN are $4.39 while 100 tablets of the regular store brand, with identical ingredients (325 mg of aspirin), are $0.99.

7) Products marketed for specific kinds of pain. DOAN'S PILLS containing magnesium salicylate has the same effect as plain aspirin, but is advertised as if it were specifically for muscular backache. DOAN'S PILLS generally cost 10 or more times as much as the equivalent amount of plain store brand aspirin. 48 tablets of DOAN'S PILLS are $4.83 ($10.36 per 100) while 100 tablets of plain store brand aspirin, which provide identical relief, are $0.99.

Once again, you will get the most effect for your money by sticking with generic aspirin for pain, fever or inflammation, and acetaminophen for pain or fever alone. Follow the guidelines discussed earlier in the chapter to choose which is appropriate for you.

---

*All prices in this section were obtained from major Washington, D.C. area drugstore chains during January and February 1983.

COUGH, COLD, ALLERGY AND ASTHMA

WHAT IS THE COMMON COLD?

The common cold is a viral infection of the upper respiratory tract (nose, throat and upper airways), resulting in inflammation of the mucous membrane lining of those areas. Common symptoms are runny nose, sneezing, sore throat and a general "achy" feeling.

HOW TO TREAT A COLD WITHOUT DRUGS

A cold is best treated by drinking plenty (at least 8-10 full glasses per day) of non-alcoholic liquids (especially warm or hot liquids), getting enough rest, and not smoking.

WHICH PRODUCTS TO USE FOR A COLD

If symptoms do not respond to the non-drug measures above and are interfering with normal activities, the following OTC products are safe and effective:

For a stuffy nose: If your nose is blocked, especially if you can't breathe through it, use nose drops or spray containing oxymetazoline hydrochloride (AFRIN, for example), xylometazoline hydrochloride (4-WAY LONG ACTING NASAL SPRAY, for example), or phenylephrine hydrochloride (NEO-SYNEPHRINE nose drops and nasal spray, for example). Buy a less expensive generic or store brand product if it is available. Do not use these drugs for more than three days.

For a runny nose: No OTC drug is appropriate. A runny nose promotes drainage and should not be treated with medication. If it lasts longer than a week, consult a health professional.

For fever, headaches, and body aches: Plain aspirin or acetaminophen, if needed. (See the chapter on Analgesics; and read the Aspirin Warning for Children, p. 20.)

For cough: A productive cough (when you are coughing something up) should not be treated. If you have an unproductive (dry) cough which keeps you from sleeping, use dextromethorphan, available in HOLD, ST. JOSEPH'S COUGH SYRUP FOR CHILDREN, or SUCRETS COUGH CONTROL FORMULA. Buy a less expensive generic or store brand dextromethorphan product if it is available.

For a sore throat: Plain aspirin or acetaminophen, swallowed whole, if needed. (See the chapter on Analgesics; and read the Aspirin Warning for Children, p. 20.)

EXAMPLES OF COLD REMEDIES NOT TO USE
Nasal Sprays

The following products contain ingredients or combinations of ingredients which an FDA panel found to lack evidence of safety, effectiveness, or both as nasal sprays: DRISTAN (Nasal Mist) DRISTAN Menthol Nasal Mist, and 4-WAY (regular) NASAL SPRAY.

Oral Nasal Decongestants (Pills or Syrup)

We do not recommend the use of any nasal decongestants which are taken by mouth for treatment of a cold, although an FDA panel has found three ingredients safe and effective. These include ingredients in: AFRINOL and SUDAFED.

Antihistamines

Although the FDA has tentatively approved these drugs, we do not recommend the use of the following drugs *for treatment of a cold,* largely because they are ineffective for this purpose: CHLOR-TRIMETON and DIMETANE.

Combination (Multi-Symptom) Cold Remedies

The following products contain ingredients which lack evidence of safety, effectiveness, or both, for treating a cold; according to an FDA panel:

DRISTAN Decongestant/Antihistamine/Analgesic Tablets and Capsules (regular and aspirin-free), NYQUIL Nighttime Colds Medicine, SINUTAB, and TRIAMINICIN tablets.

Although the FDA has tentatively approved the over the counter use of the following drug mixtures, we cannot recommend them for a cold. They contain ingredients in fixed-combination formulas which increase the possibility of side-effects, and do not necessarily make the product more effective:

ACTIFED, ALKA-SELTZER PLUS, CHLOR-TRIMETON DECONGESTANT, COMTREX, CONTAC, CONTAC SEVERE COLD FORMULA, CORICIDIN, CORICIDIN-D, CO-TYLENOL, DIMETANE DECONGESTANT, DRISTAN ULTRA COLDS FORMULA, DRIXORAL, HEADWAY, MAXIMUM STRENGTH TYLENOL SINUS MEDICINE, PYRROXATE, SINAREST, SINE-AID, SINE-OFF, SUDAFED PLUS, TRIAMINIC SYRUP, TRIAMINICIN CHEWABLES and VICKS FORMULA 44D.

Cough Remedies

Although the FDA has tentatively approved the ingredients in these products, we do not recommend the use of any of the following: CHERACOL, CHERACOL-D, FORMULA 44 COUGH MIXTURE, HEAD and CHEST, ROBITUSSIN (Plain, CF, DM, and PE) and TRIAMINIC EXPECTORANT.

Sore Throat Remedies

The following products contain ingredients which lack evidence of safety, effectiveness, or both, according to an FDA panel, as antimicrobial agents for treating a sore throat: CEPACOL Mouthwash, Throat Lozenges and Anesthetic Troches, LISTERINE Mouthwash and Lozenges, SCOPE Mouthwash, and VICKS Throat Lozenges.

WHEN TO SEEK HELP FROM A HEALTH CARE PROFESSIONAL FOR COLD-LIKE SYMPTOMS

Seek help when any of the following occur:

- A high fever greater than 101°F (38.3°C) accompanied by shaking chills and coughing up of thick phlegm (especially if greenish or foul-smelling).
- Sharp chest pain when you take a deep breath.
- Cold-like symptoms which do not improve after 7 days.
- Any fever greater than 103° F or 39.4° C.
- Coughing up of blood.
- Any significant throat pain in a child.
- A painful throat in addition to any of the following:
  1) Pus (yellowish-white spots) on the tonsils or the throat.
  2) Fever greater than 101° F or 38.3° C.
  3) Swollen or tender glands or bumps in the front of the neck.
  4) Exposure to someone who has a documented case of "strep" throat.
  5) A rash which came during or after a sore throat.
  6) A history of rheumatic fever, rheumatic heart disease, kidney disease, or chronic lung disease such as emphysema or chronic bronchitis.

WHAT ARE ALLERGIES?

Allergies are reactions caused by breathing, touching, eating or otherwise coming into contact with a substance, called an allergen, to which your body is hypersensitive. Hypersensitivity means that your body overreacts to the substance in an unpleasant or harmful way.

WHAT IS ALLERGIC RHINITIS?

Allergic rhinitis is an allergic condition causing an itchy and runny nose, sneezing, itchy and watery eyes, and a tickle in the throat. If it occurs during a particular season, due to pollens from plants such as trees, grasses, or ragweed, it is called "hay fever." Allergic rhinitis can also occur year-round in people allergic to allergens such as dust, mold, feathers, animal danders (scales from feathers, hair or skin), and occasionally food.

HOW TO TREAT ALLERGIC RHINITIS

- Find out what you are allergic to and avoid it. (See pp. 57-59.)
- If avoidance is impossible or not sufficient, and allergic symptoms interfere with normal activities, use the safe and effective OTC products listed below.

WHICH OTC PRODUCTS TO USE FOR ALLERGIC RHINITIS

Use a *single-ingredient* antihistamine product containing only brompheniramine maleate or chlorpheniramine maleate such as DIMETANE or CHLOR-TRIMETON. Buy a less expensive generic or store brand product if available. A proper dose (every 4-6 hours) is 4 mg for adults and 2 mg for children ages 6-12. Taking a smaller and/or less frequent dose may provide relief for some people.

Do not give these drugs to children under 6 years of age without first consulting a health care professional. Do not drive or operate heavy machinery if you feel drowsy while using an antihistamine. Certain people should not take antihistamines; see p. 61 for more information.

EXAMPLES OF OTC PRODUCTS NOT TO USE FOR TREATING ALLERGIC RHINITIS

Although an FDA panel has tentatively approved the use of the following drugs, we cannot recommend their use for the treatment of allergy symptoms:

All nasal sprays, including those useful for colds mentioned earlier, since they should not be used for more than 3 days; all orally administered nasal decongestants, including AFRINOL and SUDAFED, since they have a variety of side effects and are not effective in treating the major allergy symptoms; all combination allergy products, since they are more likely to cause unwanted side effects and are not more effective than antihistamines alone in treating the major allergy symptoms. The latter include ACTIFED, A.R.M., ALLEREST, CHLOR-TRIMETON DECONGESTANT, DIMETANE DECONGESTANT, DRIXORAL and SUDAFED PLUS, as well as all the combination cold remedies previously listed.

WHEN TO SEEK HELP FROM A HEALTH CARE PROFESSIONAL FOR ALLERGIC REACTIONS

Seek medical attention when:
- Recommended drugs and treatment do not give you relief.
- You experience other kinds of allergic reactions needing treatment, including skin allergies or difficulty in breathing.
- You believe you have a life-threatening allergy called anaphylaxis. (This is discussed on p. 58.)

WHAT IS ASTHMA?

Asthma is a disease in which airways in the lungs become narrow. This reversible breathing difficulty may be brought on by exposure to certain allergies or by exercise, among other causes.

HOW TO TREAT ASTHMA

The diagnosis of asthma must be made by a qualified health care professional. Treatment, whether non-drug or with OTC or prescription products, should be agreed upon by the health provider and the asthmatic. OTC products for asthma are discussed on pp. 63-66.

EXAMPLES OF DRUGS NOT TO USE FOR ASTHMA

The following products contain ingredients which lack evidence of safety, effectiveness or both, according to the FDA, for the treatment of asthma: BRONITIN Tablets, BRONKAID Tablets, BRONKOTABS, PRIMATENE (P and M) Tablets and TEDRAL Tablets and Elixir.

INTRODUCTION

Since everyone suffers from the common cold at one time or another, and many suffer from allergies or asthma, it may not be surprising that in 1981, consumers spent $1.64 *billion* on over the counter remedies for coughs, colds, allergies and asthma.[1] To generate these extraordinary sales, the drug industry spent over $150 million in 1980 advertising these products.[2]

The disturbing fact is that a large proportion of these products contain one or more ingredients that lack evidence of safety and/or effectiveness, or are composed of irrational and sometimes unsafe combinations.

The safest, best, and least expensive way to care for a cold, allergy or asthma (if attacks are usually short and go away without treatment) is to not take anything at all and let the illness run its short, *frequently self-limiting* course, or if necessary, to purchase single ingredient products to treat the individual symptoms that you have.

This chapter, divided into 5 sections (cold, cough, sore throat, allergy and asthma), will describe these ailments, the best treatment for each one and the OTC products that are currently available.

THE COMMON COLD

The viral infection we call "the common cold" can usually be treated without any professional help by rest and plenty of liquids, occasionally aided by the use of simple over the counter remedies for certain symptoms. *There are no drugs which can kill the viruses that cause colds.*

In this section of the chapter we are concerned primarily with the cold symptoms of runny or stuffy nose, as well as general aches, pain and fever. Later sections will discuss cough and sore throat, which are also part of many colds.

A cold cannot be "cured" except by time, but you are less likely to catch a cold if you do not smoke, since smoking paralyzes the hair-like structures that clean out the body's airways. Colds are usually spread by hand, more often than they are spread through the air. It's a good idea to prevent the spread of virus by trying not to touch your eyes, mouth and nose, and by washing your hands frequently when you are ill or with an ill person.

Certain other illnesses appear similar to colds, but warrant medical advice. If you have a high fever (greater than 101° F or 38.3C) accompanied by shaking chills and are coughing up thick phlegm, or if coughing or breathing deeply causes sharp chest pain, you may have pneumonia, and should consult a health care professional for diagnosis and appropriate treatment.

TREATING THE STUFFY NOSE OF A COLD OR THE FLU

It is not always necessary to treat a stuffy or congested nose. Only when your nose is so blocked that you are unable to breathe through it, or your ears are stuffed, or you are unable to sleep at night should you consider medication.

A stuffy nose can be treated with a nasal decongestant. Nasal decongestants cause narrowing of blood vessels, reducing the swelling of the mucuous membranes that line the nose. They can be useful to help breathing, clear stuffy ears, and help to avoid the drainage of nasal secretions into the throat, which can cause a sore throat or cough.

Nasal decongestants are available in topical forms (drops, sprays, nasal inhalers) or in oral forms (pills or capsules). For the treatment of short-lived congestion as with a cold or the flu, the fastest and safest relief is in the drops and sprays, applied directly to the inflamed area inside your nose.

Topical nasal decongestants should not be used for more than three days at a time. Using them for a longer period of time may cause "rebound congestion," an increase in nasal stuffiness after the medication wears off. The natural response is to apply more medication, but this can result in a serious cycle of increased nasal stuffiness, and increased use of the medicine which leads to dependence on nasal decongestants. Since this dependence can become very difficult to break, use of these decongestants should be reserved for serious congestion during a cold or the flu and should be limited to not more than three days.

If you use a nasal spray, drops, or inhaler, do not share the container. This may spread infection from one person to another.

Oral nasal decongestants (pills or liquids) should be avoided in the treatment of a disease as fleeting as a cold or the flu. The reasons for this are discussed in some detail in the section on products which follows.

OTC PRODUCTS FOR A STUFFY NOSE

Nasal sprays, drops, and inhalers are appropriate for treatment of nasal congestion which accompanies a cold or the flu. Unfortunately, some these products contain ingredients or combinations of ingredients which lack evidence of safety, effectiveness, or both as nasal decongestants.

An FDA advisory panel found the following ingredients safe and effective as topical nasal decongestants (sprays, drops or inhalers; ephedrine preparations, naphazoline hydrochloride, oxymetazoline hydrochloride, phenylephrine hydrochloride, and xylometazoline hydrochloride. In addition, propylhexedrine and 1-desoxyephedrine (alone and in combination with aromatics: camphor, menthol, methyl salicylate, bornyl acetate, and lavender oil), were found safe and effective as nasal decongestant inhalants.

A good choice for a topical nasal decongestant is a long-lasting (8-12 hour) product containing, as a single ingredient, either oxymetazoline hydrochloride, (such as AFRIN nose drops or spray, DRISTAN Long-Lasting Nasal Mist, DURATION Nasal Spray, NEO-SYNEPHRINE 12 Hour Nose Drops, SINEX Long-Acting Decongestant Nasal Spray), or xylometazoline hydrochloride, (such as 4-WAY Long-Acting — not regular — Nasal Spray, Long-Acting NEO-SYNEPHRINE II, OTRIVIN, or SINUTAB Long-Lasting Decongestant Nasal Spray).

Other effective topical nasal decongestants usually contain phenylephrine hydrochloride or ephedrine sulfate, which have a shorter duration and are taken every 4 hours. Phenylephrine is found in ALLEREST nasal spray, DURATION 4 hour nasal spray, NEO-SYNEPHRINE nasal spray and drops, and SINEX nasal spray. Ephedrine is found in VATRONOL Nose Drops.

As with other OTC products, you can often find a better bargain in less expensive generic or store brand products containing the identical active ingredient at a lower price. Many brand name products (including many Vicks products) also contain a variety of aromatic substances such as menthol, camphor, ethyl salicylate, bornyl acetate, and eucalyptus oil. These may be pleasing to some and offensive to others, but in general they do not add to the effectiveness of the product and are not worth any extra cost.

Effective nasal decongestant inhalers contain propylhexedrine (available in BENZEDREX in combination with menthol, which lacks evidence of effectiveness as a decongestant) or 1-desoxyephedrine (in VICKS inhaler). Inhalers may be less effective for some people as a nasal-inhaling effort is required to distribute the medication. It may be difficult to get the medication into a stuffed-up nose.

Some topical nasal decongestants contain ingredients or combinations of ingredients which lack evidence of effectiveness for treating nasal congestion. DRISTAN Nasal Mist and Menthol Nasal Mist both contain pheniramine maleate, an antihistamine which has no role in treating nasal congestion due to a cold.

Another example of a product which contains a combination of ingredients that lacks evidence of effectiveness is 4-WAY (Regular, not Long Acting) Nasal Spray, which contains not only phenylephrine, a safe and effective nasal decongestant, but also a second nasal decongestant, naphazoline hydrochloride, known for its uncomfortable and unsafe side effects, and pheniramine maleate, an antihistamine which does not enhance the effectiveness of the first ingredient and has many side effects. Naphazoline hydrochloride can cause rebound congestion after only one dose of this ingredient.[4] Also, there is no reason to believe that having two nasal decongestants in a product makes it any more effective than having an adequate amount of one. You're better off sticking with the single ingredient products discussed earlier.

With all topical nasal decongestants, you should be sure not to use more than the recommended dose, because this may cause side effects such as burning, stinging, sneezing, or an increase in nasal discharge. In addition, do not use these products for more than three days so as to avoid rebound congestion and drug dependence. If symptoms persist, see a health care professional.

Oral decongestants should be avoided in the treatment of nasal congestion accompanying a cold or flu. While these do not cause rebound congestion, they have the distinct disadvantage of being systemic drugs; this means they not only work much less rapidly than sprays or drops, but are also more likely to cause side effects throughout the body. Although an FDA panel found three ingredients to be safe and effective oral nasal decongestants, we cannot recommend their use in the treatment of the common cold or flu. Since nasal decongestants taken by mouth are absorbed into the blood and distributed all over the body, a very high dose (about 50 times higher than the dose that is effective in sprays, drops or inhalers) is required for them to work. These high doses are hazardous for two reasons.

- First, since oral decongestants narrow all of your blood vessels (not just those in your nose) they can increase blood pressure, even in persons with normal or low blood pressure. Both the lower doses and the more local effects of drops and sprays prevent this from being a problem with topical decongestants.

- Second, all nasal decongestants, both oral and topical, are related to a class of drugs called amphetamines ("uppers"), and like amphetamines, they may cause jitteriness and sleeplessness. These side effects are far more likely to occur with oral forms of nasal decongestants.

For these reasons, oral form nasal decongestants should be avoided by everyone, especially persons with high blood pressure, heart disease, thyroid disease or diabetes mellitus and by persons taking medication for depression that contains a monoamine oxidase (MAO) inhibitor (such as Marplan, Nardil or Parnate).

An FDA panel tentatively proposed approval of phenylpropanolamine hydrochloride (PPA), pseudoephedrine hydrochloride, and phenylephrine hydrochloride as oral nasal decongestants. These drugs are usually found in combination cold and allergy preparations which are discussed later in this chapter. An example of an oral product containing only a decongestant is SUDAFED, which contains pseudoephedrine hydrochloride.

As discussed more thoroughly in the chapter on weight control, there are a variety of serious adverse effects of PPA. (Examples of combination PPA-containing products include COMTREX, CON-TAC, FORMULA 44-D, HEAD & CHEST, SINE-OFF, and TRIAMINIC.) PPA can cause high blood pressure, even in normal people, and has been reported to cause fatal heart abnormalities, kidney disease, and muscle damage, as well as amphetamine-like nervous system effects such as rapid breathing, rapid heartbeat, tremor, restlessness, agitation, anxiety, dizziness and hallucinations. PPA is very similar to pseudoephedrine and phenylephrine in chemical structure, and it is likely that these other drugs could cause the same dangerous amphetamine-like adverse effects.

To repeat, we do not recommend the use of nasal decongestants taken by mouth for the treatment of a disease as short-lived as the common cold when safer and faster relief can be found with drops or sprays. In some cases, however, a health care professional may recommend the use of an oral decongestant in the treatment of a more prolonged illness. In these cases, a single ingredient product containing pseudoephedrine (SUDAFED is an example, but generics are available) is a better choice than a fixed combination product.

With all products containing an oral nasal decongestant, you should be sure not to exceed the recommended dose, because nervousness, dizziness, or sleeplessness may occur. If symptoms do not improve within 7 days or are accompanied by high fever, consult a health care professional.

TREATING A RUNNY NOSE

Letting your nose run, as inconvenient and uncomfortable as it may be, allows your body to remove the invading virus and correct the inflammation it has caused. Taking medication to "dry up" a runny nose, when the cause is a cold or the flu, is not wise.

Two types of medications, anticholinergics and antihistamines, are touted by the drug industry for treating a runny nose. Neither is appropriate for a cold or the flu.

Anticholinergic ingredients such as belladonna alkaloids and atropine sulfate have traditionally been included in many OTC remedies for the treatment of a runny nose. Some anticholinergic drugs have "drying" properties. According to the FDA, they lack evidence of effectiveness for treating a runny nose. In addition, they have a variety of unpleasant side effects. By drying up the air passages, they may cause a cough or cause a plug to form in the air passages which can slow down air flow to the lungs. These drugs also can cause constipation, dry mouth, sleeplessness, excitement, confusion, rapid heartbeat, and blurred vision, and they may aggravate glaucoma.

Anticholinergic drugs used to be included in OTC cold and allergy products. Many of these products, including CONTAC, have been reformulated without anticholinergics. Drugs used for colds which contain anticholinergics should not be used.

ANTIHISTAMINES: NOT FOR THE TREATMENT OF THE COMMON COLD OR FLU

Antihistamines treat the sneezing, watery itchy eyes, nasal congestion and sinus congestion caused by release of a chemical called histamine, most commonly seen in allergies such as hay fever. Although histamine release is the major cause of many common allergy symptoms, it is not a significant factor in cold symptoms. Antihistamines don't treat the symptoms of colds. Therefore, we recommend that you do not use antihistamines if you have a cold.

Many research studies have looked at the use of antihistamines in treating cold symptoms. In a review of these studies, Dr. Sheila West and her co-workers at Johns Hopkins University stated that of all the studies done, only two were adequately designed and well-controlled and that these studies "did not support the use of antihistamines to prevent or relieve the symptoms of a cold."[4]

The FDA Advisory panel also reported that antihistamines lack evidence of effectiveness in treating symptoms of a cold.

In response to the FDA Panel Report, Schering-Plough Corporation and Smith, Kline and French Laboratories, manufacturers of some of the best-selling cough and cold preparations containing antihistamines, jointly and individually submitted several studies to the FDA. As a result of these studies, the FDA appears to have started the process of reclassifying OTC antihistamines as effective for the treatment of runny nose and sneezing (though not for itchy nose or throat or itchy watery eyes caused by the common cold). We believe that these studies were seriously inadequate, and, therefore, we disagree with the preliminary decision of the FDA.*

Basically, antihistamines are good for allergies, not for colds. In addition, antihistamines have many side effects. The most frequent side effect is drowsiness, which is a problem for anyone who needs to be alert, and can be a hazard when driving or operating heavy machinery. The problem of drowsiness is so common that manufacturers of cold products without antihistamines now advertise the fact that there is "No Drowsiness" associated with their products.

Another common effect of antihistamines is the thickening of secretions in the air passages. This can make a cold or cough worse, because nasal and bronchial secretions need to be thinned to be loose enough to clear the infection.

Other side effects of antihistamines include dry mouth, nausea, upset stomach, loss of appetite, low blood pressure, blurred vision, and loss of coordination.[6]

---

* In one major study,[5] the symptomatic improvement reported by the cold sufferers and measured by the physicians was just barely better for the antihistamine users compared to those taking a placebo. In addition, no effort was made to scientifically document that study participants were all suffering from the common cold and were not actually allergy sufferers.

In addition, people with asthma, glaucoma, or difficulty urinating due to an enlarged prostate should not use antihistamines without medical supervision.

Unfortunately, nearly all OTC cold pills and liquids contain antihistamines. Common antihistamine ingredients are: chlorpheniramine maleate (in single ingredient products such as CHLOR-TRIMETON and in combination products such as COMTREX, CONTAC, CORICIDIN, CO-TYLENOL, DRISTAN ULTRA COLDS FORMULA, NOVAHISTINE, SINAREST, SINE-OFF, SUDAFED PLUS, and TRIAMINICIN), doxylamine succinate, brompheniramine maleate (in DIMETANE), dexbrompheniramine (in DRIXORAL), triprolidine (in ACTIFED), pyrilamine maleate and phenindamine tartrate.

None of these products and no other antihistamine-containing products should be used to treat the common cold. Congestion should be treated with a topical nasal decongestant if necessary, and a runny nose should be allowed to run.

Some products contain phenyltoloxamine citrate, which lacks evidence of effectiveness even as an antihistamine. SINUTAB is an example; this ingredient should be avoided. You get the drowsiness and other side effects without even the FDA's flawed promise of cold relief.

TREATING THE FEVER, HEADACHE, AND MUSCLE ACHES OF A COLD OR THE FLU

Fever, headaches, and muscle aches with a cold or flu are best treated without drugs, or should be treated with plain aspirin or acetaminophen (generic or store brand). Proper use of these pain-relievers is discussed in the Chapter on Analgesics. See p. 20 for Aspirin Warning for Children, and p. 13 for the warning signs of a headache.

If your fever climbs above 103 °F (39.4 °C), or if any fever over 100°F (38°C) lasts for more than 4 days, you should consult a health care professional. You probably don't have a cold.

If muscle aches, headache, and fever are the most prominent signs of the illness, and if a neighbor, child, or co-worker has the same symptoms, you probably have influenza. If you are otherwise in good health, you can treat this as if it were a more serious or exhausting cold, treating your symptoms as needed. Be sure to drink plenty of fluids to avoid dehydration (water loss) caused by fever-induced perspiration.

USE OF COMBINATION PRODUCTS FOR THE COMMON COLD

The vast majority of products sold as cold remedies are combination products. We cannot recommend any combination products, and we especially urge you to avoid combination cold remedies for the following reasons:

- They all contain antihistamines and/or oral decongestants; neither should be taken for the common cold.
- They all contain drug ingredients for the treatment of a wide range of symptoms; and you probably don't have all the symptoms or don't have them all at the same time. The course of a cold is varied and unpredictable, and "shotgun" treatment should not be used.
- Increasing the number of different drug ingredients increases the likelihood of unwanted side effects with no assurance that the product will be more effective.
- Even when all of the ingredients in a combination product are appropriate (which is not the case with any cold products), the fixed ratio of ingredients makes these drugs a poor choice. In other words, it is very unlikely that every ingredient is present in the correct dosage. You may overdose on one ingredient in an attempt to get enough of another one.

The combination drug products discussed here are sold primarily for cold symptoms; some are also marketed for cough or allergy, for which they are equally unwise.

The National Academy of Sciences-National Research Council conducted an exhaustive review of prescription drugs. ACTIFED and DRIXORAL (both contain an antihistamine and an oral decongestant) were studied and found ineffective for colds in this review; they are now available over the counter. Other OTC products containing combinations of antihistamines and decongestants, which should not be used to treat a cold, include: CHLORTRIMETON DECONGESTANT, CONTAC, DEMAZIN, DIMETANE DECONGESTANT, SUDAFED PLUS, TRIAMINIC SYRUP AND TRIAMINICIN CHEWABLES.

Drug makers have concocted other combinations which we do not recommend. Examples include: ALKA-SELTZER PLUS, COMTREX, CONTAC SEVERE COLD FORMULA, CORICIDIN, CORICIDIN-D, CO-TYLENOL (all), DRISTAN ULTRA COLDS FORMULA, FORMULA 44-D, HEADWAY, TYLENOL SINUS MEDICINE, SINAREST, SINE-AID, and SINE-OFF.

Some big selling combination cold remedies contain ingredients which FDA has found lack evidence of safety, effectiveness or both:

- NYQUIL, one of the most heavily advertised ($8.8 million in 1981)[7] and the best-selling of the combination cold products, contains an ingredient, ephedrine sulfate, which the FDA found lacks evidence of effectiveness as a nasal decongestant. Discussing NYQUIL, Donald C. LaBrecque, M.D., formerly Director of Clinical Research at Vick Laboratories, the manufacturer of NYQUIL, said:

48

It is a witches' brew because it contains everything under the sun. Someone sat down and said, "This is good, let us add this to it and let us add that to it," and finally, this product came out.[8]

Not only does NYQUIL contain an ingredient which lacks evidence of effectiveness (ephedrine sulfate), but it is also an irrational and potentially unsafe combination. It is 50 proof (25% alcohol). NYQUIL contains the antihistamine doxylamine succinate, the active ingredient in the sleep aid UNISOM; in our opinion, antihistamines such as doxylamine succinate are ineffective for treating the symptoms of a cold. 25% alcohol, in combination with the sedating antihisamine, makes drowsiness a major effect of this drug. You are better off with the treatment recommended earlier in this chapter.

• DRISTAN Decongestant/Antihistamine/Analgesic Tablets and Capsules, regular and aspirin free, and TRIAMINICIN tablets are examples of big-selling products that contain caffeine. Caffeine is added to these products because it allegedly "corrects" the drowsiness caused by the antihistamine (which is inappropriate for a cold in any event). The FDA Advisory panel found that evidence is lacking to prove this claim. Nonetheless you may experience the side effects of the caffeine along with the side effects of the other drugs in these irrational combinations. Whitehall Laboratories spent $23.7 million in 1981 advertising the DRISTAN line of products.[9] If you buy them, you will support this company's massive advertising budget — and probably take one or more ingredients you don't need.

• SINUTAB (pushed by a $5.87 million[10] media campaign in 1981) contains phenyltoloxamine; phenyltoloxamine lacks evidence of effectiveness as an antihistamine, according to the FDA. We would not recommend this combination (decongestant, antihistamine, analgesic), however, even if it contained an effective antihistamine. This product should not be used; according to FDA criteria for safety and effectiveness, SINUTAB, like DRISTAN tablets and capsules and NYQUIL, should not even be available.

Some of the products on the market for colds or allergy claim to be "timed-release" formulations. The idea is that one pill will last for 12 hours. Unfortunately, many of these formulations have not proven their ability to last any longer than the regular formulation, so that the action is unpredictable as well as unnecessarily expensive. Examples of products which lack evidence of effectiveness because their timed release formulations aren't proven include: C3 CAPSULES, DRISTAN 12-HOUR NASAL DECONGESTANT CAPSULES, and NEOSYNEPHRINOL DAY RELIEF CAPSULES.

COUGH

Your lungs clean themselves constantly in order to maintain efficient breathing. Mucus normally lines the walls of the lungs and captures foreign particles such as inhaled smoke and infecting virus particles. Hair-like cells push this out of the lungs. Coughing adds an additional, rapid-fire means of removing unwanted material from the lungs.

A cough is beneficial as long as it is bringing up material, such as sputum (phlegm), from your airways and lungs. This is called a "productive" cough. A dry, hacking, "non-productive"cough, on the other hand, can be irritating and keep you awake at night. Coughing can also be part of a chronic condition, such as asthma, or emphysema, or it may be caused by cigarette smoking.

A cough resulting from a chronic condition should be evaluated by a health care professional. You should also seek out medical advice: if your sputum (phlegm) becomes greenish, yellowish, or foul smelling; if your cough is accompanied by a high fever lasting several days; if coughing or breathing deeply causes sharp chest pain; or if you develop shortness of breath — you may have pneumonia. Anyone who coughs up blood should consult a health care professional.

TREATING A COUGH

A *productive cough* is useful in helping you recover from cold or flu and you should do what you can to encourage the clearance of material from your lungs by "loosening up" the mucus. This is the purpose of an expectorant, which thins secretions so that they can be removed more easily by coughing (or "expectoration"). The best expectorant is water, especially in warm liquids such as soup, which thins the mucus and increases the amount of fluid in the respiratory tract. A moist environment also helps this effort. You should drink plenty of liquids and supplement this, if you can, by moistening the air with a humidifier or plain water steamed by a vaporizer. A pan of water on the radiator can help in the winter.

A *non-productive cough* — a dry cough bringing up no mucus — may be treated with a cough suppressant, also called an antitussive. A cough which keeps you up at night or is extremely exhausting may also call for the use of one of these agents. Cough suppressants should be used in a single-ingredient product. Rest and plenty of fluids are also in order.

OTC PRODUCTS FOR A COUGH

OTC products to treat a cough contain either an expectorant or an antitussive (a cough suppressant). Of these products, the only type we recommend is a single-ingredient cough suppressant to treat a dry cough.

Expectorants

Many OTC cough remedies contain ingredients called expectorants, which are supposed to promote clearing of mucus from the lungs. In theory, this is a wonderful idea. Unfortunately, the FDA Advisory panel review of the marketed expectorants found that *ALL OTC EXPECTORANTS LACK EVIDENCE OF EFFECTIVENESS.* This includes ingredients in many widely marketed and sold products.

Guaifenesin is the most widely used of the expectorants. No well-designed study has shown that it works, despite the efforts of drug manufacturers to convince people that it does. Relying on a study recently submitted by the maker of ROBITUSSIN (performed on hospitalized patients with chronic bronchitis, rather than a self-limiting disease such as a cold), the FDA appears to have started the process of reclassifying guaifenesin as effective as an OTC expectorant.[3] In the opinion of the Public Citizen Health Research Group, the evidence upon which the FDA largely based its recent decision is inadequate,* and we urge reevaluation of this poorly done and largely irrelevant study.

Guaifenesin is the sole active ingredient in ROBITUSSIN, and an ingredient in CHERACOL, CHERACOL D, FORMULA 44-D, HEAD AND CHEST, ROBITUSSIN DM, CF, and PE, and TRIAMINIC EXPECTORANT, to name only a few. We advise you not to waste your money on these products and other products containing this ingredient, if you are looking for an expectorant.

Other expectorants which lack evidence of effectiveness are sodium citrate, ammonium chloride, eucalyptus oil, menthol, terpin hydrate preparations, and spirits of turpentine. Some ingredients. such as ipecac fluid extract (in CEROSE DM), lack evidence of safety as well.

As discussed before, there *is* one safe, effective expectorant: water, especially in warm liquids such as soup. Drink plenty of fluids as often as you can to aid clearance of the airways.

Cough Suppressants

For the occasional bothersome, unproductive cough, a variety of ingredients and combinations of cough suppressants are available. Of these, we recommend a single ingredient.

The FDA Advisory panel reviewed all of the cough suppressants in OTC products and classified only two as safe and effective: dextromethorphan hydrobromide and codeine. Through a different

---

*The information submitted to the FDA by the manufacturer (on treatment of chronic bronchitis, performed at Vercelli Pulmonary Hospital in Milan, Italy) is not sufficient to prove that guaifenesin is effective as an expectorant in the treatment of a cold. We do not believe the study was well-designed, well-controlled, or applicable to treating people with an acute disease like the common cold. For example, no studies of lung function were performed on subjects, and subjects were allowed to use various other drugs.

FDA regulatory mechanism, diphenhydramine hydrochloride is also now available as an OTC antitussive. In addition, at some point in the near future, chlophedianol hydrochloride will be marketed as an OTC cough suppresant. Finally, some aromatic compounds are sold as lozenges or chest rubs to decrease the desire to cough. Each of these ingredients is discussed below.

Dextromethorphan should be your choice if you need an over the counter medicine to stop a non-productive cough. If you can, use a product which contains dextromethorphan as a single ingredient to avoid the unpleasant side effects and expense of additional ingredients. Unfortunately, this effective product is not as readily available in the necessary dosage in many drugstores. We recommend that you buy a generic or store brand product if available; some more expensive brand name products with dextromethorphan include HOLD, ST. JOSEPH'S COUGH SYRUP FOR CHILDREN and SUCRETS COUGH CONTROL FORMULA.

Dextromethorphan acts on the cough center in the brain to suppress cough. It is a highly effective, non-narcotic drug with few side effects. Overdosing can slow breathing so you should carefully judge the amount needed. Read the label to find the concentration of the product. A proper dose is 10-20 mg every 4 hours for adults, 5-10 mg for children 6-12 years, and 2.5-5 mg for children 2-6 years. Children under 2 should not be treated with drugs for cough without medical supervision.

If you are unable to find any plain, single-ingredient dextromethorphan-containing products, and you need a cough suppressant, it may be necessary to use a product containing dextromethorphan in a combination product. If this is the case, try one with guaifenesin (it seems to us to have little or no medical action) such as COUGH CALMERS, CHERACOL D, or ROBITUSSIN DM, or a less expensive generic or store brand equivalent; and *ask your pharmacist to stock a generic, single ingredient dextromethorphan product in the future.*

Codeine is also an effective antitussive; but it is a narcotic drug with a variety of side effects, including drowsiness, constipation, lightheadedness, nausea and vomiting. It poses some hazards if taken in excessive doses: it can slow breathing and it is addictive. In proper doses, it is a safe and effective cough suppressant but we recommend that you try dextromethorphan first — it works about as well and has fewer drawbacks.

Since it is a narcotic, codeine is available in many states only by prescription. Where it is available OTC, it is usually not in a single-ingredient formulation. For these reasons, codeine is not our drug of choice as an OTC antitussive.

Diphenhydramine hydrochloride (in BENYLIN cough syrup) was approved by the FDA in September 1981 as an OTC antitussive by a process (New Drug Application) which is separate from the OTC review process. Diphenhydramine is an antihistamine also sold as a sleep aid. (It is the sole active ingredient in COMPOZ, NYTOL DPH, and SOMINEX FORMULA 2. See the chapter on sleep aids and insomnia.) It has a strong sedative effect, as well as other antihistamine side effects.

Diphenhydramine should not be used in situations where mental alertness is required, or when a drying effect (of the nose, throat and mouth) may be unwanted — as is often the case with a cold. Because of its sedative effect, it shouldn't be used with any tranquilizers, sedatives, or alcohol (which is 5% of BENYLIN Cough Syrup). We cannot recommend the use of this product. In our opinion, dextromethorphan is a safer alternative.

Chlophedianol hydrochloride is not currently in any OTC products, but appears to be targeted for a switch from prescription to OTC status.[13] The prescription product is known as Ulo, but it is not widely marketed. Until more information is available, we cannot recommend this ingredient.

Lozenges containing menthol are widely marketed for sore throats (which are discussed in the next section). An FDA Advisory panel found that these products lack evidence of effectiveness as cough suppressants. The FDA's Bureau of Drugs now appears to have started the process of reclassifying menthol in lozenges as safe and effective as a topical (on the surface) cough suppressant.[14] Menthol acts locally in the throat, rather than centrally in the brain, as do other cough suppressants. Don't take more than one menthol lozenge an hour. If you find them ineffective and are still bothered by a cough, try a medicine with dextromethorphan, discussed on p. 52. Menthol containing lozenges include HALL'S MENTHO-LYPTUS, N'ICE, and VICTOR'S; a number of generic and store-brand products are also available. For a mild cough related to a dry throat, sucking on a hard, sour candy may do as well.

Chest rubs containing menthol, camphor, eucalyptus oil, thymol, oil of turpentine, cedarleaf oil, and myristica oil (the combination in VICKS VAPORUB) have also been the subject of a recent FDA Bureau of Drugs proposal.[15] The FDA Advisory panel found these products lacking evidence of effectiveness. Based on studies of artifically-induced cough, in normal, healthy people (rather than of people with cough from colds), the FDA has started the process of reclassifying some of the ingredients in VAPORUB as safe and effective as an antitussive. Nevertheless, one ingredient, turpentine oil, is ineffective and we do not recommend the use of chest rubs like VAPORUB. A chest rub can neither soothe the throat as a sour candy does nor affect the cough center in the brain as dextromethorphan does.

Combination products for cough are not recommended to treat your ailment, for the same reasons discussed earlier in this chapter in the section on combination cold remedies. When you are unable to find the plain ingredient you are looking for, the only combination product you should consider is one which contains the single ingredient you need (such as dextromethorphan) along with a safe though ineffective ingredient (such as guaifenesin). Ask your pharmacist to stock good single-ingredient products so that you take only the medicine you need. Examples of combination cough remedies which should not be used under any circumstances include ROBITUSSIN CF, ROBITUSSIN PE, and TRIAMINIC EXPECTORANT. They all contain not only guaifenesin (discussed earlier in the this section) which in our opinion lacks evidence of effectiveness, but additional ingredients that we do not recommend.

SORE THROAT

An irritated and painful throat is often part of the common cold, but it can be part of other diseases as well. When a sore throat accompanies a cold or other viral infection, it is best treated with simple home and over the counter remedies, but when it is part of a bacterial infection, medical treatment may be required.

Strep Throat

"Strep throat" is a serious infection, because the bacteria that cause it can cause rheumatic fever, rheumatic heart disease or kidney disease. Rheumatic fever or heart disease can be avoided by taking a complete regimen of the correct antibiotic (penicillin unless you are allergic to penicillin) early in the course of the sore throat. Antibiotics are completely inappropriate, however, to treat sore throats accompanying viral infections such as a cold.

It is often very difficult, even for an experienced nurse or physician, to distinguish strep throat from any other kind of sore throat by simply looking at the throat, although a sore throat with a classic cold is unlikely to be strep. Strep throat must be diagnosed by a throat culture (results are known in two days). The culture test involves swabbing your throat and checking to see if streptococci grow from the material removed. If there's any question in your mind, it is a good idea to take advantage of this simple, risk-free form of precautionary medicine.

Several widely followed criteria are used to determine who needs a throat culture to screen for strep throat. They are listed below to help you determine whether you need one. If you have a painful throat in addition to any of the following signs, symptoms or medical problems, consult a health care professional; you probably

need a throat culture:
- Pus (yellowish-white, thick spots) on your throat or tonsils.
- Fever greather than 101 °F (38.3 °C).
- Exposure to someone with a proven strep infection.
- A rash which came with or after the sore throat.
- A history of rheumatic fever, rheumatic heart disease or kidney disease.

The cause of a sore throat in a child is difficult to judge; any significant throat pain probably should not be treated without a call to the child's doctor.

HOW TO TREAT SORE THROAT WHICH ACCOMPANIES THE COMMON COLD

If you have a mild sore throat for a few days, treat it with moisture to relieve the irritation. Warm or hot liquids (tea with honey and lemon is a favorite) are very helpful for this purpose. As with a cough, spending time in a moist environment (as provided by a vaporizer, for example) will help to prevent your throat from drying out and can prevent further irritation.

If warm liquids are not enough to relieve your sore throat pain and discomfort, we recommend plain aspirin or acetaminophen tablets, taken every four hours, which will provide effective pain relief. Because aspirin irritates the mucous membranes that line the mouth and throat, it should not not be held, dissolved, or chewed in the mouth, nor should aspirin chewing gum (such as ASPERGUM) be used. Also, aspirin chewing gum provides less effective pain relief than plain aspirin tablets swallowed whole. See the chapter on analgesics for more information on these drugs and proper use.

OTC PRODUCTS SOLD FOR SORE THROAT
Mouthwashes and Gargles

Mouthwashes and gargles are among the best selling OTC products on the market, but they play no real role in the treatment of sore throat. They are effective only as short-lived mouth "refreshers" and, in the case of one brand, as temporary pain-relievers. The use of these products for any "antibacterial" effect makes no sense because: first, all of their active ingredients lack evidence of effectiveness as antimicrobial agents; and second, a cold's sore throat is the result of a virus, not bacteria.

If you have a sore throat, we urge you not to waste your money on mouthwashes to cure the infection. None will do it. This includes the active ingredients in CEPACOL, LISTERINE and SCOPE. These products do not claim to treat a sore throat, although they list "active ingredients" on their label.

Of this type of product, the FDA Advisory Panel on OTC Oral Cavity Drug Products stated that "there were few, if any, indications justifying the use of OTC mouthwashes, mouth rinses, and gargles containing antimicrobial agents for self-medication."[16] All oral antimicrobial ingredients, including the "active ingredients" in LISTERINE (thymol, eucalyptol, methyl salicylate and menthol), lack evidence of effectiveness; but the "active ingredient" in CEPACOL and SCOPE (cetylpyridinium chloride) lacks evidence of safety as well. Cetylpyridinium chloride may have a variety of safety problems which have not been thoroughly examined; it can cause vomiting, collapse, and coma if swallowed in sufficient quantities, and its effects with long-term use or use during pregnancy are not known.

Other mouthwashes, like LISTERMINT and SIGNAL, correctly do not claim any "active ingredient." Like *all* mouthwashes and gargles, they are purely cosmetic. They will temporarily "freshen" your breath — and that is all.

CHLORASEPTIC and CHERRY CHLORASEPTIC Liquid and Aerosol Spray contain phenol and sodium phenolate. Both of these ingredients temporarily relieve pain, but neither prevents or cures infection of the mouth and throat. There is some question about the effectiveness of topical pain-killers when used in gargles, though, since little of the throat surface is actually exposed during gargling.[18]

Throat Lozenges — Some May Help

Throat lozenges are popular items for treating sore throats. As with sprays, the most they can provide is temporary pain relief; none prevent or treat infection. Some, like hard sour candy, may help keep the throat moist, and this may be their greatest value in treating a sore throat. Some lozenges contain single active ingredients and others contain combinations.

There are a number of ingredients in lozenges which the FDA Panel found safe and effective for pain relief. These include hexylresorcinol (in plain SUCRETS), phenol and sodium phenolate (in CHERRY and MENTHOL CHLORASEPTIC lozenges), benzocaine (in CHILDREN'S CHLORASEPTIC and SPEC-T SORE THROAT ANESTHETIC Lozenge), menthol (in LUDEN'S MENTHOL Lozenges) and phenol (in CEPASTAT). Generic or store brand equivalents are often available at a lower price than some of these brand names.

Care should be exercised in using throat lozenges or sprays containing pain relievers; they may mask the seriousness of an infection and delay or prevent a needed check with a health care professional. This is particularly true when caring for children, who are more likely to have strep throat or other bacterial infections requiring medical supervision. These products should not be used at all for children under 3 years.

Topical pain-relievers should not be used more often than directed on the package or for more than 2 days in any event. Discontinue use and consult a health care professional if irritation persists or increases, or if you develop a skin rash.

We do not recommend the use of throat lozenges containing decongestants, for the same reason we do not recommend pill-form decongestants (see pp. 44-45). SUCRETS Cold Decongestant Formula and SPEC-T Sore Throat/Decongestant Lozenges, for example, both contain phenylpropanolamine. SPEC-T also contains phenylephrine; together they are an irrational combination when used as nasal decongestants.

As with mouthwashes, lozenges containing antimicrobial ingredients like cetylpyridinium lack evidence of safety and effectiveness. These include CEPACOL Throat Lozenges and Anesthetic Troches, and VICKS Throat Lozenges. These should not be used.

Finally, some lozenges contain fixed combinations of drugs — products we cannot recommend, as explained under Combination Cold Remedies, p. 47. This includes products which combine pain-relievers with cough-suppressants, such as CHLORASEPTIC COUGH CONTROL LOZENGES and SPEC-T SORE THROAT/COUGH SUPPRESSANTS and LOZENGES. Cough is discussed at length earlier in this chapter (p. 50).

ALLERGIES AND HAY FEVER

If you suffer from an itchy, runny nose, watery eyes, sneezing, and a tickle in the back of your throat, then you probably have an allergy. An allergy means a "hypersensitivity" to a particular substance, called an "allergen."

Hypersensitivity means that the body's immune system, which defends against infection, disease and foreign bodies, reacts inappropriately to the allergen. Examples of common allergens are pollen from ragweed or other plants, molds, dust, feathers, cat hair, make-up, walnuts, aspirin, shellfish, poison ivy and chocolate.

Allergies reveal themselves to us in many ways. Simply speaking, there are four types of allergic responses, although many substances can cause more than one type of response in a given person. The common types of allergic reactions are:

•Itchy, runny nose, watery eyes, sneezing, and a tickle in the back of your throat. This type of allergy is sometimes called *allergic rhinitis* and is commonly caused by exposure to allergens in the air such as pollen, dust, and animal feathers or hair. It is called "hay fever" when it occurs seasonally, such as in response to ragweed in the fall.

• Hives or other skin reactions. These commonly result from something you eat or from skin exposure to an allergenic substance (such as poison ivy or chemicals on the job or in your hobby shop). Allergic skin reactions may also follow insect bites or an emotional disturbance.

• Asthma. (See section beginning on p. 62)

• Sudden generalized itching, rapidly followed by difficulty breathing and possibly shock (extremely low blood pressure) or death. This rare and serious allergic response, called *anaphylaxis,* usually occurs as a response to certain injections (including allergy shots), drugs (including antibiotics such as penicillin), and insect bites as from a bee or wasp. This reaction may become increasingly severe with repeated exposures. Anaphylaxis is a medical emergency requiring an IMMEDIATE trip to an emergency room, clinic or doctor's office. If you are likely to have an anaphylactic response to an allergen such as a bee sting, in a locale where medical attention may be out of reach, you should obtain a prescription from a physician for an emergency kit containing injectable epinephrine to keep with you, and learn how to use it.

In this section on allergy, we are concerned primarily with allergic rhinitis.

HOW TO TREAT ALLERGIC SYMPTOMS

The best way to treat an allergy is to discover the cause of your allergy, and if possible, to avoid the offending substance. Sometimes this is easy, but in many cases it is not.

If, for example, your eyes swell up, your nose runs and you break out in hives each time you are around cats, avoid cats and you've solved your problems.

If, however, you sneeze during one particular season (typically, late spring, summer or fall) each year or all year round, there is not too much you can do to avoid the pollens, dust or grass particles in the air. Some people find relief in an indoor retreat where it is cooler, closed, and less dusty, but this is not always possible.

If you can't seem to figure out the cause of your allergy, have tried eliminating most of the common allergens from your environment and are still suffering from significant discomfort, you may need to see a health care professional. It is possible that you may be an appropriate candidate for skin testing, and may be referred to a physician specializing in allergies.

In skin testing, small amounts of various allergens are placed on different spots on your skin. A day or two later, the skin is examined for signs of an allergic reaction to each of the allergens.

Skin ("patch," scratch, or injection) testing is most likely to be positive for an allergen that causes skin rashes, or contact sensitivity. Allergens that cause allergic rhinitis symptoms (runny nose, watery eyes and sneezing) may not give a "positive" result. The FDA has conducted a review of the allergenic extracts used for patch testing. The majority lack evidence of effectiveness in indicating the source of an allergy.[20]

In addition, it is common to have a positive reaction on a patch test but to have no really significant allergy when you are exposed to the particular allergen in the environment.[21] Beware of the allergist who send you home with a long list of substances to avoid because they gave positive patch tests. Even if you avoid all of them, you may be left with your allergy if none of the ones on the list is the particular one responsible for your symptoms.

When identifying the cause of your allergy is not possible, then you may choose to treat the symptoms. Because allergy symptoms are caused primarily by the release of a chemical in your body called *histamine,* a class of medication known as the *antihistamines* is the most effective initial treatment of symptoms available.

We recommend that you use antihistamines in a single-ingredient preparation to treat your symptoms. (Ingredients and products are discussed further on in the chapter.) If your allergic reactions do not respond to antihistamines, consult a health care professional to pursue other alternatives.

One treatment which a physician may offer is allergy shots. The idea of these shots is to inject you with increasingly larger amounts of an allergen to which you are allergic, in order to "desensitize" you. As these injections usually must be given year-round, even if you only have your allergy for a few months of the year, they require a major investment of time and money and are worthwhile for only a small proportion of allergy sufferers. Additionally, many of the specific, allergen extracts used for injection lack evidence of effectiveness, according to the FDA. In fact, of the hundreds of pollen extracts, only four are proven effective.[22]

Allergic rhinitis should *not* be treated with topical nasal decongestants (drops, sprays, and inhalers), which are recommended for treating the *temporary* stuffy nose of a cold. Allergies are long-term conditions, lasting for weeks, months or years, and use of these topical decongestants for more than a few days can lead to rebound congestion and sometimes permanent damage to the membranes lining the nose. If you think your congestion is caused by allergies, don't use an OTC nasal spray, or you may eventually find that you can't breathe through your nose without it.

OTC PRODUCTS FOR ALLERGY
Antihistamines

Of the products sold for allergy, we recommend that you use a single-ingredient product containing only an antihistamine. They are the most effective over the counter ingredients you can buy for treating an allergy, and you will minimize the side effects by buying the single-ingredient formulation.

The major side effect of antihistamines is drowsiness. If they make you drowsy, you should avoid driving a motor vehicle or operating heavy machinery while taking these drugs. Additionally, keep in mind that drowsiness is increased dramatically by adding other sedatives, including alcoholic beverages.

The amount of drowsiness produced by an antihistamine differs depending on the person who takes it and the antihistamine that is used. Of antihistamines classified by the FDA as safe and effective for OTC use, those causing the least drowsiness are chlorpheniramine maleate, brompheniramine maleate and pheniramine maleate.[23] For daytime use, we urge you to use one of these.

Other FDA-approved antihistamines, causing somewhat more sedation, are pyrilamine maleate and thonzylamine maleate. Those causing a great deal of drowsiness include diphenhydramine hydrochloride and doxylamine succinate, which are the ingredients in currently available OTC sleep aids.[24]

Another common side effect of antihistamines is dryness of the mouth, nose and throat. Other less common side effects include blurred vision, dizziness, loss of appetite, nausea, upset stomach, low blood pressure, headache, and loss of coordination. Difficulty in urinating is often a problem in older men with enlarged prostate glands. Antihistamines occasionally cause nervousness, restlessness, or insomnia, especially in children.

For antihistamine treatment of allergies, your first choice should be chlorpheniramine maleate or brompheniramine maleate, available in single - ingredient products such as CHLOR-TRIMETON or DIMETANE. Check the label and be sure that nothing else is in the product. CHLOR-TRIMETON DECONGES-TANT or DIMETANE EXPECTORANT both contain additional ingredients which are not necessary for the treatment of allergy. Less expensive store brand or generic equivalents are often available and should be purchased if possible. If you can't find them ask the pharmacist he or she should have it behind the counter if it is not on display. A proper dose (one to four times a day) is 2-4 mg for adults and 1-2 mg for children ages 6-12. Do not give these drugs to children under 6 years except with the advice or supervision of a physician. Time - released formulations of chlorpheniramine maleate are also available (CHLOR-TRIMETON REPETABS and TELDRIN, for example); these may be more convenient in some instances, but are considerably more expensive than store brand regular release products.

You should not use antihistamines for self-medication if you have asthma, glaucoma, or difficulty urinating due to enlargement of the prostate gland.

Nasal Decongestants

Many OTC products sold for allergies contain nasal decongestants such as phenylpropanolamine hydrochloride or pseudoephedrine hydrochloride. This type of ingredient is discussed earlier in this chapter (pp. 44-45) under OTC PRODUCTS FOR A STUFFY NOSE. They have the same disadvantages and side effects when used to treat an allergy. Some of these side effects and adverse reactions (such as jitteriness, sleeplessness, and potential heart problems) occur even more frequently when they are used to treat allergies, because allergy medication is usually taken for a longer period of time than are cold remedies.

More to the point, nasal decongestants do not treat the symptoms most frequently experienced by allergy sufferers: the runny nose, itchy and watery eyes, sneezing, cough and tickle in the back of your throat. They treat only a stuffy nose—not the major problem for most allergy sufferers.

Examples of nasal decongestant products which are labeled to treat allergy symptoms "without drowsiness" (since they don't contain antihistamines) include AFRINOL and SUDAFED. We do not recommend the use of these products for allergies.

Combination Allergy Products

As usual in the OTC market (particularly in the cold and allergy area), most products available are fixed-combination products, using a "shotgun" approach to your ailment. The majority of allergy combination products contain antihistamines *and* nasal decongestants; some also contain pain relievers. We do not recommend any of these for self-treatment.

The reasons not to take fixed-combination products are discussed on p. 47. Combinations of antihistamines and oral nasal decongestants should be avoided for the same reason. It is our opinion that nasal decongestants should not be used for allergy symptoms that are appropriate for self-treatment, since you increase the likelihood of side effects by taking a combination product and decongestants seldom address allergy symptoms.

Examples of combination drugs for allergy, which we cannot recommend, are: ACTIFED, A.R.M., ALLEREST, CHLOR-TRIMETON DECONGESTANT, DIMETANE DECONGESTANT, DRIXORAL, and SUDAFED PLUS. Many of the combination cold products listed on p. 48 (that we urge you not to use)

61

also are marketed for allergic symptoms and hay fever. We do not recommend using any of these products for allergies.

ASTHMA

Asthma is a disease characterized by hypersensitivity of the airways of the lungs to various influences; during asthma attacks, the airways narrow and breathing is made more difficult. Most asthmatics only have occasional trouble breathing; when this occurs, wheezing, chest tightness, and an unproductive cough usually accompany the sensation of shortness of breath.

Although most asthmatics are not restricted by their condition, for some the severity of the attacks can be life-threatening or can severely restrict their lifestyles.

For *all* asthmatics, however, the types of medications prescribed to treat or prevent the attacks are quite strong. If used incorrectly, these may be very dangerous — in an immediate way — to the health of the user.

For this reason, both the diagnosis and the treatment of this disorder should be supervised by a physician. Although OTC drugs are available, even these should be taken only with the advice of a physician.

Asthma attacks are commonly caused by exposure to specific allergens, air pollutants, industrial chemicals, or infection; they can be caused by exercise (especially in cold air). Asthma can be worsened by emotional factors.

Asthma is a common occupational illness (a problem related to the workplace). It frequently occurs among meat wrappers, bakers, woodworkers and farmers, and among factory workers exposed to chemicals such as TDI (used to make polyurethane foam), aminoethylethanolamine (used in soldering flux), and chemicals in the manufacture of detergents, to name only a few. An asthma-like disease called byssinosis, or "brown lung," results in Monday-morning tight chest or difficulty breathing (with the return to work after the weekend) and is common in cotton textile workers.

The shortness of breath, dry cough, and wheezing that characterize asthma are brought about by swelling of the walls of these airways, narrowing of the air passages, and accumulation of secretions along the airways. This blocks air flow in and out of the lungs.

Asthma oftens runs in families. Other ailments common to many asthma sufferers or their family members are hay fever and an allergic skin condition called eczema.

Asthma is not a diagnosis that you can make yourself, it must be diagnosed by a physician or other health care professional. It is easily confused with congestive heart failure or pneumonia, two other medical conditions that cause breathing difficulties. Both may be worsened by treatment with asthma remedies, and it is therefore extremely important that you have your condition diagnosed before starting to take asthma medication.

Although asthma can be an allergic reaction, antihistamines are not effective for asthma. They can even be harmful.

HOW TO TREAT ASTHMA

The treatment of asthma, like its diagnosis, should be determined by a physician. Asthma attacks can be very frightening, and sufferers often overtreat themselves with over the counter and/or prescription medication, especially when desired relief has not been provided by the recommended dosage.

DO NOT USE MORE THAN THE RECOMMENDED OR PRESCRIBED DOSE OF ANY ASTHMA MEDICATION WITHOUT FIRST CONSULTING YOUR PHYSICIAN.

All medications for the treatment of asthma, including those available without a prescription, should be chosen by you and a physician together.

A physician is likely to prescribe one or more prescription-only drugs for the asthmatic. The currently available OTC drugs (the subject of the discussion which follows) are not the best drugs even for the treatment of minor or infrequent asthmatic episodes. An up-to-date physician is apt to prescribe a single ingredient theophylline or aminophylline product and/or a product (tablets or inhaler) containing metaproterenol (Alupent; Metaprel), terbutaline (Brethine; Bricanyl), or albuterol (Proventil; Ventolin). All of these drugs are bronchodilators; they relax the smooth muscles of the lungs' airways to keep them open. The appropriate dose of these drugs needs to be carefully calculated by your physician; sometimes a blood test of theophylline levels is necessary.

Other prescription drugs used in asthma include cromolyn sodium (Intal), used to prevent the symptoms of asthma, and steroid hormone drugs such as prednisone tablets or a beclomethasone dipropionate inhaler (Beclovent or Vanceril), used to treat severe asthma.

OTC PRODUCTS FOR ASTHMA

It is our opinion, and your doctor will probably agree, that *CURRENTLY AVAILABLE OVER THE COUNTER PRODUCTS FOR ASTHMA ARE LESS HELPFUL AND, IN MANY CASES, LESS SAFE THAN INTELLIGENTLY SELECTED PRESCRIPTION MEDICATIONS.*

The FDA has reviewed the ingredients in OTC asthma drugs and found that many of them (including the ingredients in all currently marketed OTC asthma tablets) lack evidence of safety, effectiveness or both. Some products available now (inhalers) were found to be safe and effective, but other, safer prescription products are generally preferred by the medical profession. Additionally, the FDA switched one prescription-only ingredient to nonprescription status, but it is not yet available over the counter.

The OTC asthma products can be divided into two classes: those in inhaler form (aerosols or drops used in a spray) for use during an attack, and those in tablet or elixir form, to prevent and control symptoms.

Inhalers-Mists and Sprays

All of the OTC inhalers now available contain epinephrine (such as ASTHMAHALER, ASTHMANEFRIN, BRONKAID MIST and PRIMATENE MIST). Epinephrine sprays allow the airways to open, and the FDA has tentatively decided that these are safe and effective over the counter drug products.

Used as directed, these inhalers are safe and effective, offering fast (though not long-lasting) relief from asthma. Unfortunately, there are many drawbacks to epinephrine sprays, and doctors are increasingly warning their patients to avoid their use.

With these products, you should use as little as possible, saving them for the worst time — when the pollen count is high, or when you also have a cold or infection aggravated by asthma symptoms. Epinephrine is a short-acting drug, and when its effect wears off, the airways can narrow again by reflex action. Also, tolerance quickly develops to this medication; that is, after a few consecutive uses, the recommended dose of the drug is no longer sufficient to produce the desired effect.

In short, used correctly and only occasionally, epinephrine sprays can provide prompt and effective relief. Used excessively — and it's easy to get into the habit — ephinephrine sprays can cause even greater breathing difficulties and other very serious problems, such as nervousness, rapid heartbeat and possibly adverse effects on the heart.

Remember (with all asthma inhalers):
• Do not use these products if you have any kind of heart disease, high blood pressure, thyroid problems, diabetes, Parkinson's disease, glaucoma, or difficulty in urination due to enlargement of the prostate gland, unless directed by a health care professional.

• Do not use these products without first consulting your doctor if you are presently taking a prescription drug for high blood pressure or depression.

• Do not continue to take these products, but seek medical assistance immediately, if symptoms are not relieved within 20 minutes or if they become worse.

The FDA has proposed a prescription-to-OTC change for metered-dose inhalers containing metaproterenol sulfate. These are currently available by prescription only as Alupent and Metaprel. When this ingredient becomes available without a prescription, it will probably by a better choice than epinephrine, because it doesn't constrict blood vessels throughout the body as epinephrine does. Like epinephrine, however, this drug has side effects such as nervousness, fast heartbeat, tremor, and nausea; it can be easily overused, and should be used no more than agreed on by you and your physician.

Tablets and Elixirs

All of the widely marketed OTC tablets and elixirs for treating asthma contain combinations of ingredients which lack evidence of safety and effectivenes, according to the FDA.

BRONKAID tablets, BRONITIN tablets, BRONKOTABS tablets, PRIMATENE (P and M) tablets, and TEDRAL tablets and elixir, for example, all contain a combination of ephedrine and theophylline, with or without other ill-advised drug ingredients. The FDA did not approve any combination for OTC use and has found that theophylline (although currently in these products) is not appropriate as an OTC drug.

Theophylline alone is often the drug of choice for asthma, but the FDA has wisely proposed that it not be available over the counter. Theophylline has a very small dosage range in which it is helpful but safe. Too little theophylline (as is present in all currently available OTC products) will not work, while too much may cause side effects including headache, insomnia, nervousness, stomachache, nausea, vomiting, rapid or irregular heartbeat, and even seizures.

Ephedrine, though tentatively considered safe and effective by the FDA, is a poor drug for asthma. Ephedrine's action, unlike that of some of the newer (prescription-only) asthma remedies (terbutaline and albuterol, for example), greatly affects other parts of the body, such as the heart and nervous system. Ephedrine's major side effects are nervousness, tremor, sleeplessness, and loss of appetite. According to the reliable *Medical Letter*, "there is no longer any good reason to prescribe ephedrine."[25] There is no good reason to use it OTC either.

The combination of theophylline and ephedrine in these products causes the same problem as other fixed-ratio combination products (see p. 48). Even when all the ingredients in a combination product are advisable (which is not the case here), it is unlikely that a fixed-ratio product will provide each one in the proper amount. With these products, the amount of theophylline is too small to be effective in most cases, and you will be forced to overdose on ephedrine to get enough theophylline.

Some of the OTC asthma products contain additional ingredients which lack evidence of effectiveness.

BRONITIN and PRIMATENE M tablets both contain the antihistamine pyrilamine maleate in addition to their ill-advised combination of theophylline and ephedrine. Antihistamines have no place in the treatment of asthma, as histamine release is only a very small part of the asthma response. Further, antihistamines can dry up secretions; this may result in the formation of plugs which can block airways, making breathing more difficult, and may also make you more susceptible to lung infections. Sometimes antihistamines are added to asthma products to counteract the stimulation or "upper" effect of ephedrine. However, antihistamines lack evidence for this purpose, according to the FDA.

BRONKOTABS, PRIMATENE P and TEDRAL all contain phenobarbital in addition to the unwise combination of theophylline and ephedrine. Phenobarbital is added to products containing ephedrine to counteract its "upper" effect. Phenobarbital lacks evidence of effectiveness for this purpose. In addition, phenobarbital is a powerful and potentially dangerous barbiturate sedative which offers no therapeutic advantage. This is but another reason to avoid all irrational combinations of this sort. By adding more ingredients, the drug maker multiples the possible side effects, while producing a product which is no better and no more effective.

OVERWEIGHT

WHAT IS OBESITY?

Obesity, or being overweight, refers to an excess of body fat, or a body weight which is greater than the ideal weight. Obesity is associated with a number of serious health problems.

WHAT CAUSES WEIGHT GAIN?

Weight is gained whenever the amount of caloric energy in food eaten is greater than the amount of energy expended by the body.

HOW TO START A REASONABLE, LONG-TERM WEIGHT CONTROL PROGRAM AND LOSE ONE POUND A WEEK (see pp. 75-79)

Create a daily 500-calorie deficit:
- Evaluate your eating habits to eliminate 400 calories from each day's food intake; and
- Exercise to use an additional 100 calories each day (this can be achieved by walking 20 minutes more than you do now).

WHICH OTC DRUGS TO USE

None.

EXAMPLES OF OTC DRUGS NOT TO USE

Although an FDA panel has found ingredients in the following products to be safe and effective, we do not recommend use of any OTC diet aids, as none have evidence of effectiveness in aiding long-term weight control. Products to avoid include the following:

All products containing phenylpropanolamine, a hazardous drug, including CONTROL, DEXATRIM, DIETAC, PERMA-THENE, PROLAMINE, and THINZ-SPAN, and products containing benzocaine, including AYDS candy.

WHEN TO SEEK HELP FROM A HEALTH CARE PROFESSIONAL

Seek help when you want to lose weight, and you:

- Want to lose over 20 lbs. or 15% of your total body weight.
- Are over 60 years of age, or are over 45 years of age and have been relatively inactive in recent years.
- Have heart disease, high blood pressure, diabetes, kidney disease or any other chronic condition that is already under medical care.
- Have a family history of heart disease, diabetes or high blood pressure.
- Have chest pain, dizziness, or shortness of breath with or without exertion.

INTRODUCTION

With sales in excess of $220 million in 1981,[1] over the counter "diet pills" such as CONTROL, DEXATRIM and DIETAC are among the leaders in over the counter drug sales. Combine these figures with sales of hundreds of other diet products and diet books which flood the market each year, and the American preoccupation with slimness jumps into sharp focus.

If you are overweight, this chapter will help you to develop a weight reduction plan that works, without risking your health.

For most overweight people, a weight reduction plan is a plan to change eating and exercising habits. The use of "diet pills," over the counter or prescription, has no place in such a program. These drugs pose significant hazards to your health, and are ineffective in achieving permanent weight loss.

OVERWEIGHT

Few aspects of self-image have so totally captured and American imagination as persistently as that of weight. In a complete turn-about from the "old-fashioned" view of plumpness as a sign of prosperity, Americans have rushed to spend their money on any book, service, or product, however far-fetched, ineffective or even dangerous it may be, that promises to get rid of an extra pound or two.

Up to a point, this preoccupation has some scientific foundation. Many illnesses and life-threatening disorders are now thought to be caused or worsened, at least in part, by burdening the body with an extra load of unnecessary flesh and fat.

But while a constant barrage of movies, television programs, and advertisements presents a slim body as the ideal, nutrition experts have become increasingly doubtful about the correlation between fashion model, extra-thin looks and good health.

WHAT IS OBESITY?

The term "overweight" denotes weight exceeding an established norm or ideal. The term "obese" is commonly used to describe an excess of body fat. Obesity is also used to describe the condition of weighing from 5 to 20% over "ideal body weight."

Distinctions between these definitions are not important. The two words — obese and overweight — are used more or less inter-changeably. More important is the fact that many people, probably more than 50 million Americans,[2] weigh more than they should and consequently are at greater risk for a variety of health problems.

Generally, people have a sense of whether or not they should lose weight. Technically, though, the determination of obesity is based on the amount of total body weight which is fat. This can be measured in a variety of ways, including skinfold thickness measurements and body water-content calculation (by immersion in water), but these techniques are usually used only in research. More commonly, judgement of whether or not a person is overweight is made by comparison with ideal weight tables.

One good table is reproduced below. These are the guidelines for body weight adapted from the recommendations of a conference on obesity at the Fogerty International Center of the National Institutes of Health, and based on figures of the Metropolitan Life Insurance Company. In this table, height is without shoes, and weight is without clothes.

IDEAL WEIGHT TABLE

Height (ft, in)	Men Weight (lb) Average	Acceptable weight		Women Weight (lb) Average	Acceptable weight	
4 10				102	92	119
4 11				104	94	122
5 0				107	96	125
5 1				110	99	128
5 2	123	112	141	113	102	131
5 3	127	115	144	116	105	134
5 4	130	118	148	120	108	138
5 5	133	121	152	123	111	142
5 6	136	124	156	128	114	146
5 7	140	128	161	132	118	150
5 8	145	132	166	136	122	154
5 9	149	136	170	140	126	158
5 10	153	140	174	144	130	163
5 11	158	144	179	148	134	168
6 0	162	148	184	152	138	173
6 1	166	152	189			
6 2	171	156	194			
6 3	176	160	199			
6 4	181	164	204			

The tables were designed to give the weights which over time have resulted in the lowest mortality (death) rates. One problem with these tables is that they fail to adjust for the amount of muscle in the body: a highly muscular, well-trained athlete appears overweight in the table when he or she is not, and a middle-aged person in poor muscular condition appears at the correct weight in the table when he or she may be overweight.

Factors other than weight alone need to be considered to determine whether you definitely need to lose weight. If you get a lot of vigorous exercise regularly, weight loss may not be crucial if you are only slightly over your ideal weight and have been so for a long time. On the other hand, if you have a family history of diabetes, heart disease, or high blood pressure, weight loss is more important. Weight loss is also more important if you added your weight after age 40, especially if most of the fat is in the upper part of your body.

For most people, the weight tables *do* provide a reasonable estimate of a desirable weight. If your weight falls above this range, you should consider losing weight.

WHAT IS WRONG WITH BEING OVERWEIGHT?

People who weigh significantly more than the "ideal weight" for their height and frame are at an increased risk of developing a number of diseases. People 20% or more above their ideal weight have a significantly increased chance of getting the diseases discussed below. There is no threshold for obesity, however; even a small degree of excess fat can leave you in some danger of developing:

- **Hypertension** (high blood pressure). There seems to be an overlap between obesity (especially obesity which develops late in life and which involves the upper half of the body) and high blood pressure.
- **Diabetes** (non-insulin dependent). As with hypertension, there is an overlap between diabetes and obesity. 90% of non-insulin dependent diabetics are obese. In many cases, weight loss, or even the initiation of a weight-loss program, can improve the diabetic's blood sugar levels. In general, diet is a better approach than diabetes medication in most non-insulin dependent diabetics.[3]
- **Coronary artery disease** (blockage of blood vessels that supply the heart; the blockage causes heart attacks).
- **Hypercholesterolemia** (high levels of a fat-like substance called cholesterol in the blood) and **hyperlipidemia** (high levels of fat in the blood).
- **Stroke** (the blockage of blood vessels that supply the brain).
- **Osteoarthritis** (a debilitating form of arthritis, discussed further in the chapter on analgesics). Strain upon joints which bear body weight, such as the hips and knees, causes and worsens osteoarthritis. Excessive body weight increases this strain.
- **Pulmonary disease** (breathing difficulties). Obesity is associated with various respiratory problems, including sleep apnea (discussed further in the chapter on insomnia).
- **Other diseases,** including **hormone imbalances, gall bladder**

73

disease, and **kidney disease.** Obesity also causes increased risks to **pregnant women** and **male or female surgical patients** since it results in a higher probability of medical complications.

Some of the conditions mentioned above may result not from obesity itself, but from the kind of diet or sedentary lifestyle that leads to obesity. A sensible diet and activity plan which will help you lose weight will also help you reduce factors which may lead to other disease.

WHAT INFLUENCES BODY WEIGHT?

Several factors influence your weight:

Food intake. The more you eat, the more "fuel" you have for your body. Extra fuel which is not used in daily activities is stored in the form of fat for use another day. If that day never comes, the fat remains.

Food's energy content is measured in units of heat called calories. Despite the claims of many of the popular "fad" diets, the body, for the most part, does not distinguish between different "kinds" of calories where weight accumulation is concerned.

Activity. The more active you are, the more fuel you burn. That fuel may consist of recently eaten food, or previously stored fat.

Size and body type. The bigger and heavier you are, the more food you need just to maintain your weight. In addition, more fuel is required to maintain muscle mass and bone than to maintain fatty tissue. As a result, large boned, muscular people need to eat more just to maintain their weight than do small boned plump people.

Metabolism. This is the process by which food and stored fat are converted into energy. People with higher metabolic rates burn food and fat at a higher rate than do those with low metabolic rates.

Several factors influence metabolism. These include: sex (men tend to have higher metabolic rates than do women); age (metabolic rates tend to decrease with age); and physical activity (which increases metabolic rates). However, these metabolic differences related to sex and age appear to be largely due to differences in "lean body mass," the body's weight without fat.

A much less common cause of changes in metabolic rate is a hormonal disturbance, such as increased or decreased rates of thyroid activity.

Obviously, of all the factors influencing weight that were listed above, food intake and physical activity are the two over which you have the most direct control. A sensible weight reduction program should therefore begin with these.

WHEN TO SEEK MEDICAL ADVICE

For some, weight reduction should be supervised by a physician. People over 60 and those with heart disease, high blood pressure, diabetes, kidney disease or other chronic conditions under medical care should seek medical assistance in developing a weight reduction plan.

If your parents or other immediate family members have had heart attacks or diabetes, you should be particularly careful about weight. Such people should consider a check-up by a physician before starting a weight control program, especially if they are over 45 and have not had a check-up in the last 2 years.

Those who need to lose over 20 lbs. or 15% of their total body weight should also see a health care professional before beginning a weight control program, or before embarking on any major changes in diet or lifestyle.

HOW TO LOSE WEIGHT WITHOUT DRUGS

PRINCIPLES OF WEIGHT LOSS

The guiding principle of weight loss is simple: IF MORE CALORIES ARE EATEN THAN BURNED, WEIGHT IS GAINED; IF FEWER CALORIES ARE EATEN THAN BURNED, WEIGHT IS LOST.

Unfortunately, as most who have tried to diet can tell you, losing weight is not an easy task. In order to succeed, dieting must be a long-term process, involving permanent changes in eating habits and physical activity.

Any program which results in, or promises to result in, short-term weight loss without any dietary or lifestyle changes will typically fail after the quick success: pounds rapidly lost are rapidly gained back!

The number of people who hop from the *Last Chance Diet* to the *Scarsdale Diet* to the *Beverly Hills Diet* to the *Cambridge Diet* reveals that sustained weight loss rarely occurs with any such diets.

Diet pills, discussed later in this chapter, are similarly ineffective: they may help short-term weight loss, but they play no role in long-term weight loss. In addition, they are dangerous.

You did not gain your excess weight in just a few weeks and it hardly stands to reason that you will lose it in that time. For moderately overweight (less than 15% above ideal weight) people who are seriously interested in controlling their weight, there is no time when a "crash" diet, especially without medical supervision, is appropriate.

A REASONABLE PLAN

A sensible, safe and effective approach to weight loss is to calculate the calorie adjustment necessary to lose weight and then to make the necessary changes in diet or activity. There are no miracles. The aim is to eat less, exercise more or both; the results are slow, but safe, and effective.

Setting a calorie adjustment which will result in permanent weight loss *and* allow you to integrate these changes into your life is a considerable challenge. *The goal is to develop new, healthier diet and exercise habits, not just to lose weight fast (only to gain it back).* Minor or gradual alterations in diet are a more realistic approach to long-term weight loss than switching to a radically different diet (like a canned, reduced calorie meal program or the plans of many currently popular books).

A pound of *fat* represents an estimated 3500 calories.[4] In other words, in order to lose one pound you must use (through physical activity) 3500 more calories than you eat.

A reasonable, fairly ambitious goal is to make a calorie adjustment of 3500 calories per week. This program will *average* about one pound of weight reduction per week, assuming that your weight is now approximately constant based on your current diet and activity.

In a long-term program like this one, with a realistic calorie reduction, weight is *not* lost smoothly, constantly or evenly. Weight loss may be more pronounced in the early weeks of this reducing program as it is in any weight reduction program. During this initial period there is significant water loss as well as other body adjustments. After the initial drop in weight, your weight may level off (sometimes for a few weeks) before dropping again. This pattern of plateaus followed by drops in weight continues through a weight loss program.

A caloric adjustment of 3500 calories per week requires a net change of 500 calories each day. We recommend that you reduce 400 calories of this through a decrease in dietary intake and 100 calories in increased activity each day.

The weight loss principles that we discuss are widely applicable, but certain people (see p. 79) should be under medical supervision before embarking on any diet or exercise program.

DIET

Any effective weight control program involves changes in diet. For many people this is very difficult, especially if a diet recommends a substantial or complete departure from their accustomed food. We suggest instead that you design a reduction in calories that you can live with for good, not just for the short term.

Planning a Reduction in Calories

To reduce your daily diet by 400 calories, review the foods you eat to see what you can eliminate. You may find a "calorie counter" book helpful; they are inexpensive and available in many supermarkets and bookstores. A few suggestions which may help are:

• **Make some sensible substitutions,** using more low calorie foods in your regular daily diet. For example, if you eat a lot of meat, substitute chicken, fish or seafood for beef, lamb or pork. They have less fat and, generally, fewer calories. Eat more vegetables and less meat. Tofu (bean curd), one of a variety of vegetable protein sources becoming more widely available, has even fewer calories and is a good source of protein. Other simple substitutions can include: lowfat cottage cheese rather than other cheese; nonfat skim milk rather than whole milk; fresh fruit (more filling) rather than fruit juice; fresh vegetables rather than sweet, salty or fried snacks; and fresh fruit rather than sweet desserts.

• **Eliminate "invisible calories"** (calories which do not add to the taste, quality, or appearance of food) by trying new methods of food preparation. Several excellent cookbooks now on the market will help you prepare flavorful meals with far less fat and sugar. Trimming visible fat from meat, removing skin (a major source of fat) from poultry prior to cooking (or eating), cooking food in boullion or broth instead of butter or oil, and using lemon juice or boullion instead of butter or oil for basting or seasoning fish and vegetables will eliminate calories that you will scarcely miss.

• **Learn to be calorie-wise when dining out.** Ask the waiter or waitress to remove the tray of rolls or bread from the table, and, if possible, to bring some fresh celery or carrots. Enjoy a glass of club soda with a wedge of lime instead of a drink before dinner — alcohol is a major source of non-nutritional calories. Substitute a squeeze of lemon wedge for that heavy salad dressing and avoid fried foods.

• **Arrange for low calorie meals.** If your meals are prepared in a school dormitory, company cafeteria, or similar kind of institutional setting where you are not in control of food preparation, consult with the director of food services. Sometimes he or she will be able to help you work out a low calorie meal plan using the available food, or, depending on the size and resources of the kitchen or food source, help you to obtain specially prepared meals. Most major airlines will serve low-calorie meals if you request them a day before your trip.

• **Keep a record of what you eat and when you eat** — even checking out portion sizes with a small scale. This will help you to learn what you should avoid in order to acquire and maintain your desirable weight.

• **Learn to recognize and handle stress without responding by overeating.** Frequently people with weight problems use food as a way of coping with stress. Anxiety, anger, sadness and even boredom are feelings that at times can be attributed to stressful situations. People sometimes handle these uncomfortable emotions by seeking comfort in food, and consequently overeating. Then, after eating too much food, or the wrong kind of food, people frequently feel guilty or disappointed with themselves, which results in still more stress.

Proper Nutrition and Dieting

During a weight control program, it is especially important to provide the body with proper nutrition. A program which involves only a slight change form past habits, as described in this chapter, should not result in nutritional deficiencies, as long as those past habits were nutritionally adequate.

Basically, it is best to maintain a balanced diet, which provides adequate protein, vitamins and minerals. A diet for weight loss should also include high fiber foods, such as discussed in the chapter on constipation (see p. 93). Many of these high fiber foods and whole grain vegetables and beans are also higher in complex carbohydrates, a better source of energy than simple sugars (such as table sugar, honey, or molasses).

Many of the problems associated with the most recent "fad" diets, including liquid protein diets, "the Doctor's Quick Weight Loss Diet," "Dr. Atkins' Diet Revolution," and "The Beverly Hills Diet," have been due to inadequate allowances of vitamins or protein.[5] In a moderate, more sensible, weight loss program, you will benefit most from elimination of items containing large quantities of fats, oils, and sugar.

Elements (such as fat, alcohol, and food additives) in certain foods may be associated with particular diseases. If your weight loss program is part of a broader change to a healthier lifestyle, you might try to adjust your diet in other ways. For example, the National Academy of Sciences recently advocated a diet with the following guidelines:*

• Reduce the consumption of fat, both saturated (as in animal fat) and unsaturated (as in vegetable oil), to 30% of your total caloric intake.

• Eat fruits, vegetables and whole grain products every day, especially foods high in Vitamin C and beta-carotene, such as

---

*Although these guidelines were issued in the context of reducing cancer risks, they are useful in weight reduction as well. We would also recommend that you avoid artificially colored foods, which are usually high in calories.

citrus fruits and dark green, yellow or orange vegetables (these foods contain more valuable nutrients than other kinds of food, for each calorie of food which is consumed).

• Eat very little salt-cured, salt-pickled, or smoked foods, such as smoked sausages, smoked fish, bacon, bologna, and hot dogs. They contain salt (sodium chloride) and/or nitrites.

• Drink alcohol only in moderation, particularly if you also smoke cigarettes.[6]

There are a number of books of varying quality published on nutrition. *Jane Brody's Nutrition Book* is an up-to-date, sensible guide that we can recommend as a source for further information.

EXERCISE

As anyone who has tried it knows, losing weight *and* keeping it off by dieting alone *is very difficult.*

As an example, a woman of 120 lbs. in a sedentary job (burning about 1800 calories per day) would have to cut calories by 28% to lose one pound per week through dieting. To lose weight, she would have to cut her meals back to spartan portions (which maintain minimally adequate nutrition), with little or no leeway for fattening "treats." If, however, she walked at a brisk pace for 20 minutes (such as to and from her job) each morning and evening, she would have to cut back calories by only 17% to lose the same amount.

This example illustrates why a combination of diet *and* exercise is the most reliable and effective weight control program. Such a program will also help to reduce the loss of muscle mass that may be caused by dieting alone.

Starting a serious exercise program after years of relative inactivity can be a strain on your body, especially your heart. If vigorous exercise has not been a part of your regular activities for some time, we recommend that you start slowly with walking rather than another more strenuous form of exercise.

SEEK MEDICAL HELP BEFORE STARTING AN EXERCISE PROGRAM IF YOU:

• Are over 45 and have not had a check-up by a physician in the last year, especially if you have been fairly inactive.

• Have heart disease, high blood pressure, or are under the car of a physician for any other chronic disease.

• Have a family history of heart attacks.

• Experience any chest pain, dizziness or shortness of breath with or without physical exertion.

In all other cases, an exercise program can be part of your daily routine — an extra mile of walking instead of driving; using stairs instead of an elevator; or doing household tasks by hand instead of by machine can all contribute to an increase in calories used.

We recommend that you use *at least* an additional 100 calories *every day*. 100 calories is roughly equivalent to one of the following: 20 minutes of brisk walking (about 1 mile); 12 minutes of bicycle riding; 9 minutes of swimming; or 5 minutes of fast running. You should exercise hard enough to make yourself breathe faster. Any kind of new exercise should be preceded and followed by several minutes of stretching exercises, especially at the ankles and hips.

Depending on your physical condition, you may find that you are able to increase this amount of exercise, and hence improve upon your weight control program. Keep in mind that this increased activity should become a permanent daily activity.

Keep a log of your exercise. This can serve not only to keep you faithful to your new program, but also to encourage progress. With exercise, many people feel an increased sense of energy and a decreased desire for food.

WEIGHT CONTROL IN CHILDREN AND ADOLESCENTS

The information presented in this chapter is about weight control in adults. However, these same general principles apply to children and adolescents. Very obese children and adolescents should seek professional assistance.

Moderately overweight young people, otherwise in good health, are usually able to safely increase the calories expended by exercising more; this can be very effective when combined with a program of restrained dieting that is very careful not to sacrifice any nutritional needs. Drastic weight control programs in children and adolescents may cause a variety of health problems, including retardation of growth and development, and they are not recommended.

Some adolescents, overly concerned about weight and appearance, may be tempted to use over the counter diet aids. As with adults, these products should not be used, as they can be dangerous.

OTC WEIGHT CONTROL PRODUCTS

American drug manufacturers have been quick to capitalize on — and to promote — the public preoccupation with weight loss by filling neighborhood drugstores with prominent displays of reducing aids of every description.

Over the past few decades, a parade of diet products has been placed on the market and disappeared unnoticed over the horizon of obscurity, while others have risen to take their place. A variety of capsules, tablets, powders, liquids, gums, candies and canned low-cal meals, often with fantastic claims and prices, have been sold in recent years; some are no longer for sale, others are still available on out-of-the-way shelves, but long since replaced in prime display space by the newest craze.

An FDA Advisory Panel recently proposed rules for the marketing of over the counter weight control drug products. The only two ingredients approved for use in weight control were phenylpropanolamine hydrochloride (PPA) and benzocaine. All other drug products touted in any way for weight control lack evidence of safety, effectiveness or both.

PHENYLPROPANOLAMINE-CONTAINING PRODUCTS

Today, the most tempting items are those flat little boxes that dangle enticingly from drugstore and supermarket shelves and promise "Fast Weight Loss." These are the current aristocrats of the profit-making diet aids — the products containing the drug phenylpropanolamine hyrochloride, or PPA. Though originally marketed as a nasal decongestant, PPA is now the leading over the counter diet aid, accounting for most of the 220 million dollars in OTC diet pill sales. Products such as CONTROL, DEXATRIM (the leader in sales), DIETAC, PERMATHENE, PROLAMINE, and THINZ-SPAN contain PPA.

PPA was rated safe and effective by the FDA advisory panel for use as an anorectic (appetite suppressant) in weight control, although the agency has requested more evidence before it reaches a final decision. It is also approved in combination with caffeine to counteract the fatigue (or, more accurately, the depression) associated with dieting. Despite the panel's decision, it is our opinion that PPA poses a substantial hazard for its users, and has not succeeded in proving its effectiveness. For this reason, WE RECOMMEND STRONGLY AGAINST THE USE OF ALL PHENYLPROPANOLAMINE-CONTAINING PRODUCTS FOR USE IN WEIGHT LOSS.

No well-controlled study has shown that PPA is effective as an aid in long-term weight control. It may help you lose weight for a few days but you gain the pounds back when you stop taking it, and it won't help you make the changes in diet and exercise patterns which are needed to keep weight off.

Not only are there significant questions of PPA's effectiveness, but also serious doubts of its safety. PPA can cause hypertension (high blood pressure), even in young, healthy adults given amounts within the recommended dosage.[7] The FDA acknowledges that PPA is hazardous to a significant portion of the population[8] (at least 20%).[9] People who must avoid PPA include those with any of the following: hypertension, heart disease, diabetes, or thyroid disease. The issue is made more serious by the fact that overweight individuals (and hence people likely to use PPA as an anorectic) are more likely to suffer from all of these disorders, as discussed earlier. Additionally, it is estimated that 40% of all diabetics[10] and 30% of all hypertensives[11] are not aware of their disorders, and if they use PPA-containing products it is with an unknown and significant risk.

There have been cases of potentially fatal heart problems,[12] kidney disease and muscle damage[13] associated with the use of phenylpropanolamine-containing products, although these effects have yet to be clearly shown in healthy subjects taking the recommended doses.

There have also been reports of amphetamine ("speed")-like adverse reactions to PPA-containing products. These include accelerated pulse rate, tremor, restlessness, agitation, anxiety, dizziness and hallucinations.[14] These reactions may be aggravated by the presence of caffeine in many of these products.

For these reasons, PHENYLPROPANOLAMINE (PPA)-CONTAINING PRODUCTS SHOULD NOT BE USED FOR ANY REASON. The use of these drugs has no place in weight reduction.

As mentioned earlier, negative reactions occur with the use of PPA products in "recommended" doses. Reactions are often more severe or even life-threatening when these products are abused and overused. OTC diet aids consistently appear prominently in official statistics of drug abuse problems reported from hospital emergency rooms.[15] This fact, along with the hazards and ineffectiveness of these products in weight control, raises serious questions about the wisdom of making these products available at all.

In addition, phenylpropanolamine is a common ingredient in illicit amphetamine "look-alike" drugs.

BENZOCAINE-CONTAINING PRODUCTS

Benzocaine is an anesthetic. Contained in lozenges, chewing gum or candy (AYDS and SLIM-LINE are examples), it is sold to be used immediately prior to a meal so as to reduce sensation in the taste buds and thus lessen the desire for food. While benzocaine indeed produces a numbing of the tongue, there is little indication that this suppresses the appetite or promotes long-term weight loss in any other manner. The numbing effect of the drug tends to be fleeting, lasting only a short time after the gum or lozenge is dissolved or removed. The role of taste in appetite control is considered to be small in comparison with the role of food and the appearance of food. There is also some question of the safety of using the drug — it can sensitize some users, making them allergic to it and to other "-caine" local anesthetics, such as novocaine and lidocaine. [16,17]

This could pose problems in the event of future dental work or minor surgical procedure when these drugs are needed.

OTHER DRUG INGREDIENTS FOR WEIGHT CONTROL

A number of other ingredients were evaluated by the FDA advisory panel and found to lack evidence of safety, effectiveness or both, when used for weight control. Products containing these ingredients should not be used as diet aids: alginic acid, carrageenan, carboxymethylcellulose sodium, chondrus, guar gum, karaya gum, methylcellulose, psyllium, sea kelp, sodium bicarbonate, xanthan gum.

NON-DRUG DIET PRODUCTS

Many other products are marketed to appeal to the aspiring dieter. These include various pills, powders, measured calorie products and synthetic sweeteners. Some of these products may be harmless, if you don't mind throwing away money. Some may have a short-lived *placebo effect* (that is, they help because you take a pill, not because of the pill's contents) and thus encourage your early efforts at eating less. None have been found to have any significant success in achieving long-term weight loss, and we recommend that you avoid them all.

Starch Blockers

One example of a much-touted but worthless product is the so-called "starch blockers." An estimated one million starch blocker tablets were consumed daily in the first part of 1982.[18] These products, however, have no significant effect on the digestion and absorption of starch.[19] Starch blockers are now unavailable (or should be) due to an appropriate FDA action.

Manufacturers of starch blockers and other ineffective and possibly unsafe weight control products have attempted to keep these products on the market claiming "food" status, so that they are not regulated as "drugs." ("Drugs" are defined as products which make claims to change body function or affect a disease process, and a drug's maker is supposed to prove the product's safety and effectiveness for those claims.)

Health food stores offer their own diet products which are sold as "food", and thus have not been evaluated for safety and effectiveness by the FDA. The kelp, lecithin and Vitamin B6 preparations now appear to have yielded their popularity to a green algae named Spirulina as the "natural" way to a better figure. Glucomannan is also advertised with fabulous unsubstantiated claims.

Saccharin

So-called diet products containing sodium saccharin, such as diet soft drinks, sugar substitutes, and similar artificially sweetened products, present a different set of problems. Not only has saccharin been demonstrated to act as a carcinogen (cancer-causing agent) in laboratory animals,[20] but there have been no studies which demonstrate   that it is effective in helping to achieve long-term weight loss in overweight individuals. In other words, though you may "save" calories with saccharin diet products, you make up for those calories at another time, often hours later, by eating other foods.

A newer entry into the sugar substitute market is a chemical called aspartame. A Board of Inquiry (a panel of physicians who reviewed the scientific evidence) recomended that approval of aspartame-containing products be delayed until the chemical's association with brain cancer was resolved. This decision was overruled by the FDA, and products containing this chemical are available now or will be available soon. At this point, we recommend that you not use these products.

DOCTORS, WEIGHT CONTROL AND DIET PILLS

Certain people (see p. 75) should consult a physician before beginning a weight control program. In all probability, your doctor will approve of your decision to lose weight. The doctor may also have specific suggestions regarding your diet, and the type and amount of daily exercise you can safely handle.

In a few cases, you may still encounter a physician who prescribes "diet pills" to overweight patients. The number of prescriptions filled for anti-obesity drugs has fallen 44% in the last six years, from 19.9 million in 1975 to 11.1 million in 1981.[21]

The decreased use of these prescription appetite suppressants represents a growing awareness on the part of doctors of the capacity for addiction and abuse of these preparations, and their limitations as successful weight control agents. Unfortunately, the decrease in prescription diet pills has been more than compensated for by an increase in over the counter diet pills. All of these drugs can only help in *short-term* weight loss. Weight loss is regained quickly when the drug is stopped or tolerance is reached. In addition, these drugs can have serious side effects on the nervous system.

An ideal weight control drug would reduce the urge to overeat or alter the body's metabolism to allow weight loss, would maintain its effectiveness for the long-term, and would have few or no side effects. Unfortunately, *all* currently available weight control pills are appetite suppressants which are only effective for a short period of time and have a variety of significant problems.

The only way to lose weight is for your body to use more calories than you consume. Naturally, this involves either a reduction in calories consumed, an increase in energy expended, or, most likely, a combination of the two. While drugs are available to aid the first part of this weight-loss formula, they are potentially dangerous and are ineffective for long-term weight control. For this reason, we do not recommend their use.

CONSTIPATION

WHAT IS CONSTIPATION?

Constipation may be defined as: 1) a decrease from a person's normal number of bowel movements, 2) bowel movements occurring less than twice a week, or 3) difficulty in passing hard stools.

HOW TO TREAT SIMPLE CONSTIPATION WITHOUT DRUGS (see pp. 93-95)

- Avoid laxative drugs.
- Eat a high-fiber diet (see p. 93-94 for details).
- Drink plenty of non-alcoholic liquids (6-8 cups per day).
- Exercise regularly.
- Avoid or adjust constipating medication.
- Try to develop a regular pattern of bowel movements, whether that pattern is twice a day, twice a week, or somewhere in between.

WHICH OTC DRUGS TO USE FOR SIMPLE CONSTIPATION

None

EXAMPLES OF OTC LAXATIVES NOT TO USE

The following products contain ingredients which we and our medical consultants do not advise for self-medication, although an FDA panel found them safe and effective. The National Institute on Aging and The National Digestive Disease Education and Information Clearinghouse, for example, urge older people to "avoid taking laxatives, if at all possible."

CARTER'S LITTLE PILLS, CORRECTOL, DOXIDAN, DULCOLAX, EX-LAX, EX-LAX EXTRA GENTLE, FEEN-A-MINT, FLEET ENEMA, GLYCERIN SUPPOSITORIES, MODANE, NATURE'S REMEDY, PERDIEM, PERI-COLACE, PHILLIPS MILK OF MAGNESIA, PROMPT, SENOKOT.

WHEN TO SEEK HELP FROM A HEALTH CARE PROFESSIONAL

When any of the following occur:

- Constipation does not respond to the simple, non-drug, self-treatment plan (outlined in this chapter) within a week.
- Constipation is of a sudden and unexplained origin.
- Constipation is accompanied by considerable pain or great difficulty in passing stools.
- You notice evidence of rectal bleeding, including blood in the stools, or black tar-like stools.
- Constipation is accompanied by abdominal pain or swelling,

fever, nausea or unexplained weight loss.
- You notice a change in the thickness of stools and are now passing pencil-thin stools.
- Constipation is of long standing, particularly if it has been treated with stimulant laxatives.
- You have hemorrhoids or other anorectal disorders. (See the chapter on anorectal disorders and seek medical assistance if you have any of the signs discussed there.)

INTRODUCTION

Much of the $360 million spent on laxatives in 1981 was spent unnecessarily. Laxatives or cathartics are a category of non-prescription drugs having little, if any, place in medical self-care. They are unnecessary when a proper diet is followed and many are habit-forming, often leading to abuse. These drugs pose hazards to some people even when used infrequently — and to everyone if used repeatedly.

Many experts have noted Americans' unfounded preoccupation with a regular daily bowel movement. In fact, *perfectly healthy people may have from two bowel movements per week to three bowel movements per day.*

Although some degree of regularity may be convenient, variation in bowel habits over time is completely normal and natural. Frequency and volume of stools may change in response to amount and type of food and drink consumed, exercise performed, and individual levels of relaxation or tension. Such changes frequently take place in traveling, for example.

A decrease in frequency of stools by itself poses no threat to health. There is no scientific proof that ill health will result from "poisons" or "toxins" absorbed due to a delay in emptying the colon.[1] More serious problems involving constipation, such as intestinal blockage, make their presence known with additional symptoms such as abdominal pain or swelling, fever or nausea. If you have any of the conditions listed on p. 93, consult a health care professional.

Unfortunately, many people have enlisted the aid of various drugs to make their bodies behave more "regularly" or "normally." This does more harm than good. Laxative abuse, an unintentional and insidious habit, is a serious problem in this country. Like misuse of other drugs, laxative abuse is a result of common misconceptions regarding bodily functions, and the availability of a variety of drugs that are inappropriate for self-medication.

Understanding how the digestive system works can help you to understand why laxative products should be avoided. The following is a brief discussion of the lower digestive tract (the upper tract is discussed in the chapter on indigestion). A non-drug guide to treating occasional, simple constipation is also presented, and the chapter concludes with a section on over the counter laxatives.

THE LOWER DIGESTIVE TRACT

Partially digested food is passed from the stomach to the small intestine in a semi-liquid form. The small intestine continues to digest food, but also begins the process of food absorption. The walls of the small intestine are designed to absorb the nutrients from this material, and facilitate its movement into the bloodstream in the form of chemicals that can be converted into body tissue or energy.

Not everything we eat, however, is absorbed in the small intestine. Much indigestible matter, along with intestinal secretions and other substances, pass through the small intestine in semi-liquid form to the large intestine, also called the lower intestine or colon. Here, most of the remaining liquid is further absorbed into the body, and the remaining solid material is finally expelled in the form of a bowel movement.

The passage of food through the digestive tract is controlled by involuntary impulses from the time it is swallowed until just before the time of defecation. Rhythmic contractions of muscles pass the food through the stomach and intestines. We have virtually no control over these contractions and are generally not even aware of their occurrence.

Although the initial impetus for a bowel movement is set off by an involuntary reflex, we are normally able to exert voluntary control to prevent defecation. While the ability to control defecation voluntarily is obviously advantageous, the misuse or abuse of this power — by habitually delaying trips to the bathroom, for business, school or social reasons — may in time result in interference with normal defecation by dulling the body's natural defecatory reflex and muscular action toward this end. Similarly, the use of laxatives may create dependency on such drugs, and inhibit the ability of the body to defecate without such stimulation.

Many factors influence the amount and consistency of matter to be eliminated, which in turn influence the size, consistency and frequency of bowel movements. One factor which is important in this regard is the speed with which matter passes through the intestinal tract. Matter traveling through the large intestine has more opportunity for contact with the liquid-absorbing walls of the colon. This long period of fluid absorption may in turn result in a more solid, even rock hard, mass of fecal matter which may be more difficult to pass. On the other hand, matter traveling quickly through the large intestine may be very soft.[2]

Diets that contain ample quantities of fiber — indigestible plant cellular material found in raw vegetables, raw and dried fruits, and most beans and whole grains — tend to create a heavier mass in the large intestine. High fiber diets also tend to travel relatively quickly through the large intestine.[3]

This has two results: first, the heavier mass tends to stimulate the defecatory reflex, and second, the quick passage of this material provides less opportunity for the material to come into contact with the liquid-absorbing walls of the large intestine, so that little liquid is absorbed from the material and it remains relatively soft.

Diets that contain little fiber, on the other hand — such as those containing large quantities of refined sugar and flour products, highly cooked vegetables and fruits, and animal proteins such as meat, eggs and cheese — tend to create a smaller mass in the large intestine and travel relatively slowly through the large intestine.

This smaller mass is less efficient in stimulating the defecatory reflex, and the slower travel time provides increased opportunity for contact with the absorbent walls of the large intestine, so that much of the liquid is absorbed. The fecal mass may then become compacted, hard and difficult to pass. Ultimate passage may be uncomfortable, and may even result in painful damage to the tissue, which may further discourage regularity.

When To Be Concerned About Constipation

If bowel movements are not causing discomfort, there is no need for concern if they do not occur on a daily basis.

In order to rule out a serious disorder, you should consult a health care professional if any of the following signs characterize your constipation:

- Constipation does not respond to the simple, non-drug self-treatment plan (discussed next) within a week.
- Constipation is of a sudden and unexplained origin.
- Constipation is accompanied by considerable pain or great difficulty in passing stools.
- There is evidence of rectal bleeding, blood in the stools, or black tar-like stools.
- Constipation is accompanied by abdominal pain or swelling, fever, nausea or unexplained weight loss.
- You have noticed a change in the thickness of stools and are now passing pencil-thin stools.
- Constipation is of long standing, particularly if it has been treated with stimulant laxatives. If you need to use a laxative in order to defecate, you are dependent on laxatives, and retraining may be necessary.

HOW TO TREAT OCCASIONAL SIMPLE CONSTIPATION WITHOUT DRUGS
Diet

Make sure your daily diet includes plenty of bulk, including foods that are good sources of fiber, as well as plenty of liquid to help produce adequate bulk in the intestine.

Fiber-rich foods include whole grain breads and whole grain cereals, raw vegetables, raw and dried fruits, and beans.

One source of fiber is plain bran. Bran is the hard outer coating of cereal grains such as wheat, rice and barley, which is frequently removed in the milling process. Bran has been evaluated as a laxative by the FDA and will be discussed further under bulk-forming laxatives.

While the addition of small amounts of bran (a few teaspoonsful) to the diet may be helpful in relieving constipation, some people find it irritating. People with any kind of digestive disease, such as ulcers or intestinal obstruction, should not use it without medical supervision.

If plain bran is irritating we recommend the use of whole grain products since they include the bran part of the grain. For instance, we would suggest using whole wheat bread rather than white bread, brown rice rather than white rice, oatmeal and whole wheat cereals instead of highly processed cereals such as cornflakes, and homemade popcorn rather than highly processed snack food. These whole grain products, along with plenty of raw vegetables such as carrots and celery, and fresh and dried fruit, should supply all the fiber you need to prevent constipation from occurring, or help to correct it should it develop.

Some food manufacturers have tried to cash in on the move to high fiber food by selling products of questionable merit. An example of this is "Fresh Horizons" bread. Marketed as a "high fiber bread," this product contains by-products from wood processing, introducing a kind of "sawdust" into the bread dough. We would avoid this sort of product, in favor of food grain fiber.

While many extravagant claims have been made for the benefits of fiber in many other areas of health, we do not feel that the facts available lead to a definite conclusion other than benefits for the use discussed here. Nevertheless, we believe that a diet rich in unprocessed natural food from a wide variety of sources is desirable, and will certainly be advantageous in avoiding or correcting constipation.

Liquid

At least 6-8 glasses of water or other non-alcoholic liquids each day will help prevent painful bowel movements, by combining with fibrous matter in your colon to produce a large, soft, easy-to-pass stool.

Exercise

Regular exercise — at least half an hour per day, of cycling, swimming, jogging, or just brisk walking — will help your body maintain regularity.

Elimination or adjustment of constipating drugs

Many drugs, both prescription and non-prescription, may have a constipating effect. Some examples are:
- prescription cough medicine with codeine;
- ulcer or antacid medication containing aluminum or calcium compounds (see chapter on antacids);
- anticholinergics (prescription drugs containing atropine, like Donnatal);
- antihistamines (discussed with cough and cold preparations and with sleep-aids);
- diuretics (pills to reduce "water weight");
- muscle relaxants;
- narcotics;
- tranquilizers and sleeping pills;
- ferrous sulfate (iron supplements);
- tricyclic antidepressants (such as Elavil and Sinequan);
- phenothiazine-type antipsychotics (such as Stelazine and Thorazine);
- barium sulfate (used for some x-ray procedures); and
- drugs to lower cholesterol levels, such as cholestyramine (Questran). [4,5]

If you are having trouble with constipation and are using prescription or over the counter drugs, ask a pharmacist or doctor to review all of the medicine you use, both prescription and non-prescription, to see if any are constipating. If a suspect medication has been prescribed by your doctor for regular use, ask your doctor if it could be adjusted in some way. If you suspect a non-prescription product, consult your pharmacist and consider discontinuing use.

Regularity

Our bodies tend to function on a regular individual timetable. Whether this timetable calls for a bowel movement every three days, three times a day, or somewhere in between, a respect for your own natural bodily rhythm will help your body establish a comfortable routine. Here are some ways that you can help your body achieve reasonable regularity:

- **Heed the urge.** When you feel the need to defecate, take advantage of this promptly. Delay may permit the period of most efficient reflexive muscle activity to pass. Continued delay may impair this reflex.

- **Establish a regular time of day if possible.** There occurs, in many people, a natural reflex to defecate shortly after a meal (though usually not every meal) or at a particular time of day. If you notice such a natural cycle, cooperate with it to establish regularity.

• **Permit sufficient time.** Your body is most likely to perform best if you are not hurried. If you find that the urge to defecate often follows a particular meal, it is wise to rearrange your schedule to allow for elimination at this time, when your body is at its peak efficiency.

• **Abandon misconceptions.** Remember that people in perfectly good health may have a bowel movement as infrequently as twice a week.

LAXATIVE PRODUCTS

Many products are marketed over the counter for the treatment of constipation. These products are defined as laxatives by the FDA, and may also be known as cathartics. They may be defined by their particular modes of action, such as bulk-forming, stimulant, saline, lubricant and stool-softener laxatives. They are available in a variety of forms for both oral and rectal administration.

An FDA panel reviewed ingredients in laxative products and judged all currently available products to be safe and effective. Public Citizen Health Research Group and our medical consultants disagree: *laxative products have no place in your medicine chest.* The National Institute on Aging and The National Digestive Diseases Education and Information Clearinghouse — divisions of the National Institutes of Health — state that older people should: "Avoid taking laxatives if at all possible."[6]

There may be valid instances when your doctor may suggest that you use a laxative, stool-softener, or a related product such as a suppository or enema. These include:

• Preparation for certain diagnostic or surgical procedures;
• In connection with treatment for worms;
• In connection with treatment for certain kinds of poisoning;
• While hospitalized or otherwise incapacitated;
• While retraining to achieve normal elimination after laxative abuse has led to dependence and habituation;
• In order to avoid undue straining to defecate in conditions when this could be painful or dangerous, including hernia, anorectal disorders, certain heart or vascular conditions, such as some instances of severe hypertension, aneurysm, myocardial infarction (heart attack) and cerebrovascular accidents (strokes) as well as after certain surgical procedures.

None of these include the use of a laxative for simple constipation — or the failure to defecate regularly — which is not a disease.

If you are not experiencing discomfort, are eating a well-balanced diet with plenty of fiber and liquid and are getting exercise, you should have no need for such products whatsoever.

If changes in diet, travel, or temporary inactivity due to minor illness cause you to become constipated, your return to a diet rich in fiber and a program of regular physical activity should correct this quickly.

If it is inconvenient for you to obtain fresh fruits and vegetables and similar fiber rich food, such as when traveling, one of the bulk-forming laxatives, such as a psyllium compound, may be appropriate on an occasional basis. This is recommended only when no other source of fiber is convenient or available. No other laxative product should be used for self-medication.

THE BULK-FORMING LAXATIVES

The bulk-forming laxatives work in the same way that edible and crude fiber work in the intestine. They absorb water and soften the stool. Since the very same effect is produced by foods containing fiber, along with plenty (6 to 8 glasses per day) of non-alcoholic liquid, it would seem more sensible to avoid using a drug. Eating fiber in fresh foods, dried fruits and whole grain products is preferable and less costly.

However, if this is inconvenient for some reason — such as when traveling — the bulk-forming laxatives such as plain bran or METAMUCIL (or other less expensive bulk-forming products) may be appropriate for occasional use, and for short periods of time. Other brand-name bulk-forming laxatives include EFFER-SYLLIUM, HYDORCIL, KONSYL, L.A. FORMULA, MALTSUPEX, MITROLAN, MODANE BULK, SERUTAN, and SYLLACT. Some pharmacies carry generic or house brand bulk-forming laxative products which may be significantly less expensive than the brands listed here. A common ingredient, and the ingredient in METAMUCIL, is psyllium. If your pharmacist only carries METAMUCIL, ask him or her to stock a less expensive brand.

These products must be taken with plenty of water to prevent them from becoming dried and hence blocking the intestinal tract. Bulk-forming laxatives should never be used without medical supervision by people who have been told they have any form of intestinal blockage, diverticular disease, or similar conditions. Also, people who have a sluggish gut as a result of stimulant laxative overuse should not use these products, as blockage of the intestines can ensue.

You should also be aware of the sodium and sugar content of these bulk-forming preparations. If you need to watch the salt, calories, or sugar in your diet, check the product label. If a product is low-calorie and low-sodium, it probably will say so. If in doubt, ask your pharmacist.

Bran

Bran has recently been touted as a prevention or cure for a host of Western ills from constipation to cancer. On the other hand, large quantities of bran can be irritating to some people; and may also interfere with mineral absorption in the body.

Bran is representative of just one variety of fiber — crude fiber. Other kinds of fiber found in food products appear to differ from bran in their effect on the body.

Because complete information is not yet available, we recommend a conservative route, including a diet as well balanced as possible, using food from many sources in natural forms whenever possible (as outlined under **Diet**) to deal with simple occasional constipation (p. 93).

If you feel you would like to use small quantities of plain bran — up to a few teaspoonsful per day — this may be taken in the form of "all bran" cereals, or plain "miller's bran," available in health food stores and increasingly common in supermarkets. Some people suffer from bloating for a few weeks after adding bran to their diets. Effects are not as severe if dietary changes are made gradually.

Those under treatment for an ulcer or any kind of digestive disorder should follow their doctor's diet instructions carefully, and should not use bran without medical supervision.

WE DO NOT RECOMMEND THE USE OF ANY OF THE OTHER LAXATIVE PRODUCTS. Although effective in promoting defecation, in our opinion they are not safe and should not be used for self-medication. Each group has its significant disadvantages.

Women who are breast feeding a baby should particularly avoid all laxative products (except the bulk-forming variety) since many, if not all, of the ingredients in these products can pass into the mother's milk and affect the child.

Laxatives of the stimulant and saline groups, discussed next, tend to cause rapid and complete emptying of the lower intestine. Once this has been accomplished, it may take several days for the lower intestine to refill to the point of stimulating the urge to defecate once more. This in turn may lead to the erroneous belief that more and more laxative is needed.[7] Abuse of these drugs, leading to habituation and dependence, is very common.

STIMULANT LAXATIVES

Stimulant laxatives (including CARTER'S LITTLE PILLS, DULCOLAX, EX-LAX, MODANE, NATURE'S REMEDY, AND SENOKOT), taken over a long period of time, gradually deaden the ability of the intestine to work efficiently, causing increasing constipation, and a disease of the large intestine called "cathartic colon," in which the large intestine becomes dilated (enlarged) and will not move without chemical stimulation.[8,9] Individual ingredients in this category, such as senna, danthron, phenolphthalein, bisacodyl, and castor oil each pose additional risks to the user and can be dangerous in combination with other drugs.[10]

SALINE LAXATIVES

Saline laxatives (such as MILK OF MAGNESIA or EPSOM SALTS) contain certain drugs or chemicals that may be undesirable, are toxic in large quantities, are harmful to people with kidney problems, and may contain large amounts of sodium, undesirable to people with high blood pressure.[11]

MINERAL OIL

Mineral oil, the only lubricant laxative (and an ingredient in products such as HALEY'S M-O and AGORAL), taken over long periods of time, can interfere with nutrition. It has also been shown, in chronic use, to leak out of the rectum and cause anal irritation. Occasionally, people who are elderly or debilitated develop pneumonia as a result of accidently inhaling mineral oil.[12]

STOOL SOFTENER LAXATIVES

Stool softener laxatives include docusate sodium, docusate potassium, and docusate calcium and are found in products such as COLACE, REGUTOL and SURFAK. Stool softeners are not recommended because they have been shown to cause long-lasting undesirable changes in the cells of the intestine.[13] Stool softeners may interfere with the absorption of some nutrients. These ingredients may also enhance the absorption of other drugs.[14] Hence, they are particularly hazardous in combination with some drugs, including the lubricant laxative mineral oil and oxyphenisatin (which is chemically related to phenophthalein, a common laxative ingredient, in CORRECTOL, for example). CORRECTOL, DOX-IDAN, PERI-COLACE, and SENOKOT-S are examples of combinations of stool-softeners and stimulant laxatives. These combinations offer no advantage over the stimulant laxative alone, which we do not recommend and they should therefore be avoided.

ENEMAS AND SUPPOSITORIES

In addition to oral laxatives, laxatives are also available for rectal use such as in enema or suppository form. Although it would seem logical to favor a product that is administered closer to the site of action (in the colon), the actions of these products are *not* limited to the rectum and colon.

It is important to remember that medication contained in enemas and suppositories may be absorbed into the bloodstream in this form. In addition, the risk of irritation and damage they pose to an already irritated region outweighs any benefit they may offer for self-medication.

Many laxatives (SENOKOT, for example) are available in suppository as well as oral form, and have the same drawbacks discussed earlier. Glycerin suppositories are also available over the counter. Glycerin is a hyperosmotic laxative, which means that the presence of the drug in the rectum forces fluid to move into the rectum, attracting water to the stool. Glycerin suppositories can be irritating,[15] and we do not recommend them or any other suppositories for self-medication.

A variety of enemas are also available. These contain water, medication, or chemicals (like soapsuds) which are not normally considered drugs. Despite the attraction, for some, of using such a product just to "clean out" the system, this concept is mistaken and can be dangerous since chemicals and drugs can be readily absorbed from the rectum. Soapsuds enemas, for example, can result in severe disturbances in the body's fluid and mineral balance[16,17] and can damage the rectum and colon. A sodium phosphate biphosphate enema (such as FLEET ENEMA) can cause physical damage to the rectal area along with other adverse effects.[18,19] Use without medical direction is unwise, though they may be properly ordered by a physician for special purposes (as described on p. 96).

EXCESS ACID
AND GAS

WHAT ARE ANTACIDS?

Antacids are drugs that reduce the acidity of the stomach contents.

WHEN ARE ANTACIDS APPROPRIATE?

Antacids are appropriate for "acid ingestion," "sour stomach," and "heartburn," occurring from acidic stomach contents rising into the esophagus (the tube between your throat and stomach), causing a burning sensation. Antacids should not be used regularly without a doctor's advice. Antacids are often properly recommended by a physician for other disorders for which self-care is inappropriate.

WHICH OTC DRUGS TO USE

For infrequent self-medication: use baking soda unless you are on a salt-restricted diet (baking soda contains a large amount of sodium, like salt) or a generic or store brand liquid antacid which does not contain simethicone.

For more frequent use, *under a doctor's direction:* use an aluminum-magnesium liquid suspension product which does not contain simethicone. The most appropriate products are DELCID, MAALOX TC, or a similar product.

EXAMPLES OF AN OTC PRODUCT NOT TO USE AS AN ANTACID

Although the FDA has approved the use of ingredients in this product, we do not recommend the following as an antacid: ALKA-SELTZER EFFERVESCENT PAIN-RELIEVER AND ANTACID.

WHEN TO SEEK HELP FROM A HEALTH CARE PROFESSIONAL

Seek help when indigestion is characterized by any of the following:

- Any evidence of bleeding, such as black or bloody vomit, vomit that looks like coffee grounds, blood in stools or black tar-like stools.
- Severe heartburn or other discomfort, particularly when aggravated by exertion or accompanied by fatigue, breathlessness, perspiration, or chest pain.
- Regular or repeated stomach discomfort or pain which awakens you at night or occurs more than a few times each week and diminishes with eating.
- You are over 50 and have noticed persistent stomach-area pain.

- You have "heartburn" and there are others in your immediate family with ulcer disease.

SEEK ADVICE FROM A PHARMACIST OR PHYSICIAN BEFORE USING ANTACIDS, IF YOU:

- Are taking any prescription medication.
- Had symptoms of other digestive disorders (including nausea, vomiting, constipation or diarrhea) before suffering from "acid indigestion."
- Have, or suspect you may have, heart disease or kidney disease.

WHAT ARE ANTIFLATULENTS?

Antiflatulents are drugs to reduce the symptoms of gas. Those containing simethicone are intended to ease the expulsion of gas from the body.

WHICH OTC ANTIFLATULENT DRUGS TO USE

None. OTC antiflatulents, including those containing simethicone, are inappropriate for treating intestinal discomfort.

EXAMPLES OF OTC DRUGS WHICH SHOULD NOT BE USED TO RELIEVE INTESTINAL DISCOMFORT

The following products contain ingredients which lack evidence of safety, effectiveness or both, according to an FDA panel, for the relief of intestinal discomfort marked by bloating, distension, fullness, pressure, pain, or cramps:

ALLIMIN, CHARCOCAPS, GAS-X, MYLICON-80, PHA-ZYME.

Although an FDA panel has tentatively found certain drugs safe and effective for treatment of "over-indulgence" in food and drink, we do not recommend the use of any, including the following:

ALKA-SELTZER, BROMO-SELTZER and PEPTO-BISMOL.

INTRODUCTION

In 1981, Americans spent over $550 million on antacid products.[1] Much of this money, as well as that spent on antiflatulent products, was wasted on treating disorders that need not, cannot, or should not be treated with these products.

Massive advertising campaigns have been launched to teach us that antacids and "anti-gas" products are needed to cope with every upper digestive system upset, from a slightly queasy stomach to an inopportune belch. In fact, antacids and antiflatulents should have only very limited medical uses.

Understanding the upper digestive system and the action of these drugs can help you to decide when they should be used.

THE UPPER GASTROINTESTINAL TRACT

In this chapter we will follow the course of food from the mouth to the small intestine. The rest of its path will be picked up in the chapter on laxatives and constipation.

In the mouth, food is mashed through chewing to a semi-liquid form, combined with digestive chemicals in the saliva, and moved down the throat, through a tube called the esophagus, into the stomach. Some air is usually swallowed (this is called "aerophagia") along with this food. The amount of air swallowed increases with the use of carbonated beverages and hasty chewing. Anxiety, gum-chewing, and smoking all can contribute to aerophagia as well.

At the lower end of the esophagus, food is passed into the stomach through a circular muscle called the lower esophageal sphincter. This muscle is normally closed except when it allows swallowed food to pass down and allows swallowed air in the stomach to exit in the form of a belch.

Once in the stomach, food is combined with a variety of other digestive chemicals. Some of these chemicals — enzymes — work to digest the food so that it can be absorbed into the bloodstream from the small intestine. Other chemicals — acids — are also secreted into the stomach at this time.

Although a barrage of advertising may have convinced you otherwise, we are *not* engaged in a constant "battle against acid" in our stomach. Quite the opposite: the contents of the stomach are *normally* acidic, and this aids natural digestion.

Acid secretion into the stomach is regulated by information from the brain, stomach, and intestine that travels through the neural and hormonal channels. The amount of stomach acid is carefully controlled in response to amount and type of foods eaten.

Digestive enzymes work properly only in the correct acid-balanced environment in the stomach. This acid balance influences the breakdown and absorption not only of foods, but also of drugs.

Altering this balance by inappropriate use of antacids can result in more rapid absorption of some drugs (such as salicylates), and decreased absorption of other drugs (including tetracycline antibiotics and indomethacin (Indocin)).

From the stomach, partially digested food is emptied into the beginning of the small intestine, or duodenum. This occurs at varying rates depending on the amount, composition and acidity of the stomach contents.

At this point, any air which is swallowed and has not been released by belching is passed on to the intestine. Eventually, this gas will be released as flatus (gas passed by the rectum).

UPSET STOMACH

An "upset stomach" can mean many things. Most upset stomachs are a reaction to food or stress, and the best treatment is time and relaxation. Although antacids are often used for an upset stomach they are rarely necessary.

Upset stomachs characterized by nausea are discussed on p.127.

WHAT ANTACIDS DO: WHAT THEY SHOULD BE USED FOR

Antacids serve only one purpose — to neutralize acid in the stomach. They are used under a physician's direction for a number of disorders, such as peptic ulcer disease and gastritis, and are useful for the self-medication of one complaint: gastro-esophageal reflux, or heartburn. (This is explained on p. 107.) *Most upset stomachs are not the result of too much acid and need not be treated with antacids.*

Peptic ulcer disease is an erosion in the wall of the digestive tract, typically in the stomach or duodenum (the first part of the small intestine). Peptic ulcers are very common in this country; estimates suggest that 10% of the population will suffer from a duodenal ulcer at some point in their lives.[2]

Gastritis is an inflammation of the stomach wall, often accompanied by gastric (stomach) bleeding.

Consult a Health Care Professional When You Have Signs of Peptic Ulcer Disease or Severe Gastritis, Including:

- Digestive discomfort or pain which awakens you at night or is regular or repeated (more than a few times per week) and diminishes when you eat.
- Any evidence of bleeding, such as black, bloody or "coffee-ground" vomit, blood in stools or black tar-like stools.
- Any *severe* digestive discomfort, especially after consuming substances which can be irritating to the digestive system, including aspirin or alcohol.

Neither of these disorders is appropriate for self-treatment, although large quantities of non-prescription antacids may be recommended by a physician if you have either of them.

HEARTBURN: GASTRO-ESOPHAGEAL REFLUX

Occasional heartburn, or gastro-esophageal reflux, is the only complaint for which self-medication with antacids is appropriate. The FDA approved the terms "heartburn," "acid indigestion," and "sour stomach" as commonly used terms for this disorder.[3]

Gastro-esophageal reflux is the medical term for the reverse passage of material from the stomach through the lower esophageal sphincter (the ring-like muscle between the esophagus and the stomach) into the esophagus (the tube between the throat and the stomach). The problem often involves a weakness of the sphincter muscle. It is painful because the stomach's contents are typically highly acidic, and the esophagus (unlike the healthy stomach) may be damaged by this acid.

Heartburn, a burning feeling under the bottom of the breast-bone, usually occurs during gastro-esophageal reflux. The burning sensation spreads upward, and is aggravated by lying down or bending over. It usually occurs after meals, typically following large meals, or when lying down after a meal.

Occasional bouts of heartburn are amenable to self-treatment, but it is important to know that repeated attacks (more than a few times in a week) which do not respond to self-treatment require medical attention. ALSO, A HEART ATTACK CAN MIMIC HEARTBURN. FOR THIS REASON, IF ANY DISCOMFORT OF "INDIGESTION" IS SEVERE, ESPECIALLY IF ACCOM-PANIED BY FATIGUE, PERSPIRATION, BREATHLESS-NESS, CHEST PAIN, OR ANY SUCH PAIN MADE WORSE BY EXERTION — *IMMEDIATE MEDICAL ATTENTION IS REQUIRED.*

The discomfort of gastro-esophageal reflux can usually be prevented by eating smaller meals and not lying down after meals. If you have occasional heartburn, you shouldn't eat for 2-3 hours before going to sleep or before lying down.

If non-drug techniques fail to offer relief, antacids should help. A liquid antacid is better than a tablet because it may coat the lower esophagus and protect it from further damage; thicker suspensions may be even more useful for this purpose.

One antacid, GAVISCON, is marketed with claims that its ingre-dient alginic acid causes a "floating foam" effect that prevents heartburn. The FDA advisory panel reviewed alginic acid as an an-tacid ingredient and found that it lacks evidence of effectiveness. (Alginic acid is now listed as an inactive ingredient on GAVISCON.) Additionally, there is no evidence available to show

that GAVISCON treats heartburn more effectively than other antacids.

GAS
WHAT ANTIFLATULENTS DO

Although antiflatulent (antigas) products are a much less
popular item than antacids, they differ from antacids in that "anti-
gas" products are *never* appropriate for self-medication.

Most antiflatulent products and many antacid products contain
simethicone, which works to reduce the surface tension of gas bubbles in a solution, and therefore make large bubbles out of many
smaller bubbles. The idea is that simethicone works in your gut to
gather trapped gas bubbles together so that they are easier to expel,
either by mouth as belches or by rectum as flatus.

A physician may advise the use of an antiflatulent containing
simethicone before certain diagnostic procedures such as
gastroscopy or following certain surgical procedures such as pelvic
surgery. It is not effective in reducing the amount of gas in your
system or the discomfort of so-called "excess gas," as will be
discussed in greater detail later. Simethicone, alone or in combination with other drugs, has no place in self-medication.

"Excess gas" is a complaint commonly discussed in television
advertisements for antacids and antiflatulents. However, it is a
complaint about which there is little scientific knowledge. "Excess
gas" actually refers to two distinct conditions. One of them is not
associated with gas at all and neither should be treated with OTC
products.

"Excess Gas" 1: Bloating and Distension After Eating

An FDA advisory panel defined a syndrome called "Immediate
Post-Prandial Upper Abdominal Distress" (IPPUAD). Post-
prandial means "following a meal." The symptoms, according to
the FDA panel, are "bloating, distension, fullness, or pressure with
upper abdominal discomfort." Another syndrome called "Intestinal Distress" was described by the panel as having similar
symptoms, but occurring longer after a meal. *No OTC products
were found to be safe and effective for either of these conditions.*[4]

Despite millions of advertising dollars spent to convince us otherwise, the feeling of bloating and pain after eating is *not* caused by
gas. Recent medical evidence shows that there is no relation between these symptoms and the amount of gas in the intestinal tract.
An unusual amount of activity within the digestive tract (which occurs in some people after eating certain foods) is thought to play a
role in causing the syndrome.[5]

The use of antiflatulent products to relieve this discomfort is
therefore inappropriate, as there is no need to expel gas from the

body. Taking an antacid product is an even more irrational treatment, since the acid content of the stomach is not at fault, and should therefore not be tampered with needlessly.

There are no OTC products which are appropriate for self-treatment of bloating and distension after eating. You may find that certain foods or drinks often promote this unpleasant feeling. Individuals often discover a particular food sensitivity and are able to avoid discomfort by avoiding that item. Staying away from overly large and fatty meals can be helpful as well.

"Excess Gas" 2: Belching and Passing Flatus

This is an entirely different sort of discomfort from bloating and distension after eating, with an entirely different cause. Belching and passing flatus (gas passed by the rectum) *are* undoubtedly caused by gas.

The chief discomfort resulting from belching and passing flatus is social. The pressure to avoid embarrassment often leads people to try to reduce the amount of gas they are known to expel. No drug can reduce the volume of gas that you pass.

There are two major sources of gas in the normally functioning digestive system. One is swallowed air, which either is released in belching or continues through the intestines and must be passed as flatus. The other source of gas is produced in the intestine and must eventually leave the body as flatus. Both of these processes are *perfectly normal,* and healthy people expel a certain amount of gas each day.

Some control can be exercised over gas which is swallowed. In general, drinking carbonated beverages, swallowing after inadequate chewing, and gulping when anxious all tend to increase aerophagia (air swallowing). Avoiding these habits can decrease the amount of belching and gas that is passed as flatus.

Gas produced in the intestine is a result of fermentation of undigested sugars (as from beans, for example) and other substances and it cannot be easily controlled. The amount of gas generated in this manner varies from person to person. Production of one gas — methane — tends to stay fairly constant for each person over time, while production of another gas — hydrogen — can change considerably. Certain foods are more likely to result in hydrogen gas production. Beans, broccoli, and cabbage are notorious in this regard.

OTC antiflatulents cannot decrease the amount of gas you pass.

OVERINDULGENCE
Too Much Alcohol and Food

Overindulgence in alcohol and food is a common source of upset stomachs. Medication is not necessary to treat this sort of indigestion.

Although an FDA panel has proposed guidelines for the use of two ingredients — sodium citrate and bismuth salicylate — for the treatment of discomfort associated with "overindulgence in the combination of food and drink," we cannot recommend their use.

Sodium citrate is an antacid which is found in the solution formed when sodium bicarbonate and citric acid are dissolved in water. ALKA SELTZER and BROMO-SELTZER are examples of sodium citrate antacids. They also contain analgesics (pain-killers); ALKA-SELTZER EFFERVESCENT PAIN RELIEVER AND ANTACID contains aspirin and BROMO-SELTZER contains acetaminophen. (These pain-killers are described in greater detail in the chapter on analgesics.)

We have already outlined the only appropriate use for self-treatment with an antacid: occasional gastro-esophageal reflux (heartburn). If "overindulgence" symptoms do not include reflux, as described earlier, we do not recommend the use of antacids such as sodium citrate.

Another concern in the use of these products is the presence of aspirin, as in ALKA-SELTZER EFFERVESCENT PAIN RELIEVER AND ANTACID. The use of such a product is never recommended with an upset stomach, and is especially unwise after drinking liquor, since overindulgence in alcohol can cause damage to the stomach lining.[6] An injured stomach is especially susceptible to irritation from aspirin; the possible benefits of such a product are far outweighed by reports of massive bleeding and hemorrhage as a result of ingestion of aspirin and alcohol.[7]

Bismuth subsalicylate (the active ingredient in PEPTO-BISMOL) is a widely marketed over the counter ingredient. The manufacturer of PEPTO-BISMOL makes a number of claims for the drug, some of which are discussed under OTC diarrhea and nausea remedies.

The FDA panel based its decision to recommend approval of this drug primarily on a small scale unpublished study sponsored by PEPTO-BISMOL's manufacturer.[8] Interestingly, over half of the subjects in this study who took the placebo (a similar looking and tasting liquid but *without* the active ingredient) reported good or excellent overall relief from the symptoms of overindulgence.[9] This reinforces our belief that *no drugs are needed* for complaints of "overindulgence."

Bismuth subsalicylate also has all of the hazards of salicylates (such as aspirin) as discussed in the chapter on analgesics. If taken with other salicylates, including large dosages of aspirin, it can cause ringing in the ears, and other symptoms of overdose. Bismuth subsalicylate can also turn your stools black, thus masking an important sign of stomach or intestinal bleeding. In summary, we cannot recommend the use of PEPTO-BISMOL for self-medication of symptoms of "overindulgence," which will improve quickly without medication.

Alcoholic Hangover

An FDA panel also proposed to allow the use of a combination of ingredients already approved for certain other uses to treat the symptoms of an alcoholic hangover.

The panel proposed that ingredients from any two of the three categories — antacids, analgesics (pain-killers) and stimulants — be used together.

This proposal is not supported by scientific evidence. Very little study has been done on the treatment of alcoholic hangover. The use of these combinations for this purpose is clearly irrational.

Antacids should not be used to treat a hangover. As even the FDA panel noted in its report, excess acid is not present in an alcoholic hangover. Therefore, the use of an antacid for a hangover is inappropriate.

Aspirin, the most commonly used analgesic (pain-killer), should also be avoided in the treatment of alcoholic hangover, because it can be highly irritating and cause bleeding, particularly in a stomach injured by alcohol. If your hangover is accompanied by a headache, acetaminophen alone is your best choice. (See analgesics chapter for more information.)

Hangovers may be a result of dehydration; drinking plenty of non-alcoholic beverages may therefore be helpful as treatment and prevention.

OTC ANTACID PRODUCTS

As we have discussed, OTC antacids are appropriate for occasional self-treatment of heartburn and for professionally directed treatment of gastritis and peptic ulcer disease. For self-treatment, there are a variety of factors to consider in choosing an antacid, since the choice is yours. For ulcers or gastritis, on the other hand, your physician will probably recommend a brand name. In either case, these considerations are important to know in order to buy the most appropriate product for you.

Considerations in Choosing a Product

1) **Frequency of use.** Some ingredients in antacids are safe and effective for occasional use, but are unsafe for repeated use. As a general rule, any FDA-approved antacid is safe and effective for self-medication of occasional heartburn. For frequent or regular use of antacids, medical direction is necessary and sodium bicarbonate and calcium carbonate products should usually be avoided.

2) **Presence of non-antacid ingredients.** As we have stated throughout this book, we recommend that you use medication that contains only the ingredients that you need to treat your problem. If you need to use an antacid, we recommend that you use one containing only antacid ingredients. Check to see what other active ingredients are in an antacid product before you buy it. Unfortunate-

ly, many antacids contain other ingredients such as simethicone or aspirin.

Simethicone which is added to an antacid as an antiflatulent provides no advantage. (One study suggests that it may *reduce* the effectiveness of certain antacids containing aluminum hydroxide.[10]) Unfortunately, many otherwise good antacids, including best-sellers like DI-GEL, GELUSIL, MAALOX PLUS, MYLANTA, MYLANTA II, RIOPAN PLUS, and SIMECO, contain this unnecessary ingredient.

Among the simethicone-containing antacids which we don't recommend, are some of the brands which are often recommended by physicians for treatment of an ulcer. MYLANTA II, for example, is a high-potency antacid often used to treat duodenal ulcer. We recommend that you use another high-potency product, such as DELCID or MAALOX TC, instead of MYLANTA II. If only MYLANTA II (or another simethicone-containing antacid) is available, use it if your doctor recommends it, but ask your pharmacist to stock another high-potency antacid without the unnecessary ingredient, like DELCID or MAALOX TC.

The accompanying chart (p. 113) should allow you to compare strengths and costs of various liquid antacids to help you make a choice if your doctor recommends antacid therapy.

Aspirin as an antacid can be hazardous to an already irritated stomach. ALKA-SELTZER EFFERVESCENT PAIN RELIEVER AND ANTACID (in the blue box) should be avoided for this reason.

3) Interactions with other drugs. All antacids can either increase or decrease the effect of some other medications. For example, antacids dramatically reduce the absorption of tetracycline (an antibiotic). If you take any medicine under a doctor's direction, check with your pharmacist or doctor before taking an antacid. If you take non-prescription medicine, you may wish to consult a pharmacist before using an antacid.

4) Side effects. All antacids can have side effects. Some cause constipation, while others cause diarrhea. These side effects will be discussed under each ingredient.

5) Sodium content. If you must, for any reason, restrict your sodium (salt) intake, you should avoid sodium bicarbonate, as well as other high sodium antacids. Most products with low sodium content make this clear on their packages.

6) Sugar content. Some antacids add large amounts of sugar to make them more palatable. Carefully check the ingredients if you are diabetic or need to control your calorie intake.

7) Dosage form. Antacids are commonly available both as liquids and as chewable tablets. Some products are available as effervescing tablets or powders (these must be dissolved in water

LIQUID ANTACIDS

Antacid	Amount Needed For High Dose (Tablespoons) 1/	Sodium Per Tablespoon	Estimated $ Cost Of A Month's High Dose Therapy 2/	Comment
AlternaGel	4T	6	$125	Expensive; may be constipating
Amphojel	7⅓	21	232	Low potency; very expensive; may be constipating
Basaljel	3⅓	6	105	Expensive; may be constipating
Basaljel Extra Strength	2	69	116	Expensive; may be constipating
Camalox	2⅓	9	131	Expensive; unnecesary combination
Delcid	1	45	67	
Di-Gel	5⅓	27	136	Low potency; expensive; simethicone unneccessary
Gelusil	4	< 3	109	Contains unnecessary simethicone
Gelusil II	2	3	83	Contains unnecessary simethicone
Maalox	3⅓	3	82	Store brand or generic equivalent often available
Maalox Plus	3⅓	3	103	Contains unnecessary simethicone
Maalox TC	1⅔	< 3	69	
Mylanta	3⅔	< 3	97	Contains unnecessary simethicone
Mylanta II	2	3	77	Contains unnecessary simethicone
Phosphaljel	31	37.5	928	*Very* expensive
Riopan	3⅓	< 3	72	Riopan *Plus* contains simethicone
Simeco	2	21-42	60	Contains unnecessary simmethicone

TABLET ANTACIDS
(LIQUIDS ARE USUALLY PREFERABLE)

Antacid	Number of Tablets Needed For High Dose 1/	Sodium Per Tablet (MG)	Antacid	Number of Tablets Needed For High Dose 1/	Sodium Per Tablet (MG)
Alka-2	14	2	Maalox No. 2	8	1.8
Di-Gel*	30	10.6	Maalox Plus	16	1.4
Gelusil	13	1	Mylanta	12	1
Gelusil M	11	1.3	Mylanta II	6	1.3
Gelusil II	7	2.1	Rolaids	17½-19	53
Maalox No. 1	16	1	Tums	14	2.7

This table provides a basis for comparing the potency and value of some common OTC antacids.

1/ The first column lists how much of each antacid (liquid or tablets) must be taken to get a standard dose (enough to neutralize 140 mEq. of acid).

2/ The estimated cost of a month's high-dose therapy (140 mEq. dose 7 times daily — one and three hours after each meal and at bedtime — for 30 days), based on a shelf price 25% above wholesale price. This is the amount often used in ulcer therapy, *not* for treatment of heartburn. Your actual cost will vary depending on the amount you use and the store's profit margin.

For Occasional Heartburn: The best value is baking soda. If you are on a low-sodium diet, use a store brand (preferably liquid) aluminum-magnesium combination without simethicone.

For Antacid Therapy (under medical direction): A high potency antacid (probably an aluminum-magnesium liquid) is both more economical and more convenient. We recommend that you use one without simethicone.

The ingredients in each of these products are listed in the *Brand Name Index* of this book.

Adapted (updated and expanded) from the *Medical Letter* 1982, 24:61.
Sources: *Drug Topics Redbook* 1983, *Facts and Comparisons* May 1982
*Drake D, Hollander D., *Ann Int Med* 1981.

before they are used), or as lozenges or chewing gum. Liquids (either dissolved or effervescent solutions) are usually faster and more effective in neutralizing the liquid acid in your stomach and should be used, if convenient. Two tablespoons of MAALOX TC, for example, provide the neutralizing ability of 20 ROLAIDS tablets.[11] If a liquid is too much trouble to carry, tablets may suffice, but be sure to chew them completely.

8) Value. There is a great deal of range in price and potency of antacids. The price of the amount of antacids recommended for duodenal ulcer, for example, may range widely.[12] (See table.)

9) Taste. Preference for flavor is a personal matter, and can be a consideration in choosing an antacid, if you have been directed to use a product regularly. If you find the recommended product distasteful, ask your physician to recommend an alternative brand with similar ingredients, or use the table to find an equally effective product.

Antacid Ingredients

1) Sodium bicarbonate is a fast, effective and usually inexpensive antacid. Although it is inappropriate for repeated use (because it is absorbed and can change the acid balance of the entire body), it is perfectly good for occasional gastro-esophageal reflux unless you are restricting the salt in your diet. It is available both as baking soda and, more expensively, as an effervescing antacid without aspirin (such as ALKA-SELTZER EFFERVESCENT ANTACID, in the gold package), and as an ingredient in BISODOL powder.

Baking soda, used as directed, is one of the least expensive antacids. It should be dissolved in water before use. Another advantage is the ready availability of the product. Most kitchens already have a box.

Avoid products which needlessly combine sodium bicarbonate with other drugs. ALKA-SELTZER EFFERVESCENT PAIN RELIEVER AND ANTACID, in the blue package, contains aspirin and should not be used with stomach upset or any other abdominal discomfort.

Do not use sodium bicarbonate if for any reason you are restricting your sodium (salt) intake.

2) Calcium carbonate was the antacid of choice in years past, but it has fallen into disfavor. Like sodium bicarbonate, it is also fast and effective, but is has some disadvantages which make it less desirable. It tends to be constipating. In addition, it can cause a so-called "rebound effect," in which the stomach ultimately becomes more acidic than before the product was taken.[13] Available as a roll-pack tablet (in ALKA-2, TUMS, and CHOOZ), it can be convenient for the treatment of occasional heartburn, but it is not recommended for repeated use.

3) Aluminum salts are also effective antacids, though less so

114

than the others. They are available as aluminum-hydroxide, -carbonate, -phosphate, or -aminoacetate, although hydroxide salt is the most common form of the product. They are somewhat more expensive, as a group, than other antacids, and tend to be rather constipating.[14] Moreover, they are not as potent as other antacid ingredients. ALTERNAGEL, BASALJEL, PHOSPHALJEL and ROLAIDS are examples of aluminium salt antacids. Aluminum salts alone offer few advantages as an antacid. They are usually found in combination with magnesium salts.

4) Magnesium salts, such as magnesium-hydroxide, -oxide, -carbonate, and -trisilicate, are usually found with aluminum salts and are rarely found as a single ingredient in antacid products, although PHILLIPS MILK OF MAGNESIA (usually sold as a laxative) is one example of a single-ingredient magnesium salt antacid. Although more potent as antacids than aluminum salts, magnesium salts tend to cause diarrhea and can be hazardous to people with kidney disease.[15]

5) Aluminum-magnesium combinations have become the most popular antacid products, led by the MAALOX and MYLANTA families, and also including DELCID, DI-GEL, GAVISCON and RIOPAN. Presumably, the tendencies of aluminum and magnesium to cause constipation and diarrhea, respectively, are balanced in these products. However, it should be noted that these combinations *can* cause the side effects of either ingredient. Unfortunately, many of these products contain simethicone, which should be avoided if possible, as it is unnecessary.

6) Other combinations of antacid and non-antacid ingredients are available in over the counter antacid preparations. Some products combine more than two antacid ingredients (one example is CAMALOX). Combinations with more than two ingredients offer no advantage over an aluminum-magnesium combination or a single antacid formulation and they increase the risk of adverse effects. They should therefore be avoided.

Combinations of antacids and non-antacid ingredients are generally a waste of money and can be irrational therapy. As stated earlier, aspirin-containing products in particular should not be taken by those with a digestive upset. Aspirin causes gastric irritation and bleeding; sometimes serious bleeding and hemorrhage can result.

OTC ANTIFLATULENT PRODUCTS

Simethicone is approved as safe and effective "to alleviate or relieve the symptoms of gas.[16] Medical evidence available since this original 1974 decision, however, has shown that there is no relationship between any particular symptoms and the amount of gas in the digestive system. An FDA advisory panel which met after this evidence became available stated that simethicone lacks evidence of effectiveness in treating abdominal discomfort associated with complaints of "gas."[17]

We therefore recommend that OTC antiflatulent products not be used. This includes simethicone antiflatulents such as GAS-X and MYLICON, and antacids containing simethicone.

Other products marketed for gas or as "digestive aids" lack evidence of effectiveness and should not be used. These include charcoal products such as CHARCOCAPS, garlic powder tablets such as ALLIMIN, and products containing digestive enzymes such as PHAZYME.

DIARRHEA, NAUSEA AND VOMITING

WHAT IS DIARRHEA?

Diarrhea may be defined as a change in frequency and consistency of bowel movements, characterized by abnormally frequent passage of loose or watery stools. Acute, simple diarrhea refers to diarrhea which lasts only a few days, at the most.

COMMON CAUSES OF SIMPLE DIARRHEA

Diarrhea is often caused by a viral infection in the intestinal tract, food poisoning, anxiety or a reaction to medication, travel, food or alcohol.

HOW TO TREAT ACUTE SIMPLE DIARRHEA WITHOUT DRUGS

- Avoid milk and dairy products, fresh fruits and vegetables, coffee, spicy foods, and other foods you do not tolerate well.
- Take plenty of clear liquids (at least 4 glasses every 12 hours).
- Avoid medication not prescribed or directed by a health care professional.
- Take your temperature at least once a day.

WHICH OTC DRUGS TO USE

None.

EXAMPLES OF OTC ANTIDIARRHEAL PRODUCTS NOT TO USE

The following widely-sold drugs for treating diarrhea lack evidence of safety, effectiveness or both, according to the FDA: DONNAGEL, DONNAGEL-PG, KAOPECTATE, and PARAPECTOLIN.

Although the FDA has tentatively approved ingredients in these products, we do not recommend use of the following antidiarrheals: PEPTO-BISMOL, RHEABAN.

Advice on when to seek medical help with diarrhea is given following discussion of nausea and vomiting.

NAUSEA AND VOMITING

COMMON CAUSES OF SIMPLE NAUSEA AND VOMITING

Nausea and vomiting are often caused by an infection in the intestinal tract or a reaction to medication, food, or alcohol.

Nausea and vomiting are also common during pregnancy ("morning sickness") or they can be a part of a variety of diseases, including some infections not located in the digestive system.

HOW TO TREAT SIMPLE NAUSEA AND VOMITING WITHOUT DRUGS

- Avoid solid foods and large meals.
- Try to drink plenty of clear liquids (at least four glasses every 12 hours). Water and *flat* ginger ale or other non-cola drinks are good choices, as are diluted tea, applesauce and flavored gelatin. When nothing else will stay down, sucking on ice can work.
- Avoid medication that has not been recommended or directed by a health care professional.
- Take your temperature at least twice a day (morning and evening).
- If you can keep some food down, eat small and frequent meals.

WHICH OTC DRUGS TO USE FOR NAUSEA AND VOMITING

None.

EXAMPLES OF OTC DRUGS NOT TO USE FOR NAUSEA AND VOMITING

The following drugs contain ingredients which lack evidence of safety, effectiveness or both for the treatment of nausea and vomiting, according to the FDA: EMETROL, PEPTO-BISMOL.

WHEN TO SEEK HELP FROM A HEALTH CARE PROFESSIONAL FOR DIARRHEA, NAUSEA AND VOMITING

Get assistance when:

- Vomiting or severe diarrhea occurs in an infant less than one year of age, or an elderly or debilitated person.
- A child under age five is unable to hold down any fluids for 12 hours.
- Fever is over 101° F (38.3° C).
- There is evidence of bleeding, including any of the following: blood in vomit, black vomit or vomit that looks like coffee grounds; blood in stool; or black tar-like stools.
- Nausea, vomiting or diarrhea persists more than three days, regardless of age.
- Vomiting is very severe or violent, regardless of age.
- You suspect that a drug taken under the direction of a physician may be responsible for your complaint. See lists on pp. 124, 129.
- You are or *may be* pregnant.
- Nausea, vomiting or diarrhea is accompanied by severe, in-

capacitating abdominal pain.
- Diarrhea or vomiting results in dehydration (loss of water), characterized by dizziness while standing, confusion or unresponsiveness.
- There is vomiting in which no food is kept down, and a swollen stomach develops.

WHAT IS MOTION SICKNESS?

Motion sickness is nausea and vomiting associated with travel. Motion sickness may result from the conflict between what the individual sees and what he or she feels, when in motion.

WHICH OTC DRUGS TO USE FOR MOTION SICKNESS

Products containing cyclizine hydrochloride (such as MAREZINE), dymenhydrinate (such as DRAMAMINE), or meclizine hydrochloride (such as BONINE) can be used to *prevent* motion sickness symptoms. A less expensive generic or store brand product should be used if available. NONE SHOULD BE USED DURING PREGNANCY. If you decide to take a motion sickness drug, DON'T DRIVE. Drugs for motion sickness can make you drowsy.

HOW TO TREAT MOTION SICKNESS WITHOUT DRUGS

- Car sickness in children can be prevented by placing the child where he or she can see out of the front window of a car, such as with the help of a child's car safety seat.
- On a boat, try to move toward the center, near the water level or out on the deck, if possible.

DIARRHEA

Diarrhea may have many causes; determining the proper treatment may depend on understanding the cause of the problem. Diarrhea may be a symptom of a disease requiring a doctor's care, or it may be a temporary discomfort, due to infection from contaminated food and water. It also may result from an imbalance in the body's naturally occurring microorganism population (bacteria) caused by antibiotic treatment.

Diarrhea may be one symptom of an intestinal "flu-like" illness caused by viruses or bacteria. ("Traveler's diarrhea" from contaminated water is an example.) It may also be caused by certain medications, chemicals in foods, or by allergic reactions to food. Diarrhea may also result from emotional stress.

Mere frequency of defecation is not diarrhea, and is not in itself a cause for concern. Studies of normal populations have revealed that as many as three bowel movements per day may be normal for many individuals.[1] A *change* in bowel habits (a significant increase in number of movements per day, for example) which lasts for three or more days, however, is a cause for concern.

Diarrhea is the result of too much fluid retained in the colon (large intestine). This, in turn, can result from too much fluid entering the colon or from the failure of the colon to absorb enough fluid prior to defecation.

Acute diarrhea, characterized by sudden onset, and often accompanied by some weakness, flatulence (gas), mild cramping, fever (less than 101° F or 38.3° C) and/or vomiting, is generally self-limiting. It will typically get better in one to three days with or without medication.

Diarrhea which lasts for more than three days or which recurs on a regular basis is called chronic diarrhea. Such frequent passage of voluminous, loose, or watery stools suggests a problem requiring medical attention, especially if accompanied by severe cramping, vomiting, persistent fever (greater than 101° F or 38.3° C) or weight loss.

Any evidence of bleeding in the digestive system requires medical attention. If there is blood in the vomit, black vomit, vomit that looks like coffee grounds, blood in stools, or black tar-like stools, consult a physician.

A person with diarrhea should check his or her temperature to rule out the possibility of a more serious infection. A temperature greater than 101° F or 38.3° C accompanying diarrhea warrants checking with a doctor or other health professional.

TREAT SIMPLE DIARRHEA WITHOUT DRUGS

Since chronic diarrhea requires medical attention, we will focus only on the treatment of the acute disease. As stated before, acute diarrhea is self-limiting and will generally improve with or without treatment. Treatment (beyond switching to a bland, non-irritating diet) is chiefly intended to cut down on the number of watery stools, help you maintain sufficient body fluids and generally make you feel more comfortable while the body heals itself.

Whatever the cause of the diarrhea, the first step in treatment is to switch to a bland diet and to avoid milk and dairy products. A bland diet is one that eliminates food which may further irritate the colon. For many people, this means avoiding fresh fruits and vegetables, as well as coffee, alcohol, and spicy foods. Milk products should be avoided by everyone with diarrhea because lactose (a sugar in milk) can be difficult to digest and frequently aggravates diarrhea for many people. You may know of additional foods which you do not tolerate well.

The chief danger (though an unlikely one) of simple diarrhea is the possibility of dehydration. Drinking plenty of clear liquids, such as water or flat ginger ale, will help you to maintain body fluids. Prevention of dehydration is especially important in the care of infants (less than one year old), diabetics, and elderly or debilitated people. A severe loss of water through diarrhea, especially in these groups, warrants a call to a health care professional.

Small children may also suffer ill effects from the loss of fluids and body chemicals. While it is not usually necessary to see a physician, a child between the ages of two and five with acute diarrhea will be helped by the use of a solution which provides necessary chemicals as well as fluid. Examples are INFALYTE and PEDIALYTE, which are available without a prescription from a pharmacist.

Review the foods you ate and medications you used before the onset of diarrhea. Some people are sensitive to certain chemicals in food or drugs, and reactions to these substances are almost impossible to predict until they occur. Try to recall whether any of these foods or drugs were ever associated with an episode of diarrhea in the past, and avoid them in the future.

Some drugs are commonly associated with diarrhea. They include:
- antibiotics taken for infections;
- antacids containing magnesium (including MAALOX and MYLANTA);
- drugs for high blood pressure including guanethidine (Ismelin);
- all laxatives except the bulk-forming variety [2] (see chapter on constipation);
- drugs for irregular heartbeat such as quinidine (Cardioquin).

If you suspect that a medication used under the direction of a physician has caused diarrhea, contact your doctor. If an over the counter medication which you used without medical direction is suspect, stop using it.

OTC ANTIDIARRHEAL PRODUCTS

Although widely marketed and used, some of the products reviewed in this chapter not only lack evidence of effectiveness in treating diarrhea, but also pose significant safety hazards. None of these products actually stop or control diarrhea, and while some promise to provide relief of symptoms, we do not recommend that you use any of them.

The FDA Advisory Panel of experts that studied OTC antidiarrheal products reviewed twenty-five ingredients for safety and efficacy in treating diarrhea. Since the panel's report, the FDA has proposed changes in the panel's classification of two ingredients.

Of the twenty-five ingredients reviewed, only one ingredient available nationwide was determined by the panel to be safe and effective in the treatment of diarrhea. That ingredient is polycarbophil[3], currently marketed as calcium polycarbophil under the trade name MITROLAN. Opiates, such as opium powder and paregoric, were also found safe and effective by the panel, but widely sold products containing adequate dosages in safe preparations are currently not available without a prescription. In many states opium and paregoric are not available without a prescription in any dose.[4]

The same qualities of water absorption which make calcium polycarbophil (in MITROLAN) work as a bulk-forming laxative are also responsible for its antidiarrheal effectiveness. Because it does not slow down the expulsion of infectious agents or toxins through the intestine, calcium ploycarbophil does not interfere with the natural protective action of diarrhea.

Unfortunately, evidence of polycarbophil's effectiveness against short-lived diarrhea is meager.[5,6] For this reason, we do not recommend its use for simple, acute diarrhea.

Pepto-Bismol

Recent studies have shown that bismuth subsalicylate (in PEPTO-BISMOL) may be effective in the prevention[7] and treatment[8] of one type of diarrhea, *traveler's diarrhea*. Traveler's diarrhea is diarrhea associated with travel, particularly in areas where there are impure water supplies. Based on these studies, the FDA is in the process of reclassifying the ingredient as effective in reducing the number of bowel movements in diarrhea.[9]

Bismuth subsalicylate (PEPTO-BISMOL) has not proven its effectiveness at all for diarrhea other than that associated with travel.

Bismuth subsalicylate is not completely effective even for treating traveler's diarrhea. It has no significant effect on stool consistency, for example. Additionally, its use requires large doses (8 oz. per day) which are inconvenient when travelling in less developed areas where traveler's diarrhea is likely.

In addition, salicylates (aspirin-like substances) are readily absorbed from PEPTO-BISMOL,[10] leading to problems of salicylate side effects (including bleeding problems in some people), interaction with other drugs, and salicylate overdose (characterized by ringing of the ears and other problems) if taken with enough aspirin or other aspirin-related products.[11] Also, bismuth subsalicylate can turn your stools black and can therefore mask stomach or intestinal bleeding, which is a serious medical problem.

In summary, we do not recommend the use of PEPTO-BISMOL for self-medication of acute diarrhea, a self-limiting disease which improves quickly without medication.

Rheaban

Attapulgite (in RHEABAN, for example) was also found by the FDA panel to lack evidence of effectiveness as an antidiarrheal ingredient. The FDA now appears to be in the process of reclassifying the ingredient as "effective for reducing the number of bowel movements in diarrhea."[12]

There is no evidence that attapulgite (the active ingredient in RHEABAN) can stop or control diarrhea, or improve the consistency of stools.[13] In the opinion of the Public Citizen Health Research Group, the evidence upon which the FDA based their proposed reclassification is incomplete*, and we urge reconsideration of this decision.

In summary, we cannot recommend the use of RHEABAN for self-medication of acute simple diarrhea, a self-limiting disease which improves quickly without medication.

NO OTHER INGREDIENTS FOR THE TREATMENT OF DIARRHEA HAVE SHOWN SUFFICIENT EVIDENCE OF SAFETY AND EFFECTIVENESS to be tentatively approved by the FDA. They should not be used; they should not be sold. This includes many well-known and widely marketed products.

---

*The information submitted to the FDA by the manufacturer is not sufficient to demonstrate whether the study was well-controlled. For example, the manufacturer stated that lactose (the milk sugar that *causes* diarrhea in many people) was contained in the placebo given to the control subjects — those who did not get the attapulgite.

Kaopectate

Kaolin and pectin (the sole active ingredients in KAOPECTATE and KAOPECTATE CONCENTRATE) have failed to show evidence of effectiveness in the treatment of diarrhea. Kaolin and pectin, both alone and in combination, do not perform significantly better than a placebo (an inactive experimental "control" product) as a diarrhea remedy. Relief experienced while taking KAOPECTATE and most other OTC products can probably be attributed to the fact that simple diarrhea is self-limiting, and will usually get better in a day or two without any treatment at all.

Other products which contain kaolin and pectin include: DON-NAGEL, KAODENE, KAODENE WITH PAREGORIC and PAREPECTOLIN.

Donnagel

DONNAGEL contains not only the drugs kaolin and pectin, which lack evidence of effectiveness, but also three additional ingredients which lack evidence of safety: hyoscyamine sulfate, atropine sulfate, and hyoscine hydrobromide. These ingredients often cause blurring of vision, dryness of the mouth and throat, and hesitancy of urination. In the amounts present in DON-NAGEL, these ingredients lack evidence of effectiveness as well.

The FDA panel concluded that the combination of ingredients found in both DONNAGEL and DONNAGEL-PG (which also contains an ineffective amount of paregoric) are not safe and effective as OTC antidiarrheals. We agree; they should not be sold and they should not be used.

NAUSEA AND VOMITING

Nausea and vomiting are frequently symptoms of disorders similar to those which cause diarrhea. They may result from a self-limiting infection or a reaction to food or drugs. For the most part, nausea and vomiting, like diarrhea, need not be a cause for alarm or self-medication, and will usually stop in one to three days.

Vomiting in an infant (younger than one year) may be a sign of serious illness which requires a call or trip to the doctor. It is quite normal for babies to "spit up" a bit of food or liquid after a meal, but forceful or repeated expulsion of material, especially if accompanied by obvious discomfort, fever, or unusual behavior in the baby, may be a cause for concern. If the vomiting is not easily explained, call the doctor. Such vomiting may be the result of a serious problem, such as intolerance to a particular formula or an intestinal blockage. These and other disorders need to be diagnosed as soon as possible.

Morning Sickness

Vomiting in women who are or may be pregnant can be a cause for concern. Morning sickness (nausea and vomiting) is common in early pregnancy. A woman who may be pregnant and experiences nausea and vomiting should *not* take any kind of medication for relief. Small, frequent meals, soda crackers, drinking hot or cold (non-alcoholic) liquids and avoiding foods you do not tolerate well can help. If this brings no relief, and you are extremely uncomfortable, or if you have lost a great deal of fluid through vomiting, seek prompt medical attention. One OTC product, EMETROL, is marketed for nausea and vomiting, including morning sickness. The ingredients in EMETROL lack evidence of effectiveness according to the FDA, and we do not recommend its use.

Causes for Concern

Nausea and vomiting may be a symptom of one of a number of serious diseases, including an intestinal blockage or a body-wide infection such as Reye's Syndrome (in children under 18) or Toxic Shock Syndrome. For this reason it is important to consult a health care professional if:

• Nausea or vomiting is accompanied by a fever greater than 101 °F(38.3 °C). Take your temperature in the morning and evening each day to rule out the possibility of a more serious infection.

• Nausea or vomiting is accompanied by severe tiredness, sleepiness, exhaustion or lethargy or any other unusual symptom, especially in a child or adolescent who is recovering from a viral infection such as flu or chicken pox.

• Vomiting is black or looks like coffee grounds. This is a sign of bleeding.

• Vomiting in a small child (under the age of five) is so severe that no fluids can be held down for 12 hours. Dehydration may develop quickly in such a child.

• No fluids are held down due to vomiting and a swollen stomach area develops. An intestinal blockage may have developed.

• Vomiting is accompanied by severe abdominal pain.

• Vomiting is severe or violent. Physical damage to the throat may occur.

A short uncomplicated bout of nausea and vomiting poses no threat to a healthy adult, although vomiting in a child or elderly or debilitated person can be dangerous. Dehydration can rapidly result. For this reason, it is important to try to replace liquids lost by drinking clear liquids and to stop triggering further vomiting spells by avoiding solid foods and dairy products.

As with diarrhea, certain foods and drugs can cause nausea and vomiting in sensitive people. Common offending drugs are:

- antibiotics;
- heart drugs containing digitalis glycosides such as digoxin (Lanoxin);
- narcotic pain-killers such as codeine;
- female hormones — including most birth control pills, containing estrogen;
- prescription drugs used to treat asthma, such as aminophylline and theophylline;
- salt substitutes such as potassium chloride; and
- iron preparations.[14]

Nausea caused by some drugs, including aspirin and iron preparations, can be avoided by taking them with meals. However, some drugs such as the antibiotic tetracycline should *not* be taken with meals since doing so decreases absorption of the drug to a point where it is ineffective. Consult a physician if you suspect that a drug used under medical direction has caused nausea and vomiting. If you suspect that nausea and vomiting were caused by a drug that you used without medical direction, stop using it.

There are no OTC drugs generally recognized as safe and effective for the treatment of nausea and vomiting.[15] Although marketed for vomiting, as well as diarrhea and indigestion, bismuth subsalicylate (in PEPTO-BISMOL), like levulose, fructose, and orthophosphoric acid (the ingredients in EMETROL), lacks evidence of effectiveness for this purpose.

MOTION SICKNESS

Nausea and vomiting which is associated with car, boat, or air travel is commonly called *motion sickness.* Although not thoroughly understood, it is the only variety of nausea and vomiting for which self-medication is appropriate and prevention using an OTC product is possible. Sensitive individuals can prevent and treat motion sickness with certain precautions, using over the counter products if necessary.

Though commonly known as "carsickness," "seasickness," or "airsickness," motion sickness can be experienced in any situation in which movement confuses your body. One current theory explaining motion sickness is referred to as "neural mismatch."[16] Neural mismatch is characterized by conflicts between the information of two sensory systems.

In motion sickness, it is thought that information derived from sight does not "match" information derived from other senses, including the sense of motion perceived by the inner ear and the body-location sense of the muscles and joints.[17]

Often motion sickness can be prevented and treated with a few simple techniques. Carsick children have been cured when they are allowed to see out of the *front* window of the car so that what they see matches what they feel.[18] Regardless of any accomodations that are made to permit children to see out of the front window, appropriate seat belts or safety seats must be used for the safety of children.

Seasickness and airsickness can often be prevented by moving to the center of the ship near the water line or over the wing of the plane. This can decrease the body's sensation of movement by reducing actual motion. Once nausea of motion sickness has set in, it often can be diminished by lying down with the eyes open. Airsickness may be reduced by gazing at a point on the distant horizon, since this helps to decrease the perception of motion.

If these non-drug techniques fail, and you frequently suffer from motion sickness, you should consider one of the three OTC drug ingredients — cyclizine, dimenhydrinate, and meclizine — available for this complaint. All three are antihistamines, which cause drowsiness, and so they should never by used if you are driving or operating heavy machinery or if you need to be alert for any other reason. Other side effects of these drugs are discussed in the chapters on sleep-aids and cough and cold remedies. (See pp. 46, 160 for side effects and a list of drugs with which they may interact.) *They should not be used by pregnant women* or people with asthma or glaucoma or people who have difficulty urinating due to an enlarged prostate. Nor should they be used in combination with alcohol.

The three ingredients found to be safe and effective by the FDA for prevention and treatment of motion sickness are cyclizine hydrochloride (in MAREZINE, for example), dimenhydrinate (in DRAMAMINE, for example), and meclizine hydrochloride (in BONINE, for example).[16]

They should be used only as directed. You may find any one of the three to be most effective for you. As with other over the counter products, you should buy generic or house brands of these ingredients, if possible, since they are less expensive.

HEMORRHOIDS

WHAT ARE HEMORRHOIDS?

Hemorrhoids are enlarged (inflamed and uncomfortable) blood vessels and surrounding tissue in the anorectal area. Hemorrhoids and other anorectal disorders can cause pain, burning and itching. Some hemorrhoids and other anorectal disorders require medical attention; others can be treated without medical supervision.

HOW TO TREAT HEMORRHOIDS AND OTHER ANORECTAL DISORDERS WITHOUT DRUGS
(See pp. 139-140)
- Improve bowel habits with a high fiber diet.
- Keep anorectal area clean and dry, washing with clear, warm water after each bowel movement, and/or take sitz baths (see pp. 140) and apply moist heat several times a day.
- Avoid irritating the anorectal area with unnecessary products, devices or scratching.

WHICH OTC DRUGS TO USE

Petroleum jelly or zinc oxide applied externally as a protectant.

EXAMPLES OF OTC ANORECTAL PRODUCTS NOT TO USE

The following products contain ingredients that lack evidence of safety, effectiveness, or both, according to the FDA:

ANUSOL, DIOTHANE, EPINEPHRICAINE, HEMORRIN, NUPERCAINAL, PAZO, PONTOCAINE, PREPARATION H, PROCTODON, RECTAL MEDICONE, TANICAINE, TRONOLANE SUPPOSITORIES, and WYANOID OINTMENT and SUPPOSITORIES.

In addition, although the FDA has tentatively found ingredients in these products safe and effective, we do not recommend the use of the following: LANACANE CREAM and TRONOLANE CREAM.

WHEN TO SEEK HELP FROM A HEALTH CARE PROFESSIONAL

Consult a health care professional when anorectal discomfort is accompanied by any of the following:
- Severe pain, inflammation or swelling.
- Pain, swelling or severe itching which does not improve in one week using the simple measures discussed in this chapter.
- Rectal bleeding. Some bleeding may be quite harmless, but it

should *always* be evaluated by a health care professional.
- Material seeping from the affected area.
- Anything that protrudes through the body surface in the anorectal area, such as a prolapsed hemorrhoid, that does not return to normal in several days.

INTRODUCTION

Anorectal disorders are conditions that cause pain and discomfort in the lower six inches of the digestive tract. These disorders include hemorrhoids (or piles) and other conditions that result in pain, severe itching, bleeding, seepage, or swelling. Discomfort can also be caused by pinworms and other infections.

In 1981 Americans spent over $110 million on over the counter hemorrhoidal preparations.[1] These figures do not include preparations that were not sold specifically for hemorrhoidal relief, such as hydrocortisone products, petroleum jelly, and zinc oxide ointment.

Disorders of this region are among the most uncomfortable known and account for millions of lost hours on the job as well as hours of sleepless shifting in bed.

To deal with this discomfort, many sufferers turn to a variety of OTC products touted to relieve the pain, swelling and itching of anorectal disorders. Unfortunately, there is little evidence that most of these drug products are necessarily better for promoting relief than cleanliness, improved bowel habits and other non-drug techniques, or the use of simple, inexpensive generic products such as petroleum jelly or zinc oxide preparations.

Self-treatment of most anorectal disorders should center upon making discomfort tolerable while allowing the body to heal itself.

THE ANORECTAL REGION

Some understanding of the structure and function of the anorectal area will help you decide how to approach disorders in this region.

Health professionals divide the region into three areas: the peri-anal area, the anus, and the rectum.

The peri-anal area is an area of skin about 2½ inches in diameter which surrounds the opening of the anus. This is a very sensitive area with many pain-sensing nerves. The skin in this area is moister than skin of other parts of the body, and is easily irritated.

The anus, or anal canal, is the lowest portion of the digestive tract. It is just over an inch in length and lined with skin. Highly sensitive nerves within the skin of the anal canal are capable of transmitting feelings of pain, discomfort and distension. Most pain from anorectal problems is focused in this area.

Above the anus lies the rectum. This portion of the intestinal tract is about 5-6 inches long, and connects the large intestine, or colon, with the anus. The rectum is lined with *mucous membrane* that contains nerves but cannot sense pain. Mucous membrane is the smooth lubricated surface which lines the inside of body openings. Another example of mucous membrane is the inside of the mouth.

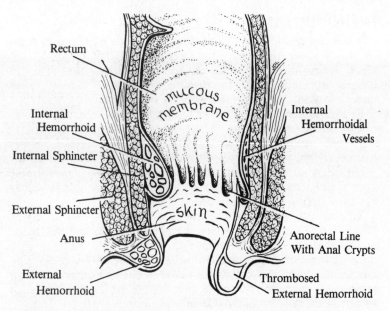

Anorectal region. Adapted by permission from *Handbook of Nonprescription Drugs,* 7th ed., p. 642, © 1982 American Pharmaceutical Association.

Between the anus and the rectum is an area called the anorectal line. Anal crypts are pocketlike formations in the area of the anorectal line. These crypts can trap bits of fecal matter, resulting in irritation and, occasionally, infection.

Interconnecting networks of blood vessels, much like the vessels in the lips, lie under the surface of the skin and mucous membrane of the anus and rectum. These networks of vessels join to form the hemorrhoidal blood vessels, which are often the center of discomfort.

Skin and mucous membrane make up the wall of the anal canal and rectum, respectively. When intact, they form a barrier to protect the body from infection and injury. Skin and mucous membrane have different abilities to absorb substances, including medication; some drugs may be absorbed more easily through the skin, others more easily through mucous membrane. A broken barrier, such as injured, irritated or diseased skin or mucous membrane, allows microorganisms such as bacteria, as well as increased amounts of other materials, including drugs, to enter the body.

DISORDERS OF THE ANORECTAL REGION

Many disorders affect the anorectal area. Due to the ample nerve supply of the anal and peri-anal area, these disorders can be quite painful. Some kinds of discomfort in this region are not appropriate for self-treatment. If you have any of the possible danger signs listed below, you should consult a health care professional:

- Any *severe* pain, inflammation or swelling.
- Any pain, swelling or severe itching that does not improve, using the simple measures discussed in this chapter, after one week.
- Any rectal bleeding. Some bleeding may be quite harmless, but it should *always* be evaluated by a health care professional.
- Any material seeping from the affected area.
- Anything that protrudes through the body surface in the anorectal area, such as a prolapsed hemorrhoid, that does not return to normal in several days.

The only disorders which are appropriate for self-care are mild anal itching and simple, uncomplicated inflammation of hemorrhoids.

HEMORRHOIDS

These swellings, sometimes known as "piles," are the result of enlargement of hemorrhoidal blood vessels and the surrounding tissue. Hemorrhoids arising from the skin below the anorectal line are called *external hemorrhoids*. Those arising from the mucous membrane above the anorectal line are called *internal hemorrhoids*.

Occasionally, internal hemorrhoids become so enlarged that they protrude below the anorectal line and through the anal opening. These are known as prolapsed hemorrhoids. Anyone having a prolapsed hemorrhoid should seek medical attention.

The cause of hemorrhoidal disease is not entirely understood. Hemorrhoid formation is partially controlled by hereditary factors beyond our control but is also thought to be related to factors such as occupation, posture and diet.

The likelihood of hemorrhoids is increased with a variety of circumstances, including pregnancy, long periods of standing or sitting, coughing, sneezing, vomiting, and physical exertion[2]. Hemorrhoids may also occur because of constipation or diarrhea. Straining occurring with constipation or diarrhea, and passage of hard stools in constipation, can cause and irritate hemorrhoids. Constipation may result from insufficient fiber and liquid in the diet. Congestion in blood vessels, as well as excessive tension in the anal sphincter muscles (the ring-like muscles which control the size of the anal opening), play a role in development of painful hemorrhoids. Infection in the anal crypts may also cause the inflammation of hemorrhoids.

In general, hemorrhoids cause discomfort, but not excruciating pain. Because of their ample pain-sensing nerve fibers, external hemorrhoids are more painful than internal hemorrhoids, although a prolapsed internal hemorrhoid can be painful. Uncomplicated, external hemorrhoids, though uncomfortable, usually will heal themselves or be significantly reduced within two weeks. All that is necessary is to try to eliminate unnecessary irritation and allow healing to progress. If healing does not occur in two weeks, you may have internal hemorrhoids.

Some hemorrhoids may cause complications requiring medical attention. Internal hemorrhoids often bleed. Blockage of the blood supply in the affected blood vessel(s) may result in *strangulated* or *thrombosed* (clotted) hemorrhoids. These are very painful and require medical attention.

Pruritis Ani or Anal Itching

Anal itching is a common and very annoying symptom of many anorectal disorders. It may be the result of infection (including pinworms, discussed next), allergy, irritation from body secretion or clothing, psychological reasons, or certain drugs (such as some antibiotics). It can also be a symptom of hemorrhoidal disease.

Uncomplicated itching, unaccompanied by warning signs listed at the beginning of the chapter, is appropriate for self-care. Like other itching, it is made worse by scratching; this can lead to the "itch scratch" cycle, as well as to physical damage to this sensitve area.

Pinworms

Enterobiasis, or pinworms, is an intestinal infection estimated to affect 30 to 40 million people in the United States and Canada.[3] Pinworms are one cause of anal itching.

Pinworms live in the large intestine. The adult female worm (about 0.4 inches or 1 cm. long) ventures out at night to lay eggs in the perianal area. This causes intense anal itching (pruritis ani), and can, on occasion, lead to vaginal infection in women.

The worm enters the body when a person swallows worm eggs, which may be found on contaminated fingers. The infection spreads readily in the home between members of the family and may also be spread from child to child at play. A child or adult who is bothered early in the night with intense rectal itching is likely to have pinworms.

Sometimes pinworms can be detected by placing a small piece of double stick tape on the skin around the anus and leaving it there overnight. If there is a pinworm infection, a worm can be caught on the tape. Most people do not have the equipment or expertise, though, to make a *definite* diagnosis of a pinworm infection, so you should consult a health care professional if you suspect pinworms.

The FDA has proposed that pinworm infections could be safely and effectively self-treated with a drug called pyrantel pamoate[4] (currently available by prescription as Antiminth). This drug is not yet available without a prescription, but it may be by 1984.[5] Even when such a product becomes available, however, you should seek medical advice for diagnosis and treatment of this disorder.

HOW TO CARE FOR ANORECTAL DISORDERS, SUCH AS HEMORRHOIDS, WITHOUT DRUGS

While self-care techniques and products discussed in this chapter may not cure your disorder, some may safely be used to make you feel more comfortable and protect the affected area from further irritation while natural healing occurs.

In general, OTC products such as petroleum jelly and zinc oxide may ease the pain or itching of anorectal disorders (including hemorrhoids), although neither they nor any other OTC product can treat the underlying problem. On the other hand, non-drug self-treatment, especially changes in hygiene and diet, can in many cases actually correct the causes of this discomfort. We therefore suggest that you pursue non-drug techniques before resorting to medication.

Bowel Habits

If you are suffering from constipation, diarrhea, or any difficulty in passing stools, it is important to remedy these sources of irritation to the anorectal area. Otherwise, the body's healing abilities can not work effectively.

Refer to appropriate sections of this book (pp. 93, 123) for self-treatment of these problems. A high fiber diet (p. 93), which helps to soften the stool and relieve occasional constipation, is especially important in preventing future irritation.

Cleanliness

One source of anal itching and irritation is traces of body secretions and stool in and around the anal and peri-anal area. These may be very irritating; they can make the skin more subject to damage by scratches or cracking and less able to fight off infection.

Cleaning the area with mild soap and water on a daily basis is helpful. It is important not to dry the area too much, and a gentle soap is essential. Try to avoid rubbing the anorectal area; blotting or patting with toilet paper — moistened if necessary — is preferable to wiping, for example. Cleaning with warm water after each bowel movement is very helpful.

In cleaning the anorectal area, there is no need to use any special antiseptic or lubricant. In fact, some of these chemicals may only weaken or irritate the skin. Moisture trapped in non-porous undergarments (underwear that can't "breathe") can cause irritation as well.

Sitz Baths and Other Forms of Moist Heat

Simple hemorrhoids often respond to sitz baths. Sitz baths simply involve sitting in warm water (110-115°F., or 43-36°C., very warm but not painfully hot to your hand), 2-3 times a day, for 15 minutes at a time. Products are available that fit over the toilet for easy sitz baths. Applications of other forms of moist heat, including warm, damp towels, are helpful as well.

Rest

With certain disorders, walking can be irritating to the anal area, as can prolonged standing and sitting. For severe discomfort from hemorrhoidal disease, a day or more of bed rest (lying down) may be necessary, to take the pressure off the hemorrhoidal veins.

OTC PRODUCTS FOR ANORECTAL DISORDERS

Many products are sold without prescription for the relief of anorectal disorders. Some are heavily advertised. Many contain ingredients that may provide some relief, but these are frequently in combination with ingredients that are ineffective or unsafe. Effective ingredients are frequently available *generically* at a much lower cost than that of heavily advertised products.

Before taking any drugs for anorectal disorders, keep in mind that topically applied medication (that is, medication applied directly to the skin or other affected surface) may be absorbed into the general body circulation. Most products are more easily absorbed by mucous membrane than by skin. For this reason, some of these products are safe for use only on skin, and should not be allowed *into* the rectal area.

The FDA Advisory Panel on OTC Hemorrhoid Products reviewed ingredients used in over the counter anorectal products. These ingredients were divided into nine categories, which will be defined and discussed below. Six categories (protectants, astringents, counter-irritants, local anesthetics, vasoconstrictors and keratolytics) contained some safe and effective ingredients. Three categories (antiseptic, anticholinergics, and wound healing agents) contained no ingredients with evidence of safety and effectiveness. This panel did not consider hydrocortisone products, yet these products are widely marketed for anal itching and will be discussed later in the chapter.

Some ingredients were considered in more than one category, and all ingredients were considered for appropriateness externally (for the anal and peri-anal areas) and intrarectally (in the rectum). As a result, some ingredients were found to be safe and effective for more than one use. Calamine and zinc oxide, for example, were determined safe and effective both as astringents and as protectants.

Some ingredients were found to be safe and effective for one use, but not for another. Cod liver oil and shark liver oil, for example, were determined safe and effective as protectants, but were found to lack evidence of effectiveness as wound-healing agents.

Finally, some ingredients were found to be safe and effective when applied externally (to the anal and peri-anal skin) but not when taken intrarectally. This is due to differences in absorption, as was previously discussed. Those anesthestics, counter-irritants, or keratolytics, for example, that were found to be safe and effective for external use, were *not* determined to be safe and effective for intrarectal use. The difficulty of confining these ingredients to the anal and peri-anal skin and preventing their spread to the rectal wall leads us to recommend that you not use these ingredients in anorectal products.

For most simple disorders (those that you can safely treat yourself), when an ointment is desired, use of a protectant is all that is necessary. We cannot recommend the use of other products.

Following is a discussion of the categories of anorectal ingredients.

Categories of Ingredients Containing Some Ingredients Considered Safe and Effective by the FDA Panel

Protectants are agents that are applied to form a physical barrier as a protective coating. They often are used as a base for other ingredients. Those most commonly encountered in anorectal products are cocoa butter, cod liver oil, lanolin, mineral oil, shark liver oil, white petrolatum (petroleum jelly) and zinc oxide.

According to the FDA Panel, these are all safe and effective as protectants for internal and external use, as long as the protectants in a product total at least 50 percent of the product. In addition, glycerin is safe and effective, but for external use only. Protectants can protect the region against further irritation. There is no evidence that any product containing a combination of these ingredients is more effective than any one ingredient alone.

There is some evidence that the most effective ingredient is white petrolatum.[6] This is available, inexpensively, in generic or house-brand form, as well as in more costly, advertised brand-name products. Petrolatum, or petroleum jelly, is marketed as VASELINE, for example. There is no reason to purchase more expensive and exotic ingredients such as shark liver oil (an active ingredient in PREPARATION H) as they appear to have no advantage over basic petroleum jelly or zinc oxide ointment. Finally, because many people are allergic to wool alcohol and lanolin,[7] it is best to avoid these ingredients, particularly if your skin has shown sensitivity to any skin lotion in the past. (Many lotions contain lanolin.)[8]

Bismuth subgallate (in ANUSOL and NUPERCAINAL) was found to lack evidence of effectiveness as a protectant.

141

Astringents are agents that have something of a "puckering" effect on skin and mucous membrane. Through an unknown mechanism, they provide temporary relief of burning, itching and irritation. These ingredients cannot reduce swelling, however.[8]

The safe and effective astringents are calamine, witch hazel (or hamamelis water), and zinc oxide. Witch hazel is appropriate only for external use, while the others may be used intrarectally as well.

Tannic acid (in TANICAINE, available until recently) is not safe for use, and should no longer be available in anorectal products; its potential to cause liver damage is well documented.

Counter-irritants are agents that produce a sensation to distract from pain, burn or itching. Typically, these products make skin feel cool when applied.

The only safe and effective counter-irritant is *menthol* in a water base for external use only. Large amounts, if absorbed, can have serious adverse effects, so intrarectal use (where it is more readily absorbed) can be dangerous. It would be impractical to try to confine this ingredient to the external area once applied. Therefore, we do not recommend its use.

Camphor (in PAZO, for example), hydrastis, turpentine oil, and juniper tar are not generally recognized as safe and effective for anorectal use.

Local Anesthetics are agents that produce a temporary disappearance of sensation in the area applied. This is accomplished by blocking the capacity of the nerve to send information about discomfort. They play no role whatsoever in promoting healing. They provide temporary relief from symptoms; but they can be sensitizing or irritating, and may even prolong healing. *We do not recommend the use of local anesthetics for anorectal disorders.*

The FDA Panel found benzocaine and pramoxine hydrochloride to be safe and effective local anesthetics *for external use only* for anorectal discomfort. Intrarectal application of an anesthetic is irrational, as there is little or no actual pain sensation in the mucous membrane above the anorectal line.

Benzocaine (found in many products, including AMERICAINE and LANACANE) can cause sensitization, so that the user becomes allergic not only to it, but also to other "-caine" anesthetics (such as novocaine and lidocaine).[9,10] Pramoxine hydrochloride (found in TRONOLANE) is less likely to be sensitizing.[11]

All other anesthetics were found by the FDA Panel to lack evidence of safety and effectiveness. These include diperodon (in DIOTHANE and PROCTODON), phenacaine (in TANICAINE, available until recently), dibucaine (in NUPERCAINAL), tetracaine (in PONTOCAINE), as well as benzyl alcohol, cyclonine, and lidocaine.

142

Vasoconstrictors are agents that cause temporary narrowing of the blood vessels. Presumably, they function to reduce congestion in hemorrhoidal blood vessels. Vasoconstrictors will not permanently stop bleeding; if bleeding is present, medical attention is required. Conclusive evidence that vasoconstrictors reduce swollen hemorrhoids does not exist. For this reason, we do not recommend the use of vasoconstrictors for anorectal disorders.

Products containing vasoconstrictors are not widely marketed. The FDA has tentatively approved as vasoconstrictors the ingredients ephedrine sulfate and phenylephrine hydrochloride, both in water-based solution, for intrarectal and external use, and epinephrine hydrochloride in water-base solution for external use only. Epinephrine (in EPINEPHRICAINE) lacks evidence of safety and effectiveness for anorectal use.

Keratolytics are agents that produce loosening and shedding of surface layers of skin. Keratolytics in products containing a combination of ingredients are designed to remove the outside (keratin) layer of skin in order to allow the other therapeutic ingredients to be effective. We do not recommend the use of these products. Since no topically applied ingredients can speed healing, it is irrational to use a product that is supposed to aid the action of other ingredients. If a drug is ineffective, no amount of "aid" will make it effective. Also, keratolytic products are not harmless; they are by nature potentially irritating. There is no keratin layer in the rectum, so intrarectal use is even more irrational.

Alcloxa (called allantoin in PERIFOAM) and resorcinol (in LANACANE) were determined to be generally recognized as safe and effective keratolytics. For the reasons stated above, however, we do not recommend their use.

Categories of Anorectal Ingredients Containing No Safe and Effective Ingredients

Antiseptics are agents that will inhibit the growth and development of microorganisms (bacteria), while not necessarily destroying them. None are needed for care of simple anorectal discomfort.

Some antiseptics are toxic and should not be used for anorectal disorders. Boric acid, found in WYANOID Ointment and WYANOID Suppositories, is an example. The FDA Panel found boric acid not to be safe or effective in OTC anorectal preparations; it is toxic when absorbed, and lacks clinical evidence of effectiveness.

Anticholinergics are agents designed to inhibit or prevent the transmission of some nerve impulses. They are not effective in the relief of any anorectal symptoms, however, and should be avoided. They pose a hazard due to possible toxicity when absorbed.

Atropine (in TANICAINE Ointment and Suppositories,

available until recently), and belladonna extract (in WYANOID Suppositories) are anticholinergics. Products such as these should not be used.

Wound-healing agents are ingredients intended to accelerate tissue repair or wound healing. Such agents would be helpful if they worked, but unfortunately, no ingredients are generally recognized as safe and effective wound-healing agents. Some heavily advertised products contain ingredients purported to be wound-healing agents, but none have been found safe and effective by the FDA.

The following ingredients lack evidence of effectiveness as wound-healing agents; some lack evidence of safety as well: cod liver oil, live yeast cell derivatives (in PREPARATION H), Peruvian balsam (in ANUSOL, RECTAL MEDICONE, WYANOID Ointment and Suppositories, and HEMORRIN), shark liver oil (in PREPARATION H), Vitamin A and Vitamin D (both in EPINEPHRICAINE).

Preparation H

The most widely used anti-hemorrhoidal product is PREPARA-TION H, which now holds an estimated 56% share of the more than $100 million hemorrhoid product market. Its producer, American Home Products' Whitehall Laboratories, spent $14.6 million in 1981 to convince people of PREPARATION H's ability to "shrink swelling of hemorrhoidal tissue."[12] As discussed above, the product's active ingredients are unconvincing in their effectiveness, despite their popularity.

PREPARATION H contains live yeast cell derivative and shark liver oil as active ingredients. Live yeast cell derivative is without evidence of effectiveness for any anorectal use. Shark liver oil is *not* a safe and effective wound-healing agent, but, in adequate amounts (more than currently found in PREPARATION H), it is an effective — though expensive — protectant.

But PREPARATION H contains only 3% shark liver oil; in order to be an effective protectant ingredient, shark liver oil would need to constitute 50% of the product. PREPARATION H, THEREFORE, DESPITE ITS PRICE AND POPULARITY, IS NOT GENERALLY RECOGNIZED AS SAFE AND EFFEC-TIVE AS AN OTC ANORECTAL PRODUCT.

For anorectal discomfort, first try the non-drug approached described on pp. 139-140. If you then want to use an over the counter drug, try petroleum jelly; it is much less expensive (especially when purchased generically) and has more evidence of safety and effectiveness than PREPARATION H.

Hydrocortisone Products

Hydrocortisone products are widely marketed for rectal itch. Examples are CORTEF, CORTAID, LANACORT, PREPCORT CALDECORT, and DERMOLATE. The use of 0.50% hydrocortisone for anorectal discomfort has not been fully evaluated for safety and effectiveness,[13] and we therefore do not recommend this use.

Hydrocortisone was not considered by the FDA panel that reviewed over the counter anorectal drugs. The panel on external analgesics (pain-killers), however, proposed rules under which 0.25%-0.50% concentrations of hydrocortisone or hydrocortisone acetate can be used over the counter as an anti-pruritic (anti-itch) product. This tentative approval is for hydrocortisone products for a variety of indications involving itching, including "itchy anal areas."[14]

The panel that approved the topical use of hydrocortisone did not cite any well-controlled studies in which anal itching was successfully treated with 0.50% hydrocortisone.[15] Until products containing 0.50% hydrocortisone are shown to be effective, we do not recommend their use.

Hydrocortisone should not be used carelessly. This type of medication (a steroid hormone) can mask signs of infection and of other diseases, delaying necessary treatment.[16] Long-term use of topical hydrocortisone products can also cause a variety of skin disorders.[17]

Severe itching requires medical attention to determine the cause of the itching. Mild itching does not require treatment, other than the self-care outlined earlier in the chapter.

Dosage Forms and Applications

Anorectal products are sold in many different forms and applications. Creams, gels and ointments (both oil- and water-based solutions) for application by hand, spray, application "pipe" or suppository are available.

Some forms of application are more appropriate for certain products and conditions than others. Ointments and creams are easily applied by hand to anal and perianal areas.

Suppositories generally remain in the rectum where they are in contact with the mucous membrane. Suppositories are therefore inappropriate, for example, for products containing anesthetics, counter-irritants, or keratolytics which should not be used inside the rectum. TRONOLANE suppositories, for example, contain an anesthetic which is not safe and effective for intrarectal use. These, and all other suppositories, should not be used.

In addition, plastic applicator "pipes" may cause damage to delicate inflamed tissue. Pipes used to apply ointment or cream should be flexible and well-lubricated, and have side openings as well as a hole in the end.

Plan of Treatment for Hemorrhoids

A standard medical text[18] recommends conservative treatment for hemorrhoids, and we agree. If diet, rest and moist heat do not provide relief, a protectant such as petroleum jelly or zinc oxide may be helpful. If there is no sign of relief within a week, consult a health care professional. Among the therapies which may be applied *under medical direction* are tying off hemorrhoids with a rubber band, injections, and anal dilation (stretching of the anus). As a last resort, surgery may be considered.

SLEEPING PROBLEMS

WHAT IS INSOMNIA?

Insomnia refers to perceived sleeping problems, with difficulty falling and staying asleep. Insomnia can result in excessive tiredness during waking hours. There is no need for concern as long as waking hours are not affected. Some people need only 7, 6 or even 5 hours of sleep per night. An occasional restless night is not unusual or unhealthy, especially during times of stress.

WHICH OVER THE COUNTER DRUGS TO USE

None.

EXAMPLES OF OTC DRUGS NOT TO USE

The following products are formulated with ingredients lacking evidence of effectiveness, according to an FDA advisory panel: EXCEDRIN P.M., NERVINE, QUIET WORLD, Q-VEL, and SLEEP-EZE.

Although the FDA has tentatively approved ingredients in the following products as nighttime sleep-aids, we do not recommend any of these. These are all antihistamines, may be dangerous to certain people, and are associated with a myriad of side effects, of which drowsiness is only one: COMPOZ, NYTOL DPH, SOMINEX FORMULA II, UNISOM.

HOW TO TREAT OCCASIONAL INSOMNIA WITHOUT DRUGS

- Evaluate your sleeping problem by keeping a sleeping log.
- Discover and eliminate factors which may interfere with sleep, such as irregularity of sleeping hours, environmental factors, physical and mental factors, and substances in food, drinks and drugs.
- Establish patterns which can help you sleep, such as daytime exercise, nighttime routines, relaxation techniques, and other strategies for coping with sleepless nights.

WHEN TO SEEK HELP FROM A HEALTH CARE PROFESSIONAL

When any of the following occur:

- Insomnia does not respond to the non-drug techniques described in this chapter after 2-3 weeks, and activities during waking hours are seriously affected.
- You suspect that sleeplessness or excessive daytime drowsiness may be due to an underlying physical disorder or emotional problem.
- Depression may be present, characterized by all or some of the following: insomnia (especially early awakening), feelings

149

of sadness and worthlessness, loss of appetite, weight loss, constipation, listlessness, change in sexual behavior, inability to concentrate and poor job performance. Other psychological problems, such as dramatic mood swings, can also cause insomnia and also indicate the need for professional help.

• You, your family or your friends suspect sleep apnea may be present. Sleep apnea is usually characterized by pronounced next-day drowsiness, and by loud snoring punctuated by brief halts in breathing.

INTRODUCTION

In 1981, Americans spent over $30 million on non-prescription sleep-aids.[1] Was this money well spent? We do not believe so.

We do not recommend the use of non-prescription sleeping pills. Many sleep problems respond well to the simple non-drug techniques described in this chapter.

Severe or chronic insomnia may require professional help, but such help should *not* consist of routine or long-term prescriptions for sleeping pills.

WHAT IS INSOMNIA?

One-fourth to one-third of American adults claim to experience some difficulty in falling or remaining asleep. This difficulty, known as insomnia, troubles most people at some time.

Insomnia may be of short duration and traceable to some specific cause — unusual stress or great excitement — or it may be severe, lasting for a long period of time and seriously interfering with normal daily activities.

Unless your sleep problem is causing significant difficulties in your daily life, it is no cause for concern. Your health will not suffer from occasional bouts of poor sleep.

Some people need only 7, 6 or even 5 hours of sleep per night. An occasional restless night is not unusual or unhealthy, especially during times of stress.

Scientific studies have consistently shown that people who complain of insomnia are poor judges of their own sleep. In several studies, people complaining of insomnia were asked to estimate how long they slept while being monitored in a laboratory. They usually underestimated the amount of time they actually slept.

Since it is very difficult for most people to tell when they fall asleep or judge the quality of their sleep without sophisticated laboratory equipment, how then can you tell if you have a sleep problem?

The best test is how you feel. If you are able to carry out your daily activities without feeling drowsy, chances are excellent that you are getting all the sleep you need. No matter how many hours you have slept — or think you have slept — the most desirable sleep duration is that which allows you to stay active all day.

COMMON CAUSES OF OCCASIONAL INSOMNIA

An occasional bout with sleeplessness, resulting in excessive daytime drowsiness, can be caused by a variety of factors. Insomnia may result from environmental factors (including an uncomfortable bed, noise or excessive light), irregular sleeping hours, tension or anxiety, a physical disorder, or substances in food, drink or drugs. All of these will be discussed later in this chapter under HOW TO TREAT INSOMNIA WITHOUT DRUGS.

Special Sleep Problems

A number of other problems can disturb sleep. These include sleep apnea, snoring, sleepwalking, and muscle twitching or cramping.

Sleep apnea causes the affected person to temporarily stop breathing during sleep. This is a serious problem requiring medical attention. Knowledge of the disorder is just beginning to become widespread, and the number of sufferers is still unknown.

Sleep apnea is the sudden cessation of breathing during sleep. This may occur from a few times per night to several hundred times per night. Heavy snoring is also a common characteristic of sleep apnea. The cause of sleep apnea is not known in many cases. In some overweight victims, though, weight loss can correct the symptoms.

Frequently the person with sleep apnea does not realize that he or she suffers from this disorder. People with this problem may feel very tired during the day even after sleeping for 8 or more hours without understanding the cause of the exhaustion. While some people with sleep apnea awaken feeling breathless or unable to breathe, many perceive themselves as sleeping normally at night. Others are aware of waking, but do not realize that these episodes are caused by breathing difficulties; as soon as they awaken, normal breathing resumes.

Sometimes the individual's sleep-mate discovers the problem by noticing the characteristic heavy snoring or interruption of breathing.

Sleep apnea is not an appropriate condition for self-treatment. If you suspect that you are having breathing difficulties associated with sleep, if you awaken breathless during the night, or if your bed-partner or roommate tells you that you snore very heavily and that your breathing seems to stop at times during sleep, you should definitely seek medical advice. Sleep centers are located throughout the United States. Your physician can refer you to one if this seems appropriate for you.

The use of sleeping pills — prescription *or* OTC — can be *very* dangerous to anyone with sleep apnea. These drugs depress the respiratory system and can cause breathing to stop more often and for longer periods of time. Many sleep experts believe that the use of sleeping pills in such cases may kill many people each year. Sleeping pills and other central nervous system depressants, including alcohol or antihistamines (found in cold and allergy drugs, as well as OTC sleep-aids) should be carefully avoided in all people who may have sleep apnea.

Snoring is the noise produced by air passing through a partially closed airway. In some cases, but not usually, it may be a sign of sleep apnea. Snoring, even loud snoring, unaccompanied by a stop in breathing, is not sleep apnea. Changing positions sometimes stops snoring. Rolling from the back to the stomach, for example, may silence the snore.

Because snoring indicates some degree of breathing difficulty during sleep (even when it is not accompanied by sleep apnea) and, again, because sleeping pills depress breathing, snorers should not use sleeping pills.

Nightmares may interfere with sleep, leaving the dreamer awakened and frightened. They are often caused by internal stress or conflict which the person may not even recognize. Frequently, a mental health professional can help the person troubled by nightmares to understand and express the source of the stress or conflict so that the pressure which finds its outlet only in dreams may be relieved.

Some regularly prescribed drugs (as well as some illegal "recreational" drugs) may cause bad dreams. If you are taking any prescription medication and are regularly troubled by nightmares, check with your physician. If you use "recreational" drugs such as marijuana, cocaine, LSD, PCP, etc., and have nightmares, you should reevaluate your use of these substances.

Nighttime muscle twitching is a fairly frequent occurrence. Repeated twitching, unnoticed by the victim, can cause frequent awakening and fragmented sleep, which leads to daytime sleepiness. This is most common in middle-aged people. If these symptoms are causing repeated loss of sleep which interferes with daytime activities, consult a physician. No medication available without a prescription is safe and effective for treatment of this problem. Q-VEL, containing quinine sulfate, is marketed for nighttime muscle cramps, but an FDA panel found that this ingredient lacks evidence of effectiveness.

Serious Sleep Problems and When to Seek Professional Help

For most instances of insomnia, we recommend that you first try the non-drug self-treatment plan which follows this section. If, after giving these suggestions a reasonable trial period — at least two or three weeks — you are still experiencing sleeping problems and, as a result, are unable to go about your daily tasks efficiently, you may need professional help.

Sleep problems that do not respond to simple self-care and do not seem to have a psychological component may be the result of a physical disorder, such as the pain caused by arthritis. In this case, you should contact a health care professional.

A sleep problem that is not the result of an identifiable medical problem may require the help of a sleep specialist. Sleep disorder centers have been created around the country in recent years, and a physician may refer you to such a special clinic if appropriate. You should be aware that this specialized care can be expensive and may not be covered by your health insurance.

You should also seek professional help if you suspect you have depression or narcolepsy.

Depression is a common cause of insomnia, daytime drowsiness, or excessive sleep. Some of the symptoms of depression are: sadness, feelings of worthlessness, loss of appetite, weight loss, constipation, listlessness, changes in sexual behavior, inability to concentrate, and poor job performance. Not all of these signs need be present. If you or someone you know is having problems with severe insomnia and has any of these other symptoms, then he or she should consult a mental health professional — a psychiatrist, clinical psychologist, or licensed psychiatric social worker.

Narcolepsy is a disorder which causes irresistable attacks of sleepiness during the day. This disorder involves much more than daytime drowsiness. Attacks of sleep are sudden, can occur at inopportune moments, and often are accompanied by a loss in muscle tone. This can have serious consequences, as when driving, and should not be taken lightly. If you think you have narcolepsy, consult a health care professional.

HOW TO TREAT INSOMNIA WITHOUT DRUGS
STEP 1: EVALUATING YOUR SLEEP PATTERN: KEEPING A SLEEP DIARY

If you believe that difficulty in sleeping is interfering with your daily activities, it may help to keep a sleep diary. This will help you to identify patterns of sleep difficulties, so that you can find the source of the problem in order to correct it. Such a record will also help you determine whether the suggestions on the following pages will be useful to you.

In your log, you should record a number of factors along with the day of the week and date of each entry. Useful factors include: 1) the time you go to bed, 2) the time you arise, 3) the type of sleep problem you experience, 4) foods or drinks consumed after 5 p.m. which may cause sleeplessness (see pp. 156-157), 5) any drugs (including alcohol) taken after 5 p.m., 6) how you feel the next day, and other factors which may affect sleep, including anxiety producing events during the day.

One problem with keeping this kind of log is that it can focus your attention on the number of hours that you sleep or spend trying to sleep. Do not count hours while you lie in bed. Needless attention to time spent awake can cause additional sleeplessness. *Remember, your watch or clock is not the best guide to whether you are getting enough sleep. You are. If you feel adequately rested during the day, and are able to accomplish your daily tasks with reasonable efficiency, you are almost certainly getting enough sleep.*

154

STEP 2: DISCOVERING AND ELIMINATING FACTORS WHICH MAY INTERFERE WITH SLEEP
Regularity of Sleeping Hours

Do you go to bed and arise at regular hours? Regularity is of prime importance in sleeping well. Our bodies operate on finely tuned internal clocks which are set to a daily cycle. This cycle is sometimes known as our circadian (meaning "about a day") rhythm.

Helping your body achieve a regular daily sleep/wake cycle may alleviate your sleeping problem. One way to do this is to set your alarm clock for the same time each day (even on weekends) and then arise at that time, no matter how late you fall asleep. This will help establish a more regular circadian rhythm.

Going to sleep or waking at a different time on different days of the week can upset your sleep rhythm. For example, if you switch to later hours on weekends, you can set your internal clock "forward" and cause trouble when you need to awaken early on Monday. This may be a cause of your sleeping problems.

If your job or social commitments make sleeping regular hours difficult, you may develop sleep problems. Split-shift workers may have a particularly difficult time in this regard. Long distance air travelers are acquainted with the disruption of their circadian clocks known as "jet-lag." If you can possibly readjust your employment or other commitments to permit regularity, you should notice a significant improvement in your sleep problems.

People caring for infants and young children may have similar difficulties in establishing and maintaining a regular sleep cycle and should try to find someone to share some of the late-night duties if possible.

Naps. Sometimes, especially as we grow older, we tend to nap during the day and sleep less at night. As long as you feel well rested, there is nothing wrong with this. If you feel tired during the day and sleep poorly at night, however, you may wish to eliminate naps from your daily routine or set a time to be awakened from your nap, to see if this improves your sleep at night.

Environmental Factors

Do you have a consistently quiet, dark place in which to sleep? Some people can "sleep through anything," but if you have a sleep problem, you may need to adopt special measures to make sure your sleeping place is dark and quiet, at least until you establish a good sleeping pattern.

Examine your surroundings for light and noise. Do you need to cover a window against the glare of a street light or early morning sun? Does a dripping faucet, barking dog, or loud radio or television interrupt your sleep? Does your sleep-partner have habits, such as stealing the covers, tossing or snoring, which make sleeping difficult?

Use any variety of methods to deal with these annoyances. If all else fails, earplugs, the "white noise" of a television set tuned to a non-broadcasting channel, or eyeshades may help.

Good ventilation and a comfortable temperature are also important for good sleep, as is comfortable, loose-fitting bed clothing.

Physical and Mental Factors

Many common physical and mental disorders or problems can interfere with sleep.

Pain is one of the most common causes of sleeplessness. Pain from a headache, an ulcer, a toothache, a muscle ache, arthritis, or any other source may prevent restful sleep. Occasional minor pain may respond to one of the non-prescription pain-killers discussed in the chapter on analgesics. Backache may be helped by a bed board, a firm mattress, or by sleeping on your side, with a bend at your hips and knees.

If your pain is severe, or if it has been troubling you for several days or more, you may need appropriate treatment from a health care professional.

Physical conditions without pain such as enlargement of the prostate or a urinary track infection or inflammation may cause you to awaken at night in order to urinate. Many other physical conditions may cause insomnia, but usually there are other symptoms as well. A health care professional can help you if any of these conditions are interfering with your sleep.

Psychological factors often play a large role in sleeplessness and excessive tiredness. Wide mood swings from overactive "highs" to deep inconsolable "lows" can result in poor sleep, as can depression, discussed earlier. The help of a mental health professional may be necessary to break out of a cycle of sleeplessness. Anxiety caused by worrying about falling asleep often exacerbates and continues insomnia which originally had another cause.

Substances in Foods, Beverages and Drugs

Foods. Many people find that a heavy or highly-spiced meal eaten close to bedtime may cause digestive distress and interfere with sleep. Also there is a caffeine-like stimulant in chocolate that can cause sleep problems.

Beverages containing stimulants. Many common beverages contain stimulant drugs which prevent or disturb sleep. These drugs include caffeine and its chemical relations (xanthines). Caffeine (and these closely related chemicals) may be found in coffee, tea and many soft drinks including both cola and some non-cola drinks. Caffeine and related stimulants interfere with sleep by stimulating the central nervous system.

If you have a sleeping problem, and if you drink beverages containing caffeine and related chemicals, try cutting down on the use of these beverages, especially in the afternoon, evening, or night, or eliminate them entirely. (If you decide to cut them out, do so gradually, perhaps over a period of two or three days, to avoid annoying caffeine withdrawal headaches.)

Alcoholic beverages. Although alcohol is a central nervous system depressant, many people find that it has a disturbing effect on their sleep. While an alcoholic beverage may initially cause drowsiness, the resulting sleep is often disturbed and intermittent.

Some people find drinking a "nightcap" helps them sleep. Others following this practice awaken a short time later and find it difficult to fall asleep again. Alcohol is *not* effective in long- term treatment of insomnia.

Alcoholics and many chronic alcohol users tend to have highly disturbed sleep patterns which can require medical treatment.

Non-prescription medication. Many products sold over the counter may affect sleep. Many products sold for the relief of pain (including ANACIN and EXCEDRIN) contain small amounts of caffeine, the stimulant in coffee. If you wish to use a non-prescription product for pain relief, see the chapter on analgesics, and avoid products containing caffeine.

Products sold as non-prescription appetite suppressants for weight control (such as DEXATRIM) usually contain a stimulant known as phenylpropanolamine (PPA), and often contain caffeine as well. Both of these stimulants can cause sleeplessness. This is one of the many drawbacks of these products. (See pp. 81-82 for more information.)

Certain pills or liquids sold without a prescription for the relief of colds contain both caffeine and/or other ingredients such as phenylpropanolamine, ephedrine, and pseudoephedrine which are included as nasal decongestants. OTC asthma products contain theophylline, ephedrine, epinephrine, or metaproterenol sulfate. All of these ingredients may interfere with sleep.

Prescription medication. Many widely prescribed drugs interfere with sleep. These include medications which contain stimulants, medications which interfere with the quality of sleep and, finally, sedative medications which help you sleep while you use them but result in sleeplessness when you stop.

Prescription drugs stimulating the nervous system include drugs for asthma (such as theophylline and aminophylline), many cough and cold remedies, drugs in the amphetamine family (Benzedrine, Dexedrine, and others) and related families of drugs such as those contained in diet pills (Ionamin, Preludin, and Tenuate, to name a few).

Medications which may interfere with quality of sleep include thyroid preparations (such as Euthroid and Synthroid), monoamine oxidase inhibitors (such as Marplan, Nardil, and Parnate), propranolol (Inderal), and many others.

Medications used to help you sleep can cause sleeplessness after their use is discontinued. This most insidious cause of insomnia can result following use of tranquilizers, anti-anxiety drugs, illicit sleeping pills (illegally distributed tranquilizers and sedatives containing any of a number of ingredients), and tricyclic antidepressants (such as Elavil, Sinequan, and Tofranil).

If you are having a sleeping problem and are using prescription drugs, tell your doctor. It may be possible to change your drug or adjust your dosage. Be sure to let your doctor know *all* the drugs you are taking from any source, including prescription drugs from another doctor and non-prescription OTC ones, so that their total effect upon your sleep may be evaluated.

Recreational drugs. It is not the purpose of this chapter to discuss the many health and legal hazards of these drugs, but rather to alert you to the possibility that they may cause sleep problems.

All so-called "recreational drugs" have the capacity to disturb or prevent sleep. Some, such as amphetamines ("speed") and cocaine, are stimulants and will obviously affect sleep, but any drug which has any sort of mind- or mood-altering effect may easily disturb sleep patterns. Use of marijuana, opiates (heroin, etc.), LSD, PCP, and any other substance should be reconsidered as a possible cause of insomnia.

In addition, nicotine in cigarettes is a stimulant which may affect sleep.

STEP 3: ESTABLISHING PRACTICES WHICH HELP YOU SLEEP
Exercise

Many people find that physical activity, especially out of doors, contributes to better sleep. If you find that such activity is too stimulating when carried out just before bedtime, select an exercise period earlier in the day or evening. Running, swimming, cycling or just brisk walking for at least half an hour a day on a regular basis can improve your sleep.

Relaxation

Sometimes — particularly in periods of high stress — you may become too tense and anxious to permit sleep to occur naturally. There are many excellent relaxation techniques described in books or taught in community centers which may help you.

We do not endorse any one method specifically, and would caution against any "course" sold at a high price, or "technique" making extravagant claims. We would similarily discourage expenditure of great sums of money on commercially marketed programs involving meditation, biofeedback, or similar methods, since their effectiveness in helping poor sleepers has not been conclusively proven.

Deep muscle relaxation and some yoga techniques are useful for some people for general relaxation and can reduce the tension which causes occasional insomnia. Their effectiveness in treating chronic insomnia has yet to be proven in rigorously controlled scientific studies.

Nighttime Routines

Bedtime should be a time for relaxing, enjoyable routines. A quiet, pleasant bedtime period free of arguments or excessive worry about the events of the day, a light snack of simple, bland food, a pleasant book, television show, record or radio broadcast can help induce relaxation and natural sleep. A warm bath may also be used to induce relaxation so you can sleep, but the water should not be too hot, because some people find a hot bath stimulating.

The area in which you sleep should be for sleeping, and not for activities which create undue tension or worry. If you have difficulty sleeping, try to keep work-related material away from your sleeping area, and do not work in bed.

Developing Strategies for Sleepless Nights

Do not try to sleep if you are not sleepy. If you are lying in bed wide awake, get up, read, go to another part of the house, answer mail, or find some other way to occupy your time until you are sleepy. Keeping this schedule will help you to associate your bed with sleep.

Be sure to set your alarm clock for your normal time of awakening, and get up at that time, no matter how little you have slept. While you may feel somewhat tired the next day, it will help you establish a better sleep-wake cycle.

OTC NIGHTTIME SLEEP-AIDS

Although several products sold without a prescription claim to aid sleep, we do not recommend the use of any of them.

These products contain either doxylamine succinate, diphenhydramine hydrochloride or pyrilamine maleate.

In 1978, the FDA published its report on over the counter nighttime sleep-aids. The FDA Commissioner concluded that all of the active ingredients in currently marketed medications lack evidence of safety, effectiveness or both as OTC nighttime sleep-aids. (The same conclusion had been reached by an FDA advisory panel in a report published in 1975.) Although diphenhydramine hydrochloride (in COMPOZ, NYTOL DPH and SOMINEX FOR-

MULA 2, among others) and doxylamine succinate (in UNISOM) have recently undergone a change in legal status so that they may be sold over the counter,* we remain unconvinced of their safety *and* effectiveness as sleep-aids and recommend strongly against their use.

According to the FDA panel, pyrilamine maleate, found in products such as EXCEDRIN P.M., NERVINE, QUIET WORLD and SLEEP-EZE, lacks evidence of safety and effectiveness as a nighttime sleep-aid.[2] Since the FDA advisory panel recommendation was published, many of the OTC sleep-aids containing pyrilamine maleate have been reformulated to use the FDA-sanctioned ingredient, diphenhydramine hydrochloride. To date, COMPOZ, NYTOL, and SOMINEX have been reformulated in this manner. Other OTC sleep aids which contain pyrilamine maleate may do the same. However, this in no way changes our advice against their use.

All of the active ingredients currently marketed as over the counter sleeping medicines are antihistamines. These drugs are primarily used to treat allergic reactions. Drowsiness is one common side effect of antihistamines. In this case, drug manufacturers are making use of this side effect and marketing the drug for this purpose. In addition to drowsiness, however, these drugs also have many other side effects, such as thickening of bronchial secretion, dizziness, excessive dryness of the mouth, nose and throat, blurred vision, stomach or intestinal problems (especially with pyrilamine), mental confusion, loss of appetite, ringing in the ears, and, less commonly, nervousness, insomnia, muscle spasm, tremors, headache, palpitation of the heart, restlessness, or even convulsions. Dizziness, mental confusion and feeling faint are more likely in the elderly. Nervousness, restlessness and insomnia are more likely in children. At higher dosages, the chance of these side effects and of other serious problems increases.

These antihistamines are also hazardous for a large number of people, including those with asthma, glaucoma, or difficulty urinating due to prostate enlargement. Antihistamines can interact dangerously with other drugs, especially other sedatives and depressants, including alcohol and medications for seizures. If taken by a pregnant woman, antihistamines may cause birth defects. Antihistamines also should not be used by mothers who are breast feeding because the drug may pass into the breast milk and cause unwanted effects in the infant.

---

*Doxylamine succinate (in UNISOM) is considered safe and effective as a result of a New Drug Application (an alternative approval process for drugs). The FDA has now found diphenhydramamine safe and effective as an OTC sleep-aid.

One danger in the use of these drugs is that if they fail
there may be a natural temptation to take lar
recommended dosages, resulting in severe adverse
especially when alcohol is taken as well.

Products containing ingredients such as bromides, scopolamine,
and an antihistamine known as methapyrilene are associated with
severe hazards and should no longer be available in over the
counter sleeping pills. *Check all products in your medicine cabinet
and do not use any containing these ingredients.*

Some OTC sleep-aids also contain pain-relievers such as aspirin
or acetaminophen in combination with one of the antihistamines (EXCEDRIN P.M., QUIET WORLD). If you believe
that occasional insomnia may be due to pain which can be treated
successfully with aspirin or acetaminophen, buy a generic brand of
the pain-reliever (without additional ingredients) and leave the
sleeping pills on the drugstore shelf. (See the chapter on analgesics
for more information on aspirin and acetaminophen.)

Several other preparations sold without prescription are claimed
to have sleep inducing properties. These include certain mineral
combinations, herbal preparations and, more recently, a substance
known as l-tryptophan, which is an amino acid (a building block
for protein). While optimistic claims are made for these preparations by their manufacturers and some of the publications in which
they advertise, their safety and efficacy have not been determined
by the FDA.

L-tryptophan. There have been some studies carried out on
l-tryptophan to determine safety and effectiveness, but the results
have been inconclusive and somewhat disappointing. Since
l-tryptophan is not sold as a drug, though, the manufacturer need
not prove conclusively that it is safe or effective. We do not
recommend that you use l-tryptophan to induce sleep.

All in all, there are a large number of products available to aid
the insomniac, but we do not advise the use of any of them. For the
chronic or severe case, none of the over the counter drugs (and in
most cases, none of the prescription ones, either) are appropriate.
For mild and occasional bouts of insomnia, we advise you to avoid
drugs and to try the self-help techniques described earlier in this
chapter. This should save you money and protect your health at the
same time.

OTC DAYTIME SEDATIVES

On June 22, 1979, the FDA published regulations stating that no
ingredients are safe and effective for OTC use as daytime sedatives
for nervousness, tension or irritability. In response, some products
(such as COMPOZ, NERVINE, and QUIET WORLD) were

repackaged and/or reformulated for use as nighttime sleep-aids. No daytime sedatives are currently available over the counter. None are safe and effective.

DOCTORS, INSOMNIA AND PRESCRIPTION SLEEPING PILLS

As we discussed earlier in this chapter, some sleep problems respond to professional help which addresses the underlying conditions which interfere with sleep or helps to establish positive sleep enhancement routines.

Unfortunately, some physicians are not well informed or are unwilling to take the time to address an individual patient's sleep problem. Frequently, such physicians resort almost immediately and exclusively to prescribing sleeping pills.

Many prescription sleeping pills are currently available. Some of the most commonly prescribed pills are members of a family called the benzodiazepines, popularly known as "minor tranquilizers." Drugs in this category include flurazepam (Dalmane), temazepam (Restoril) and, a new member of the group, triazolam (Halcion). Other benzodiazepines such as diazepam (Valium) and chlordiazepoxide (Librium) are often prescribed for people with sleeping problems, although they are not specifically marketed for this use. Other drugs, now less frequently prescribed as sleeping pills, include the barbiturates (Seconal, phenobarbitol, etc.), ethchlorvynol (Placidyl), glutethimide (Doriden), methyprylon (Noludar), methaqualone (Quaalude), and chloral hydrate (Noctec, Somnos).

All of these drugs are addictive.[3] Occasional use can easily become regular use. Discontinuing regular use may cause a return to insomnia (since dependence develops and the underlying problem has not been solved) and the beginning of withdrawal symptoms (withdrawal from benzodiazepines frequently causes anxiety, restlessness, headache, muscle twitching and pain, shaking, and changes in vision).[4, 5] Low doses may not suffice after a few weeks' use, and may result in ever increasing levels of drug use. After using many of these pills (Dalmane, for example), you may build up drug metabolites (active ingredient by-products of the drug) in your body, which over time may cause a slowing of reactions during the day and result in a kind of "hangover."[6] This build-up is intensified in older people. The regular use of sleeping pills, for the same reason, may make older people less alert and lively, and aggravate memory loss and other manifestations of aging.[7] The effects of some of these drugs may even be confused with senility.

Sleeping pills may react harmfully — even fatally — with other prescription drugs, narcotic drugs, and alcohol.

Sleeping pills slow down respiratory function in some individuals. Unfortunately, there may be no way to identify these people in advance. Sleep apnea — the cessation of breathing during sleep — can become life-threatening when sleeping pills are taken by susceptible people.

Sleeping pills pose special hazards for people with certain health problems, including those with kidney or liver disease. In addition, sleeping pills should not be taken by pregnant women.

In conclusion, we do not recommend the use of prescription sleeping preparations as routine or long-term remedies for sleeplessness.

SOURCES

INTRODUCTION

[1] LaBrecque DC. Testimony before the Subcommittee on Monopoly of the Senate Select Committee on Small Business, Dec. 7. 1972. *Advertising of Proprietary Medicines,* part 3, 1972:1003. The product described in this testimony contained additional ingredients.

[2] *American Druggist,* March 1979, page 22.

[3] *Executive Health,* 13, March 1977.

[4] *Advertising Age,* September 9, 1982.

[5] *American Druggist,* February 1983, page 10.

[6] *American Druggist,* September 1982. page 33

[7] *American Druggist,* September 1982

[8] *American Druggist,* February 1983.

[9] *Resident & Staff Physician,* December 1982.

[10] *Pharmacy Times,* January 1983.

PAIN, FEVER AND INFLAMMATION

[1] Consumer expenditure study. *Product Marketing/Cosmetic and Fragrance Retailing.* August 1982:42.

[2] Woods NF, Most A, and Dery GK. Prevalence of perimenstrual symptoms. *Am J Public Health.* 1982; 72:1257-64.

[3] 42 *Federal Register* 35390. July 8, 1977.

[4] *Evaluations of Drug Interactions,* 2nd Ed. Washington DC: American Pharmaceutical Association, 1976; Supplement, 1978.

[5] 42 *Federal Register* 35480. July 8, 1977.

[6] Ibid.

[7] 47 *Federal Register* 22802. May 25, 1982.

[8] 42 *Federal Register* 35412, 35416. July 5, 1977.

[9] 47 *Federal Register* 34636. Aug. 10, 1982.

[10] Beaver WT. Aspirin and acetaminophen as constituents of analgesic combinations. *Arch Intern Med.* 1981; 141:293.

[11] 47 *Federal Register* 55076. Dec. 7, 1982.

[12] 44 *Federal Register* 36378. June 22, 1979.

[13] Korberly BH, Sohn CA, Tannenbaum RP. Menstrual products. In: *Handbook of Nonprescription Drugs.* 7th Ed. Washington DC: American Pharmaceutical Association, 1982:364.

[14] *Advertising Age.* September 9, 1982:164.

[15] Ibid, p. 111.

[16] Ibid, p. 22.

COUGH, COLD, ALLERGY AND ASTHMA

[1] *Wall Street Journal.* January 13, 1983:33.

[2] *Product Marketing.* August 1981:26.

[3] 41 *Federal Register* 38397. September 9, 1976.

[4] West S, et al. A review of antihistamines and the common cold. *Pediatrics.* 1975; 56:100-7.

[5] Howard JC, et al. Effectiveness of antihistamines in the symptomatic management of the common cold. *JAMA.* 1979; 242:2414-7.

[6] *About Your Medicines.* Rockville, MD: United States Pharmacopeial Convention, Inc., 1981.

[7] *Advertising Age.* September 9, 1982:156.

[8] LaBrecque DC. Testimony before the Subcommittee on Monopoly of the Senate Select Committee on Small Business, Dec. 7, 1972. *Advertising of Proprietary Medicines,* part 3, 1972:1033.

[9] *Advertising Age.* September 9, 1982:22.

[10] *Advertising Age.* September 9, 1982:184.

[11] Finiguerra M, Morandini G. Guaifenesin vs. placebo in chronic bronchitis. Unpublished report submitted to the FDA by A.H. Robins Company, September, 1982.

[12] Dec. 22, 1982 letter from William Gilbertson, Director of OTC Drug Evaluation, FDA, to Robert E. Keenan of A.H. Robins Company.

[13] April 20, 1982 letter from William Gilbertson, Director of OTC Drug Evaluation, FDA, to Thomas C. McPherson of Riker Laboratories.

[14] January 29, 1981 letter from William Gilbertson, Director of OTC Drug Evaluation, FDA, to Joseph D. Clark of Warner Lambert Company.

[15] April 22, 1982 letter from William Gilbertson, Director of OTC Drug Evaluation, FDA, to George F. Hoffnagle of Richardson-Vicks, Inc.

[16] 47 *Federal Register* 22779. May 25, 1982.

[17] 47 *Federal Register* 22865. May 25, 1982.

[18] 47 *Federal Register* 22779. May 25, 1982.

[19] 47 *Federal Register* 22911. May 25, 1982.

[20] Final Report, Panel on Review of Allergenic Extracts. Bureau of Biologics, FDA, DHHS, Rockville, MD. PB81-182115. March 13, 1981.

[21] Berkow R, ed. *The Merck Manual,* 14th Ed., Vol. I. Rahway, NJ: Merck Sharpe and Dohme Research Laboratories, 1982:193.

[22] Final Report, Panel on Review of Allergenic Extracts.

[23] 41 *Federal Register* 38380. September 9, 1976.

[24] Ibid.

[25] *Medical Letter.* 1982; 24:83.

LOSING WEIGHT

[1] *Drug Topics.* July 5, 1982:79.

[2] Anderson L, et al. *Nutrition in Health and Disease.* Philadelphia: Lippincott, 1982:467.

[3] Warner R. Wolfe SM, Rich R. *Off Diabetes Pills: A Diabetic's Guide to Long Life.* Washington, DC: Public Citizen's Health Research Group, 1978.

[4] Williams SR. *Nutrition and Diet Therapy.* St. Louis: Mosby, 1981:536.

[5] Friedman RB, et al. What to tell patients about weight-loss methods, 1. Diets. *Postgraduate Medicine.* 1982; 72:73-80.

[6] *Diet, Nutrition and Cancer.* National Academy of Sciences, 1982.

[7] Horowitz JD, et al. Hypertensive responses induced by phenylpropanolamine in anorectic and decongestant preparations. *Lancet.* 1980; 1:60-1.

[8] 47 *Federal Register* 8475. Feb. 26, 1982.

[9] 35 million *adults* alone have definite hypertension (greater than 160/95 or taking medication). From: *The Public and High Blood Pressure,* NIH Publication #81-2118, September 1981.

[10] Personal communication. Diabetes Clearinghouse, DHHS, September 14, 1982.

[11] *Hypertension in Adults, 25-74 yrs of age, USA, 1971-1975.* DHHS, PHS, #81-1671, April 1982.

[12] Pentel PR, Mikell FL, Zavoral JH. Myocardial injury after phenylpropanolamine ingestion. *Br Heart J. 1982; 47:51-4.*

[13] Swenson, RD, *Golper TA, Bennett WM.* Acute renal failure and rhabdomyolysis after ingestion of phenylpropanolamine-containing diet pills. *JAMA.* 1982; 248:1216.

[15] *Drug Exception Reporting System, Jan. 1980-Mar. 1982.* Drug Abuse Warning Network. US National Institute on Drug Abuse, 1982.

[16] Fisher A. *Contact Dermatitis,* 2nd Ed. Philadelphia: Lea and Febiger, 1973:42, 312, and 313.

[17] North American Contact Dermatitis Group. Epidemiology of contact dermatitis in North America: 1972. *Arch of Dermatol.* 1973; 108:537-40.

CONSTIPATION

[1] Davenport H. *Physiology of the Digestive Tract,* 5th Ed. Chicago: Year Book Medical Publishers, 1982:234.

[2] Goldfinger SE. Constipation, diarrhea, and disturbances of anorectal function. In: Isselbacher KJ, et al., eds. *Harrison's Principles of Internal Medicine,* 9th Ed. 1980:199.

[3] Ibid.

[4] Douglas AP. Gastrointestinal disorders. In: Davies DM, ed. *Textbook of Adverse Drug Reactions.* New York: Oxford University Press, 1977:136.

[5] Wood AJ, Oates JA. Adverse reactions to drugs. In: Isselbacher KJ, et al., eds. *Harrison's Principles of Internal Medicine,* 9th Ed. New York: McGraw-Hill, 1980:388.

[6] National Institute on Aging, National Digestive Diseases Educational Information Clearinghouse, Constipation. *Age Page.* U.S. Department of Health and Human Services, September 1982.

[7] *AMA Drug Evaluations,* 3rd Ed. Chicago: American Medical Association, 1977:1071.

[8] Rawson MD. Cathartic colon. *Lancet.* 1966; 1:1121.

[9] Rutter K, Maxwell D. Diseases of the alimentary system: constipation and laxative abuse. *Brit Med J.* 1976; 2:997-1000.

[10] Thompson WG. Laxatives: clinical pharmacology and rational use. *Drugs.* 1980; 19:49-58.

[11] 40 *Federal Register* 12911. March 25, 1975.

[12] Fingl E. Laxatives and cathartics. In: Gilman AG, Goodman LS, Gilman A, eds. *Goodman and Gilman's The Pharmacological Basis of Therapeutic,* 6th Ed. New York: Macmillan, 1980:1009.

[13] Thompson, 1980.

[14] 40 *Federal Register* 12912. March 25, 1975.

[15] 40 *Federal Register* 12911. March 25, 1975.

[16] Pike BF, et al. Soap colitis. *N Engl J Med.* 1971; 285:217-8.

[17] Young JS, et al. Enema shock in Hirschsprung's disease, *Dis of Colon and Rectum.* 1968; 11:391-4.

[18] Turrel R. Laceration to anorectum incident to enema. *Arch of Surgery.* 1960; 81:953.

[19] Meisel JL. et al. Human rectal mucosa: proctoscopic and morphological changes caused by laxatives. *Gastroenterol.* 1977; 72:1274-9.

EXCESS ACID AND GAS

[1] Consumer expenditure study. *Product Marketing/Cosmetic and Fragrance Retailing.* August 1982:38.

[2] McGulgan JE. Peptic ulcer. In: Isselbacher KJ, et al., eds. *Harrison's Principles of Internal Medicine,* 9th Ed. New York: McGraw-Hill, 1980:1373.

[3] 21 *Code of Federal Regulations* 331.30(a).

[4] 47 *Federal Register* 486. January 5, 1982.

[5] Lasser RB, et al. The role of intestinal gas in functional abdominal pain. *N Engl J Med.* 1975; 293:524-6.

[6] Davenport HW. Ethanol damage to canine oxyntic glandular mucosa. *Proc Soc Exp Biol Med.* 1962; 126:657-62.

[7] Gottfried EB, et al. Alcohol-induced gastric and duodenal lesions in man. *Am J Gastroenterol.* 1978; 70:587-92.

[8] Needham CD, et al. Aspirin and alcohol in gastrointestinal hemorrhage. *Gut.* 1971; 12:819-21.

[9] 47 *Federal Register* 43548. October 1, 1982.

[10] Berkowitz JM. Bismuth subsalicylate in excessive alcohol/food intake. FDA Docket No. 82N-0166. OTC Volume 170208: 11-15.

[11] Stead JA, et al. In vitro and in vivo defoaming action of three antacid preparations. *J Pharm Pharmacol* 1978; 30:353-8.

[12] Drake D, Hollander D. Neutralizing capacity and cost effectiveness of antacids. *Ann Intern Med.* 1981; 94:215-7.

[13] Ibid.

[14] Harvey SC. Gastric antacids and digestants. In: Gilman AG, Goodman LS, Gilman A, eds. *Goodman and Gilman's The Pharmocological Basis of Therapeutics,* 6th Ed. New York: Macmillan, 1980:988.

[15] Antacids. *Medical Letter.* 1982; 24:61.

[16] Harvey, 1980:993.

[17] 21 *Code of Federal Regulations* 332.30 (Final rule published in 39 *Federal Register* 19877. June 4, 1974).

[18] 47 *Federal Register* 454-86. January 5, 1982.

DIARRHEA, NAUSEA AND VOMITING

[1] 40 *Federal Register* 12924. March 21, 1975.

[2] Douglas AP. Gastrointestinal disorders. In: Davies DM, ed. *Textbook of Adverse Drug Reactions.* New York: Oxford University Press, 1977: 134.

[3] 40 *Federal Register* 12924. March 21, 1975.

[4] Ibid.

[5] Antidiarrheal product table. *Handbook of Nonprescription Drugs,* 7th Ed. Washington DC: American Pharmaceutical Association, 1982:66-7.

[6] Calcium polycarbophil (Mitrolan). *Medical Letter.* 1981; 23:52.

[7] Dupont HL, et al. Prevention of traveler's diarrhea (emporiatic enteritis). *JAMA.* 1980; 243:237-41.

[8] Dupont, HL, et al. Symptomatic treatment of diarrhea with bismuth subsalicylate among students attending a Mexican University. *Gastroenterol.* 1977; 73:715-8.

[9] August 19,1982,letter from William Gilbertson, Director of OTC Drug Evaluation, FDA, to Sal Mercurio of Norwich-Eaton.

[10] Feldman S, et al. Absorption of salicylate from a bismuth sub-salicylate antidiarrheal preparation (Pepto-Bismol). *Clin Pharmacol Ther.* 1980; 27:252.

[11] Salicylate in Pepto-Bismol. *Medical Letter.* 1980; 22:63.

[12] October 14,1982,letter from William Gilbertson, Director of OTC Drug Evaluation, FDA, to David C. Openheimer of Pfizer Pharmaceuticals.

[13] Ibid.

[14] Douglas, 1977.

[15] 44 *Federal Register* 41068. July 13, 1979.

[16] Reason JT. Motion sickness adaptation: a neural mismatch model. *J R Soc Med*. 1978; 71:819-29.

[17] Jay WM, et al. Visual suppression of motion sickness. *N Engl J Med*. 1980; 302:1091.

[18] Schor EL. Prevention of "car sickness" in children. *N Engl J Med*. 1979; 301:1066.

HEMORRHOIDS

[1] Consumer expenditure study. *Product Marketing/Cosmetic and Fragrance Retailing*. August 1982:40.

[2] Hodes B.. Hemorrhoidal products. *Handbook of Nonprescription Drugs,* 7th Ed. Washington, D.C.: American Pharmaceutical Association, 1982:643.

[3] Plorde JJ. Intestinal nematodes. In: Isselbacher KJ, et al., eds. *Harrison's Principles of Internal Medicine,* 9th Ed. New York: McGraw-Hill, 1980:899.

[4] 47 *Federal Register* 37062. August 24, 1982.

[5] Phone conversation with representative of Pfipharmecs, October 22, 1982.

[6] Steigleder GK, Raab WP. Skin protection affected by ointments. *J Invest Dermatol*. 1962; 38:129.

[7] 45 *Federal Register* 35632, 35635. May 27, 1980.

[8] 45 *Federal Register* 35645. May 27, 1980.

[9] Fisher A. *Contact Dermatitis,* 2d Ed. Philadelphia: Lea and Febiger, 1973:42, 312, and 313.

[10] North American Contact Dermatitis Group. Epidemiology of contact dermatitis in North America: 1972. *Arch Dermatol*. 1973; 108:537-40.

[11] Ritche JM, Cohen PJ. Cocaine, procaine and other synthetic local anesthetics. In: Goodman LS, Gilman A, eds. *Goodman and Gilman's The Pharmacological Basis of Therapeutics,* 5th Ed. New York: Macmillan, 1975:391.

[12] *Advertising Age.* September 9, 1982:22.

[13] Hodes B, 1982:648.

[14] 44 *Federal Register* 69813. December 4, 1979.

[15] 44 *Federal Register* 69822. December 4, 1979.

[16] Lundsgaard-Hansen P. Masking effects of drugs. In: Meyler L, Peck HM, Eds. *Drug-Induced Diseases,* Vol. 4. Amsterdam, 1972:213.

[17] Guin J.D. Complications of topical hydrocortisone. *J Am Acad Dermatol.* 1981; 4:417-22.

[18] LaMont J, Isselbacher JK. Diseases of the Colon and Rectum. In Isselbacher KJ, et al. eds. *Harrison's Principles of Internal Medicine,* 9th Ed. New York: McGraw-Hill, 1980:1436.

SLEEPING PROBLEMS

[1] *Drug Topics.* July 5, 1982:79.

[2] 43 *Federal Register* 25544. June 13, 1978.

[3] Mendelson WB. *The Use and Misuse of Sleeping Pills.* New York: Plenum Medical Books, 1980:127.

[4] Maletzky BM, Klotter J. Addiction to diazepam. *Int J Addictions.* 1976; 11:95-115

[5] Tyrer P. et al., Benzodiazepine withdrawal symptoms and propranolol. *Lancet.* 1981; 1:520-22.

[6] Solomon F, White CC, Parron DL, et al. Sleeping pills, insomnia and medical practice. *N Engl J Med.* 1979; 300:803-8.

[7] Committee on the Review of Medicines. Systematic review of the benzodiazepines. *Br Med J.* 1980; 280:910.

OTHER SOURCES ON SLEEPING PROBLEMS

Further information can be obtained from:

Project Sleep, National Program on Insomnia and Sleep Disorders, Room-17-60, 5600 Fishers Lane, Rockville, MD 20857.

Institute of Medicine. *Sleeping Pills, Insomnia and Medical Practice.* Washington DC: National Academy of Sciences, 1979.

Bargmann E, Wolfe SM, Levin J. *Stopping Valium (and Ativan, Centrax, Dalmane, Librium, Paxipam, Restoril, Serax, Tranxene, Xanax).* Washington DC: Public Citizen's Health Research Group, 1982. (A book on the use of benzodiazepines available in bookstores or directly from the Health Research Group.)

PART II:
INGREDIENTS INDEX, BRAND NAME INDEX, GLOSSARY, HOW THIS BOOK WAS COMPILED AND HISTORY OF OTC REVIEW

INGREDIENTS INDEX

The following table represents the current status of ingredients in the FDA's ongoing OTC Drug Review. Each ingredient and use is followed by an evaluation published in the *Federal Register,* and made by an FDA Advisory Panel or the agency itself. If the most recent *Federal Register* notice indicates that an ingredient-use is "generally recognized as safe and effective," this is noted by "yes"; otherwise it is noted by "no."

Most of these designations are based on reports of the FDA Advisory Panels which will be re-evaluated by the FDA at some future date and, therefore, are subject to change. However, in the past, the FDA has agreed with the findings of its OTC Review Advisory Panels a very high percentage of the time.

At the time of publication, this current list was not available in a single place. This table was compiled using a printout from the FDA dated November 13, 1980, and updated by combing numerous *Federal Register* notices published since that date. The list is as accurate as possible given the number of separate notices which it was necessary to review, and includes changes through December 31, 1982.

INGREDIENT	USE	SAFE AND EFFECTIVE
Acetaminophen	Sedative	No
Acetaminophen (with Antacid and/or Caffeine)	Hangover	Yes
Acetaminophen	(Internal) Analgesic	Yes
Acetaminophen	Antipyretic	Yes
Acetaminophen	Antirheumatic	No
Acetaminophen	Premenstrual Tension, Menstrual Pain	Yes
Acetaminophen	Sleep Aid	No
Acetaminophen	Fever Blisters	No
Acetanilid	(Internal) Analgesic	No
Acetanilid	Antipyretic	No
Acetanilid	Antirheumatic	No
Acetic Acid	Alters Vaginal PH	No
Acetic Acid, Glacial	Wart Remover	No
Acetic Acid, Glacial	Corn and Callus Remover	No
Acetone	Astringent (External)	No
Acidulated Phosphate Fluoride	Anticavity Dental Rinse	Yes
Agar	Bulk Laxative	No
Alcloxa	Antifungal (Skin)	No
Alcloxa	Acne	No
Alcloxa	(Anorectal) Keratolytic (External)	Yes
Alcohol	Acute Toxic Ingestion	No
Alcohol	(Skin) Antiseptic (60-95% V/V)	Yes
Alcohol	Weight Control	No
Alcohol	Smoking Deterrent	No
Alcohol	Astringent (External)	No
Alcohol	Insect Bite Neutralizer	No

177

INGREDIENT	USE	SAFE AND EFFECTIVE?
Alcohol	IPPUAD	No
Alfalfa	Weight Control	No
Alfalfa Leaves	Premenstrual Tension, Menstrual Pain	No
Alginic Acid	Antacid	No
Alginic Acid	Anorectic (Bulk)	No
Alkaloids of Sabadilla	Pediculicide	No
Alkyl Aryl Sulfonate	Lowers Surface Tension and Produces Mucolytic Effects (Vaginal)	No
Alkyl Isoquinolinium Bromide	Acne	No
Alkyl Isoquinolinium Bromide	Dandruff	No
Allantoin	Corn and Callus Remover	No
Allantoin	Wound-Healing Agent (Skin)	No
Allantoin	Sunscreen (Combined with Aminobenzoic Acid)	No
Allantoin	Skin Protectant	Yes
Allantoin	Dandruff, Seborrheic Dermatitis, Psoriasis	No
Allantoin	Minor Irritations (Vaginal)	No
Allyl Isothiocyanate	Nasal Decongenstant (Topical Inhalant)	No
Allyl Isothiocyanate	Counterirritant	Yes
Almadrate	Antacid	Yes
Almadrate Sulfate	IPPUAD	No
Aloe	Stimulant Laxative	Yes
Aloes	Premenstrual Tension, Menstrual Pain	No
Aloe Vera Stabilized	Minor Irritations (Vaginal)	No
Aloe Vera	Minor Burn, Cut, and Abrasion	No
Aloin	Stimulant Laxative	No
Aloin	Smoking Deterrent	No
Alum	Astringent (Oral)	Yes
Alum	Astringent (Vaginal)	No
Alum	Astringent (External)	No
Alumina Powder, Hydrated	Antidiarrheal	No
Aluminum Acetate	Wet Dressing, Astringent (External)	Yes
Aluminum Bromohydrate	Antiperspirant	No
Aluminum Carbonate	Antacid	Yes
Aluminum Carbonate	Hyperphosphatemia	No
Aluminum Chlorhydroxy Complex	Astringent (External)	No
Aluminum Chloride	Antiperspirant (Alcoholic Solutions)	No
Aluminum Chloride	Antiperspirant (Aerosol) (15 percent or less aqueous solution)	No

178

INGREDIENT	USE	SAFE AND EFFECTIVE
Aluminum Chloride	Antiperspirant (Nonaerosol) (15 percent or less aqueous solution)	Yes
Aluminum Chlorohydrate	Antiperspirant (Aerosol)	Yes
Aluminum Chlorohydrate	Antiperspirant (Nonaerosol)	Yes
Aluminum Chlorohydrex	Acne	No
Aluminum Chlorohydrex Polyethylene Glycol Complex	Antiperspirant (Aerosol)	No
Aluminum Chlorohydrex Polyethylene Glycol Complex	Antiperspirant (Nonaerosol)	Yes
Aluminum Chlorohydrex Propylene Glycol Complex	Antiperspirant (Aerosol)	No
Aluminum Chlorohydrex Propylene Glycol Complex	Antiperspirant (Nonaerosol)	Yes
Aluminum Dichlorohydrate Propylene Glycol Complex	Antiperspirant (Aerosol)	No
Aluminum Dichlorohydrate Propylene Glycol Complex	Antiperspirant (Nonaerosol)	Yes
Aluminum Dichlorohydrex Polyethylene Glycol Complex	Antiperspirant (Aerosol)	No
Aluminum Dichlorohydrex Polyethylene Glycol Complex	Antiperspirant (Nonaerosol)	Yes
Aluminum Dichlorohydrexpropylene Glycol Complex	Antiperspirant (Aerosol)	No
Aluminum Dichlorohydrexpropylene Glycol Complex	Antiperspirant (Nonaerosol)	Yes
Aluminum Hydroxide	Antacid	Yes
Aluminum Hydroxide	Acne	No
Aluminum Hydroxide	(Anorectal) Protectant (External)	Yes
Aluminum Hydroxide	Protectant (Intrarectal)	Yes
Aluminum Hydroxide	IPPUAD	No
Aluminum Hydroxide	Hangover	Yes
Aluminum Hydroxide	Intestinal Distress	No
Aluminum Hydroxide	Skin Protectant	Yes
Aluminum Hydroxide	Smoking Deterrent	No
Aluminum Hydroxide Gel Dried	Analgesic Adjuvant (Antacid or Buffering)	Yes
Aluminum Hydroxide-Hexitol Stabilized Polymer	Antacid	Yes
Aluminum Hydroxide-Magnesium Trisilicate Co-Dried Gel	Antacid	Yes
Aluminum Hydroxide -Magnesium Carbonate, Co-Dried Gel	Antacid	Yes
Aluminum Hydroxide-Sucrose Powder Hydrated	Antacid	Yes
Aluminum Oxide	Acne	No
Alumnium Phosphate (Gel)	Antacid	Yes
Aluminum Phosphate (Gel)	Hypophosphatemia	No
Aluminum Sesquichlorohydrate	Antiperspirant (Aerosol)	No

INGREDIENT	USE	SAFE AND EFFECTIVE ❓
Aluminum Sesquichlorohydrate	Antiperspirant (Nonaerosol)	Yes
Aluminum Sesquichlorohydrate Polyethylene Glycol Complex	Antiperspirant (Aerosol)	No
Aluminum Sesquichlorohydrate Propylene Glycol Complex	Antiperspirant (Aerosol)	No
Aluminium Sesquichchlorohydrate Propylene Glycol Complex	Antiperspirant (Nonaerosol)	Yes
Aluminum Sulfate	Antifungal	No
Aluminum Sulfate	Antiperspirant	No
Aluminum Sulfate	Astringent, as Styptic Pencil	Yes
Aluminum Sulphate Buffered	Antiperspirant (Aerosol)	No
Aluminum Sulphate Buffered	Antiperspirant (Nonaerosol)	Yes
Aluminum Zirconium Pentachlorohydrate	Antiperspirant (Aerosol)	No
Aluminum Zirconium Pentachlorohydrate	Antiperspirant (Nonaerosol)	Yes
Aluminum Zirconium Octachlorohydrate	Antiperspirant (Aerosol)	No
Aluminum Zirconium Octachlorohydrate	Antiperspirant (Nonaerosol)	Yes
Aluminum Zirconium Octachlorohydrex Glycine Complex	Antiperspirant (Aerosol)	No
Aluminum Zirconium Octachlorohydrex Glycine Complex	Antiperspirant (Nonaerosol)	Yes
Aluminum Zirconium Octachlorohydrate Glycine Complex	Antiperspirant (Nonaerosol)	Yes
Aluminum Zirconium Pentachlorohydrex Glycine Complex	Antiperspirant (Aerosol)	No
Aluminum Zirconium Pentachlorohydrex Glycine Complex	Antiperspirant (Nonaerosol)	Yes
Aluminum Zirconium Trichlorohydrate	Antiperspirant (Aerosol)	No
Aluminum Zirconium Trichlorohydrate	Antiperspirant (Nonaerosol)	Yes
Aluminum Zirconium Trichlorohydrex Glycine Complex	Antiperspirant (Aerosol)	No
Aluminum Zirconium Trichlorohydrex Glycine Complex	Antiperspirant (Nonaerosol)	Yes
Amino Acids	Hair Grower	No
Aminoacetic Acid	Antacid	Yes
Aminoacetic Acid	Antidiarrheal	No
Aminoacetic Acid	Anitemetic	No
Aminoacetic Acid	Analgesic Adjuvant (Antacid or Buffering)	Yes
Aminoacridine Hyrochloride	Boil	No

INGREDIENT	USE	SAFE AND EFFECTIVE ❓
Aminobenzoic Acid	Analgesic Adjuvant	No
Aminobenzoic Acid	Antipyretic Adjuvant	No
Aminobenzoic Acid	Antirheumatic Adjuvant	No
Aminobenzoic Acid	Sunscreen	Yes
Aminophylline	Bronchodilator	No
Ammonia Water Stronger	Counterirritant (Skin)	Yes
Ammoniated Mercury	Skin Bleaching Agent	No
Ammonium Bromide	Sedative	No
Ammonium Bromide	Sleep-Aid	No
Ammonium Chloride	Expectorant	No
Ammonium Chloride	Diuretic For Premenstrual And Menstrual Period	Yes
Ammonium Chloride	Expectorant	No
Ammonium Chloride	Smoking Deterrent	No
Ammonium Chloride	Stimulant	No
Ammonium Hydroxide	Insect Bite Neutralizer	No
Amylase	Intestinal Distress	No
Amyl Salicylate	Foot Preparation	No
Amyltricresol, Secondary	Antimicrobial (Oral)	No
Amyltricresol, Secondary	Antifungal	No
Anise Oil	Weight Control	No
Anise Seed	IPPUAD	No
Antimony Potassium Tartrate	Expectorant	No
Antipyrine	(Internal) Analgesic	No
Antipyrine	Antipyretic	No
Antipyrine	Antirheumatic	No
Antipyrine	(Eye) Anesthetic, Analgesic	No
Antipyrine	Otic Analgesic	No
Aqua Ammonia	Insect Bite Neutralizer	No
Arginine	Weight Control	No
Aromatic Powder	IPPUAD	No
Aromatics	Astringent (External)	No
Asafetida	IPPUAD	No
Asclepias Tuberosa	Menstrual Cramps	No
Ascorbic Acid	Weight Control	No
Ascorbic Acid	Treatment of "Common Cold"	No
Ascorbic Acid	Hair Grower	No
Ascorbic Acid	Hair Remover	No
Ascorbic Acid	Corn and Callus Remover	No
Ascorbic Acid	Wart Remover	No
Asparagus	Premenstrual Tension Menstrual Pain	No
Aspergillis Oryza Enzymes	Intestinal Distress	No
Aspirin	Sedative	No

181

INGREDIENT	USE	SAFE AND EFFECTIVE ∎
Aspirin	Analgesic, Anesthetic Antipruritic (Skin)	No
Aspirin (With Antacid)	Hangover	Yes
Aspirin	(Internal) Analgesic	Yes
Aspirin	Antipyretic	Yes
Aspirin	Antirheumatic	Yes
Aspirin	Analgesic (With Buffering)	Yes
Aspirin	Premenstrual Tension Menstrual Pain	Yes
Aspirin	Sleep-Aid	No
Aspirin	Anesthetic, Analgesic (Oral)	Yes
Atropine	(Anorectal) Anticholinergic (External)	No
Atropine	Anticholinergic (Intrarectal)	No
Atropine Sulfate	Antidiarrheal	No
Atropine Sulfate	Anticholinergic	No
Attapulgite Activated	Antacid	No
Attapulgite Activated	Antidiarrheal	No*
Bacillus Acidophilus	Intestinal Distress	No
Bacitracin	Skin First Aid Antibiotic	Yes
Bacitracin Zinc	Skin First Aid Antibiotic	Yes
Basic Fuchsin	Antifungal	No
Bean	IPUUAD	No
Bearberry	Diuretic	No
Beeswax	Toothache-Relief Agent	No
Belladonna Alkaloids	IPPUAD	No
Belladonna Alkaloids	Anticholinergic	No
Belladonna Alkaloids	Corn and Callus Remover	No
Belladonna Alkaloids	Bronchodilator (Inhalation)	No
Belladonna Alkaloids	Foot Preparation	No
Belladonna Extract	(Anorectal) Anticholinergic (External)	No
Belladonna Extract	Anticholinergic (Intrarectal)	No
Belladonna Leaves, Extract of	Smoking Deterrent	No
Belladonna Leaves, Extract of	IPPUAD	No
Benzalkonium Chloride	Dandruff	No
Benzalkonium Chloride	Surgical Hand Scrub	No
Benzalkonium Chloride	Skin Wound Cleanser	Yes
Benzalkonium Chloride	Skin Antiseptic	No
Benzalkonium Chloride	Health Care Personnel Handwash	No
Benzalkonium Chloride	Skin Wound Protectant	No

*Attapulgite. Athough no change has been published in the *Federal Register,* the FDA appears to have started the process of reclassifying this ingredient as a safe and effective anti-diarrheal ingredient. However, we do not recommend that you use it. See p. 126.

INGREDIENT	USE	SAFE AND EFFECTIVE **?**
Benzalkonium Chloride	Patient Preop. Skin Prep.	No
Benzalkonium Chloride	Insect Bite Neutralizer	No
Benzalkonium Chloride	Antimicrobial (Oral)	No
Benzalkonium Chloride	Minor Irritations (Vaginal)	No
Benzalkonium Chloride	Astringent (External)	No
Benzethonium Chloride	Antimicrobial Soap	No
Benzethonium Chloride	Antifungal	No
Benzethonium Chloride	Surgical Hand Scrub	No
Benzethonium Chloride	Skin Wound Cleanser	Yes
Benzethonium Chloride	Skin Antiseptic	No
Benzethonium Chloride	Dandruff, Cradle Cap	No
Benzethonium Chloride	Health Care Personnel Handwash	No
Benzethonium Chloride	Skin Wound Protectant	No
Benzethonium Chloride	Patient Preop. Skin Prep.	No
Benzethonium Chloride	Antimicrobial (Oral)	No
Benzethonium Chloride	Minor Irritations (Vaginal)	No
Benzethonium Chloride	Astringent (External)	No
Benzocaine	Anesthetic Combined With An Antifungal Agent	No
Benzocaine	Smoking Deterrent	No
Benzocaine	Acne	No
Benzocaine	(Anorectal) Anesthetic (External) (In Polyethylene Glycol Ointment)	Yes
Benzocaine	Anesthetic (Intrarectal) (In Polyethylene Glycol Ointment)	No
Benzocaine	Analgesic, Anesthetic, Antipruritic (Skin)	Yes
Benzocaine	Male Genital Desensitizer	Yes
Benzocaine	Anesthetic, Analgesic (Oral)	Yes
Benzocaine	Oral Mucosal Analgesic	Yes
Benzocaine	Toothache-Relief Agent	No
Benzocaine	Otic Analgesic	No
Benzocaine	Poison Oak and Ivy (Greater Than 5%)	No
Benzocaine	Minor Irritations (Vaginal)	No
Benzocaine	Pediculicide	No
Benzocaine	Anorectic, Anesthetic (In Gum, Lozenge, or Candy)	Yes
Benzocaine	Wart Remover	No
Benzocaine	Boil	No
Benzocaine	Psoriasis	No
Benzocaine	Astringent (External)	No
Benzoic Acid	Antifungal	No
Benzoic Acid	Acne	No
Benzoic Acid	Foot Preparation	No

INGREDIENT	USE	SAFE AND EFFECTIVE ?
Benzoic Acid	Kidney and Bladder Irritation	—
Benzoic Acid	Antimicrobial (Oral)	No
Benzoic Acid	Hair Grower	No
Benzoic Acid	Astringent (External)	No
Benzoin Tincture, Compound	Expectorant	No
Benzoin Tincture, Compound	Expectorant (Inhalant)	No
Benzoin Tincture, Compound	Oral Mucosal Protectant	Yes
Benzoxiquine	Antifungal	No
Benzoyl Peroxide	Acne	Yes
Benzyl Alcohol	(Anorectal) Anesthetic (External)	No
Benzyl Alcohol	Skin Antimicrobial	No
Benzyl Alcohol	Anesthetic (Intrarectal)	No
Benzyl Alcohol	Antiseptic	No
Benzyl Alcohol	Analgesic, Anesthetic Antipruritic (Skin)	Yes
Benzyl Alcohol	Pediculicide	No
Benzyl Alcohol	Anesthetic, Analgesic	Yes
Benzyl Alcohol	Toothache-Relief Agent	No
Benzyl Alcohol	Oral Mucosal Analgesic	No
Benzyl Benzoate	Pediculicide	No
Betaine Hydrochloride	Hydrochlorhydria, Achlorhydria	No
Betaine Hydrochloride	Intestinal Distress	No
Bile Salts	Stimulant Laxative	No
Biotin	Weight Control	No
Birch	Diuretic	—
Bisacodyl	Stimulant Laxative	Yes
Bismuth Aluminate	Antacid	Yes
Bismuth Carbonate	Antacid	Yes
Bismuth Oxide	(Anorectal) Protectant (External)	No
Bismuth Oxide	Protectant (Intrarectal)	No
Bismuth Sodium Tartrate	Intestinal Distress	No
Bismuth Subcarbonate	Antacid	Yes
Bismuth Subcarbonate	(Anorectal) Protectant (External)	No
Bismuth Subcarbonate	Protectant (Intrarectal)	No
Bismuth Subcarbonate	IPPUAD	No
Bismuth Subgallate	Antacid	Yes
Bismuth Subgallate	Protectant (External)	—
Bismuth Subgallate	Protectant (Intrarectal)	No
Bismuth Subgallate	IPPUAD	No
Bismuth Subgallate	Ostomy Odor	No
Bismuth Subnitrate	Antacid	Yes
Bismuth Subnitrate	Antidiarrheal	No
Bismuth Subnitrate	Protectant (External)	No

INGREDIENT	USE	SAFE AND EFFECTIVE ?
Bismuth Subnitrate	Protectant (Intrarectal)	No
Bismuth Subnitrate	Boil	No
Bismuth Subnitrate	Skin Protectant	No
Bismuth Subsalicylate	Antidiarrheal	No*
Bismuth Subsalicylate	Overindulgence in Alcohol and Food	Yes
Bismuth Subsalicylate	Antiemetic	No
Black Radish Powder	Intestinal Distress	No
Blessed Thistle	Intestinal Distress	No
Blue Century	Diuretic	—
Boldo	Appetite Stimulant	—
Bone-Marrow Red-Glycerin Extract	Weight Control	No
Borate Preparations	Dandruff, Seborrheic Dermatitis	No
Borax	Astringent (External)	No
Boric Acid	Antifungal	No
Boric Acid	Acne	No
Boric Acid	(Anorectal) Antiseptic (External)	No
Boric Acid	Antiseptic (Intrarectal)	No
Boric Acid	Antimicrobial (Oral)	No
Boric Acid	Anti-Infective (Eye)	No
Boric Acid	Skin Protectant	No
Boric Acid	Skin Healing	No
Boric Acid	Alters Vaginal PH (Greater Than 1% Boron)	No
Boric Acid	Lowers Surface Tension and Produces Mucolytic Effects (Vaginal) (Greater Than 1% Boron)	No
Boric Acid	Minor Irritations (Vaginal) (Greater Than 1% Boron)	No
Boric Acid	Astringent (Vaginal) (Greater Than 1% Boron)	No
Boric Acid	Astringent (External)	No
Bornyl Acetate	Nasal Decongestant (Topical/Inhalant)	No
Boroglycerin	Antiseptic (External)	No
Boroglycerin	Antiseptic (Intrarectal)	No
Boroglycerin	Alters Vaginal PH (Greater Than 1% Boron)	No
Boroglycerin	Lowers Surface Tension and Produces Mucolytic Effects (Greater Than 1% Boron)	No
Boroglycerin	Astingent (Vaginal) (Greater Than 1% Boron)	No

*Bismuth subsalicylate. Although no change has been published in the *Federal Register,* the FDA appears to have started the process of reclassifying this ingredient as a safe and effective antidiarrheal ingredient. We do not recommend that you use it. See p. 125.

INGREDIENT	USE	SAFE AND EFFECTIVE ❓
Boroglycerin Glycerite	Antimicrobial (Oral)	No
Bran Tablets	Bulk Laxative	No
Bran Dietary	Bulk Laxative	Yes
Brompheniramine Maleate	Antihistamine	Yes
Buchu	Weight Control	No
Buchu, Potassium Extract	Weight Control	No
Buckthorn	Intestinal Distress	No
Buffered Resin of Cation and Anion Exchange Resins	Prevention of Poison Ivy Dermatitis	No
Butaben Picrate	Analgesic, Anesthetic, Antipruritic (Skin)	Yes
Butacaine Sulfate	Oral Mucosal Analgesic	Yes
Butacaine Sulfate	Toothache-Relief Agent	No
Para-Tertiary-Butyl-Meta-Cresol	Astringent (External)	No
Caffeine	Stimulant Corrective	No
Caffeine	Diuretic for Premenstrual and Menstrual Periods	Yes
Caffeine	Analgesic Adjuvant	No
Caffeine	Antipyretic Adjuvant	No
Caffeine	Antirheumatic Adjuvant	No
Caffeine	Premenstrual Tension, Menstrual Pain	No
Caffeine	Stimulant	Yes
Caffeine	Fever Blisters	No
Caffeine	Hangover Due to Over-Indulgence In Alcohol	Yes
Caffeine, Citrated	Analgesic Adjuvant	No
Caffeine, Citrated	Antipyretic Adjuvant	No
Caffein, Citrated	Antirheumatic Adjuvant	No
Calamine	Astringent (Anorectal)	Yes
Calamine	(Anorectal) Protectant (External)	Yes
Calamine	Protectant (Intrarectal)	Yes
Calamine	Skin Protectant	Yes
Calamine	Insect Bite Neutralizer	No
Calcium	Weight Control	No
Calcium Acetate	Foot Preparation	No
Calcium Acetate	Astringent (External)	No
Calcium Carbaspirin	(Internal) Analgesic	Yes
Calcium Carbaspirin	Premenstrual Tension Menstrual Pain	Yes
Calcium Carbaspirin	Antipyretic	Yes
Calicum Carbaspirin	Antirheumatic	Yes
Calcium Carbonate	Weight Control	No
Calcium Carbonate, Precipitated	Antidiarrheal	No
Calcium Carbonate, Precipitated	IPPUAD	No

INGREDIENT	USE	SAFE AND EFFECTIVE ?
Calcium Carbonate, Precipitated	Corrective (Antacid or Buffering)	Yes
Calcium Caseinate	No	
Caffeine, Citrated	Analgesic Adjuvant	No
Caffeine, Citrated	Antipyretic Adjuvant	No
Caffein, Citrated	Antirheumatic Adjuvant	No
Calamine	Astingent (Anorectal)	Yes
Calamine	(Anorectal) Protectant (External)	Yes
Calamine	Protectant (Intrarectal)	Yes
Calamine	Skin Protectant	Yes
Calamine	Insect Bite Neutralizer	No
Calcium	Weight Control	No
Calcium Acetate	Foot Preparation	No
Calcium Acetate	Astringent (External)	No
Calcium Carbaspirin	(Internal) Analgesic	Yes
Calcium Carbaspirin	Premenstrual Tension Menstrual Pain	Yes
Calcium Carbaspirin	Antipyretic	Yes
Calicum Carbaspirin	Antirheumatic	Yes
Calcium Carbonate	Weight Control	No
Calcium Carbonate, Precipitated	Antacid	Yes
Calcium Carbonate, Precipitated	Antidiarrheal	No
Calcium Carbonate, Precipitated	IPPUAD	No
Calcium Carbonate, Precipitated	Corrective (Antacid or Buffering)	Yes
Calcium Caseinate	Weight Control	No
Calcium Chloride	Replacement of Minerals Lost in Diarrhea	—
Calcium Gluconate	Intestinal Distress	No
Calcium Hydroxide	Antidiarrheal	No
Calcium Iodide Anhydrous	Expectorant	No
Calcium Lactate	Premenstrual Tension Menstrual Pain	No
Calcium Lactate	Weight Control	No
Calcium Pantothenate	Wart Remover	No
Calcium Pantothenate	Premenstrual Tension Menstrual Pain	No
Calcium Pantothenate	Weight Control	No
Calcium Phosphate	Antacid	Yes
Calcium Phosphate Dibasic	Corrective (Antacid or Buffering)	Yes
Calcium Polysulfide	Acne	No
Calcium Propionate	Minor Irritations (Vaginal)	Yes
Calcium Sucrose Phosphate	Anticavity Agent	No
Calcium Thiosulfate	Acne	No
Calcium Undecylenate	Antifungal	Yes
Calomel	Stimulant Laxative	No

INGREDIENT	USE	SAFE AND EFFECTIVE ❓
Calomel	Topical Antimicrobial	No
Camphor	Antifungal	No
Camphor	Acne	No
Camphor	(Anorectal) Counterirritant (External)	No
Camphor	Expectorant (Topical/Inhalant)	No
Camphor	Nasal Decongestant (Topical/Inhalant)	No
Camphor	Expectorant (Lozenge)	No
Camphor	Antitussive (Topical/Chest Rub)	No*
Camphor	Antitussive (Inhalant Room Spray)	No
Camphor	Nasal Decongestant (Lozenge)	No
Camphor	External (Greater Than 2.5%)	No
Camphor	Counterirritant (3% to 11%)	Yes
Camphor	Analgesic, Anesthetic, Antipruritic (0.1% to 3%)	Yes
Camphor	Insect Bite Neutralizer	No
Camphor	Antimicrobial (Oral)	No
Camphor	Anesthetic, Analgesic (Oral)	No
Camphor	Oral Mucosal Analgesic	No
Camphor	Boil	No
Camphor	Wart Remover	No
Camphor (Gum)	Astringent (External)	No
Camphor Gum	Foot Preparation (Skin)	No
Camphorated Metacresol	Analgesic, Anesthetic Antipruritic (Skin)	No**
Camphorated Oil	Withdrawn From All Sale and Use	No
Candictoin	External Feminine Itching	No
Cantharides	Aphrodisiac	No
Capsaicin	Counterirritant	Yes
Capsicum	IPPUAD	No
Capsicum Fluid Extract of	IPPUAD	No
Capsicum Oleoresin	Counterirritant	Yes
Capsicum	Counterirritant	Yes
Capsicum	Toothache-Relief Agent	No

*Camphor. Although no change has been published in the *Federal Register,* the FDA appears to have started the process of reclassifying this ingredient as a safe and effective anititussive, when used as a chest rub. However, we do not recommend that you use it. See p. 53.

**Camphorated metacresol. Although no change has been published in the *Federal Register,* the FDA appears to have started the process of reclassifying this ingredient as a safe and effective skin analgesic, anesthetic, and antipruritic.

INGREDIENT	USE	SAFE AND EFFECTIVE **?**
Capsicum	Smoking Deterrent	No
Captan	Dandruff	No
Caramiphen Edisylate	Antitussive	No
Carbamide Peroxide	Antimicrobial (Oral)	No
Carbamide Peroxide	Debriding Agent (Oral)	Yes
Carbamide Peroxide in Anhydrous Glycerin	Wound Cleanser (Oral Injury)	Yes
Carbamide Peroxide in Anhydrous Glycerin	Ear Wax Softening Agent	Yes
Carbetapentane Citrate	Antitussive	No
Carbon	IPPUAD	No
Carboxymethylcellulose Sodium	Antidiarrheal	No
Carboxymethylcellulose Sodium	Bulk Laxative	Yes
Carboxymethylcellulose Sodium	Demulcent (Eye)	Yes
Carboxymethylcellulose Sodium	Anorectic (Bulk)	No
Carboxymethylcellulose	Antacid	No
Carrageenan	Anorectic (Bulk)	No
Carrageenan (Degraded)	Stimulant Laxative	No
Carrageenan (Native)	Bulk Laxative	No
Casanthranol	Stimulant Laxative	Yes
Cascara Fluid Extract Aromatic	Stimulant Laxative	Yes
Cascara Sagrada Bark	Stimulant Laxative	Yes
Cascara Sagrada Extract	Stimulant Laxative	Yes
Cascara Sagrada Extract	IPPUAD	No
Cascara Sagrada Extract	Smoking Deterrent	No
Cascara Sagrada Fluid Extract	Stimulent Laxative	Yes
Castor Oil	Stimulent Laxative	Yes
Castor Oil	Emollient (Skin)	No
Castor Oil	Wart Remover	No
Catechu Tincture	Intestinal Distress	No
Catechu Tincture	IPPUAD	No
Catnip	IPPUAD	No
Cedar Leaf Oil	Nasal Decongestant (Topical)	No
Cellulase	Intestinal Distress	No
Cellulase	IPPUAD	No
Cetalkonium Chloride	Antimicrobial (Oral)	No
Cetyl Alcohol	Chafing and Chapping	No
Cetylpyridinium Chloride	Antimicrobial (Oral)	No
Chamomile Flowers	IPPUAD	No
Charcoal, Activated	Antacid	No
Charcoal, Activated	Antidiarrheal	No
Charcoal, Activated	Adsorbent (For Acute Toxic Ingestion)	Yes
Charcoal, Activated	IPPUAD	No

INGREDIENT	USE	SAFE AND EFFECTIVE ?
Charcoal, Activated	Intestinal Distress	No
Charcoal, Activated	Ostomy Odor	No
Charcoal, Activated	Minimize Hangover	No
Charcoal, Wood	Intestinal Distress	No
Chlophedianol Hydrochloride	Antitussive	•
Chloral Hydrate	Counterirritant	No
Chloral Hydrate	Analgesic, Anesthetic Antipruritic (Skin)	No
Chlorhydroxyquinoline	Acne	No
Chlorobutanol	Analgesic, Anesthetic, Antipruritic (Skin)	No
Chlorobutanol	Skin Antimicrobial	No
Chlorobutanol	Corn and Callus Remover	No
Chloroform	Expectorant	No
Chlorophyll	IPPUAD	No
Chlorophyll	Antimicrobial (Oral)	No
Chlorophyllins	Wound-Healing Agent (Skin)	No
Chlorophyllins	Smoking Deterrent	No
Chlorophyllins, Water-Soluble	Wound Healing Agent (Oral Injury)	No
Chlorophyllins, Water-Soluble	Ostomy Odor, Urinary and Fecal Incontinence	No
Chlorothymol	Antifungal	No
Chloroxylenol	Antifungal	No
Chloroxylenol	Acne	No
Chloroxylenol	Antimicrobial Soap	No
Chloroxylenol	Surgical Hand Scrub	No
Chloroxylenol	Skin Wound Cleanser	No
Chloroxylenol	Skin Antiseptic	No
Chloroxylenol	Health Care Personnel Handwash	No
Chloroxylenol	Skin Wound Protectant	No
Chloroxylenol	Patient Preop. Skin Prep.	No
Chloroxylenol	Foot Preparation	No
Chlorpheniramine Maleate	Antihistamine	Yes
Chlorpheniramine Maleate	Fever Blisters	No
Chlorprophenpyridamine Maleate	Menstrual Pain	No
Chlortetracycline Hydrochloride	Skin First Aid Antibiotic	Yes
Cholesterol	Boil	No
Choline	Weight Control	No
Choline Salicylate	(Internal) Analgesic	Yes
Choline Salicylate	Antirheumatic	Yes

*Chlophedianol hydrochloride. Although this drug was not reviewed by the FDA Panel and no change has been published in the *Federal Register*, the FDA appears to have started the process of reclassifying this prescription-only ingredient as a safe and effective OTC antitussive ingredient. See p. 53.

INGREDIENT	USE	SAFE AND EFFECTIVE ?
Choline Salicylate	Antipyretic	Yes
Choline Salicylate	Premenstrual Tension Menstrual Pain	Yes
Chondrus	Anorectic (Bulk)	No
Cimicifuga	Smoking Deterrent	No
Cimicifuga Racemosa	Menstrual Cramps	No
Cinnamedrine Hydrochloride	Premenstrual Tension/Menstrual Pain — Smooth Muscle Relaxant	No
Cinnamon Oil	Intestinal Distress	No
Cinnamon Oil	IPPUAD	No
Cinnamon Tincture	IPPUAD	No
Cinoxate	Sunscreen	Yes
Citric Acid	Antacid	Yes
Citric Acid	IPPUAD	No
Citric Acid	Intestinal Distress	No
Citric Acid	Weight Control	No
Citric Acid	Analgesic Adjuvant (Antacid or Buffering)	Yes
Citric Acid	Alters Vaginal PH	No
Citric Pectin	Intestinal Distress	No
Cloflucarban	Antimicrobial Soap	No
Cloflucarban	Skin Wound Cleanser	No
Cloflucarban	Skin Antiseptic	No
Cloflucarban	Health Care Personnel Handwash (For Bar Soap Use Only)	No
Cloflucarban	Skin Wound Protectant	No
Cloflucarban	Patient Preop. Skin Prep.	No
Cloflucarban	Surgical Hand Scrub	No
Cloves, Ground	Smoking Deterrent	No
Coal Tar	Antifungal	No
Coal Tar	Acne	No
Coal Tar (Shampoo)	Dandruff, Seborrheic Dermatitis, Psoriasis	No
Co-Carboxylase	Smoking Deterrent	No
Cocoa Butter	(Anorectal) Protectant (External)	Yes
Cocoa Butter	Protectant (Intrarectal)	Yes
Cocoa Butter	Skin Protectant	Yes
Coconut Oil	Pediculicide	No
Cod Liver Oil	(Anorectic) Protectant (External)	Yes
Cod Liver Oil	Protectant (Intrarectal)	Yes
Cod Liver Oil	(Anorectal) Wound Healing Agent (External)	No
Cod Liver Oil	Wound Healing Agent (Intrarectal)	No

191

INGREDIENT	USE	SAFE AND EFFECTIVE ?
Cod Liver Oil	Antitussive	Yes
Codeine	Antitussive	Yes
Codeine	(Internal) Analgesic	No
Codeine	Premenstrual Tension Menstrual Pain	No
Codeine Alkaloid	Antitussive	Yes
Codeine Phosphate	Antitussive	Yes
Codeine Phosphate	(Internal) Analgesic	No
Codeine Sulfate	Antitussive	Yes
Codeine Sulfate	Analgesic	No
Collinsonia Extract	(Anorectal) Miscellaneous (External)	No
Collinsonia Extract	Miscellaneous (Intrarectal)	No
Colloidal Oatmeal	Dandruff	No
Colloidal Oatmeal	Itching	Yes
Colloidal Oatmeal	Astringent (External)	No
Colocynth	Stimulant Laxative	No
Compound White Pine Syrup	Expectorant	No
Conicus Benedictus	Weight Control	No
Copper	Weight Control	No
Copper Gluconate	Weight Control	No
Copper Oleate	Pediculicide	No
Copper Undecylenate	Antifungal	Yes
Coriander, Ground	Smoking Deterrent	No
Corn Oil	Weight Gain	—
Corn Oil, Aqueous Emulsion	Gall Bladder Diagnostic Agent	Yes
Corn Silk, Potassium Extract	Weight Control	No
Corn Starch	Smoking Deterrent	No
Corn Starch, Partially Hydrolyzed	Glucose Tolerance, Postprandial Testing	—
Corn Syrup	Weight Control	No
Cottonseed Oil	Lubricant	No
Creosote	Toothache-Relief Agent	No
Creosote, Beechwood	Antitussive	No
Creosote, Beechwood	Expectorant	No
Creosote, Beechwood	Nasal Decongestant	No
Cresol	Psoriasis	No
Cresol	Antifungal	No
Cresol	Antiseptic (Skin)	No
Cresol	Antimicrobial (Oral)	No
Cresol	Anesthetic, Analgesic (Oral)	No
Cresol	Oral Mucosal Analgesic	No
Cresol	Toothache-Relief Agent	No
Cresol	Astringent (External)	No

INGREDIENT	USE	SAFE AND EFFECTIVE ?
Cresol Saponated	Antiseptic (Skin)	No
Cupric Sulfate	Astringent (External)	No
Cupric Sulfate	Weight Control	No
Cyanocobalamin	Weight Control	No
Cyclizine Hydrochloride	Antiemetic (Motion Sickness)	Yes
Cyclomethycaine Sulfate	Analgesic, Anesthetic Antipruritic (Skin)	No
Cystine	Weight Control	No
D-Calcium Pantothenate	Stimulant Laxative	No
Dandelion	Appetite Stimulant	—
Danthron	Stimulant Laxative	Yes
Dehydrochloric Acid	IPPUAD	No
Dehydrochloric Acid	Intestinal Distress	No
Dehydrochloric Acid	Stimulant Laxative	Yes
Denatonium Benzoate	Nailbiting and Thumbsucking Deterrent	No
Dequalinium Chloride	Antimicrobial (Oral)	No
Dextran 70	Demulcent (Eye)	Yes
Dibucaine Hydrochloride	Analgesic, Anesthetic, Antipruretic (Skin)	Yes
Dextromethorophan	Antitussive	Yes
Dextromethorphan Hydrobromide	Antitussive	Yes
Dextrose	Hangover	No
Dibenzothiophene	Acne	No
Dibucaine	(Anorectal) Anesthetic (External)	No
Dibucaine	Anesthetic (Intrarectal)	No
Dibucaine	Analgesic, Anesthetic, **Antipruretic** (Skin)	Yes
Dibucaine	Anesthetic, Analgesic (Oral)	No
Dibucaine Hydrochloride	(Anorectal) Anesthetic (External)	No
Dibucaine Hydrochloride	Anesthetic (Intrarectal)	No
Dibucaine Hydrochloride	Analgesic, Anesthetic, **Antipruretic** (Skin)	Yes
Dibucaine Hydrocloride	Anesthetic, Analgesic (Oral)	No
Dicalcium Phosphate Dihydrate	Anticavity Agent (Any Dosage Form)	No
Dichlorophen	Antifungal	No
Dichlorophenyl Trichloroethane	Foot Preparation	No
Diethanolamine P-Methoxycinnamate	Sunscreen	Yes
Digalloyl Trioleate	Sunsreen	Yes
Dihydroxyaluminum Aminoacetate	Antacid	Yes
Dihydroxyaluminum Aminoacetate	Analgesic Adjuvant (Antacid or Buffering)	Yes
Dihydroxyaluminum Sodium Carbonate	Antacid	Yes
Dihydroxyaluminum Sodium Carbonate	IPPUAD	No

INGREDIENT	USE	SAFE AND EFFECTIVE ?
Dihydroxyaluminum Sodium Carbonate	Analgesic Adjuvant (Antacid or Buffering)	Yes
Dimenhydrinate	Antiemetic (Motion Sickness)	Yes
Dimethicone	Skin Protectant	Yes
Dimethisoquin Hydrochloride	Analgesic, Anesthetic, Antipuritic (Skin)	Yes
Dioctyl Calcium Sulfosuccinate	Stool Softner Laxative	Yes
Dioctyl Potassium Sulfosuccinate	Stool Softner Laxative	Yes
Dioctyl Potassium Sulfosuccinate	Lowers Surface Tension and Produces Mucolytic Effects	Yes
Dioctyl Sodium Sulfoscuccinate	Stool Softner Laxative	Yes
Dioxybenzone	Sunscreen	Yes
Diperodon	(Anorectal) Anesthetic (External)	No
Diperodon	Anesthetic (Intrarectal)	No
Diperodon Hydrochloride	Corn and Callus Remover	No
Diphenhydramine Hydrochloride	Antiemetic	No
Diphenhydramine Hydrochloride	Antihistamine	No
Diphenhydramine Hydrochloride	Antitussive	No*
Diphenhydramine Hydrochloride	Sedative	No
Diphenhydramine Hydrochloride	Analgesic, Anesthetic, Antipuritic (Skin)	Yes
Diphenhydramine Hydrochloride	Sleep Aid	Yes
Dipropylene Glycol Salicylate	Sunscreen	No
Disaccharide	Hangover	No
Docusate Calcium	Stool Softner Laxative	Yes
Docusate Potassium	Stool Softener Laxative	Yes
Docusate Sodium	Stool Softner Laxative	Yes
Docusate Sodium	Pediculicide	No
Docusate Sodium	Weight Control	No
Dodecaethyleneglycol Monolaurate	Contraceptive	No
Dog Grass	IPPUAD	No
Domiphen Bromide	Antimicrobial (Oral)	No
Don Qual	Aphrodisiac	No
Doxylamine Succinate	Antihistamine (No More Than 7.5 mg)	Yes
Doxylamine Succinate	Sedative	No
Doxylamine Succinate	Sleep-Aid	No**
Duodenal Substance	Intestinal Distress	No

*Diphenhydramine hydrochloride. The FDA has found diphenhydramine hydrochloride to be safe and effective as an antitussive, and has approved the license application submitted by the manufacturers of BENYLIN. However, we do not recommend that you use it. See p. 53.

**Doxylamine succinate. The FDA has found doxylamine succinate to be safe and effective as a nighttime sleep-aid, and has approved the license application submitted by the manufacturers of UNISOM. However, we do not recommend that you use it. See p. 159.

INGREDIENT	USE	SAFE AND EFFECTIVE ❓
Dyclonine Hydrochloride	(Anorectal) Anesthetic (External)	No
Dyclonine Hydrochloride	Anesthetic (Intrarectal)	No
Dyclonine Hydrochloride	Analgesic, Anesthetic, Antipuritic (Skin)	Yes
Dyclonine Hydrochloride	Anesthetic, Analgesic (Oral)	Yes
E. Coli Vaccines	(Anorectal) Miscellaneous (External)	No
E. Coli Vaccines	Miscellaneous (Intrarectal)	No
Ededate Disodium	Tooth Desensitizer	No
Edetate Disodium	Minor Irritations (Vaginal)	No
Edetate Sodium	Minor Irritations (Vaginal)	No
Elaterin Resin	Stimulant Laxative	No
Elecampane	IPPUAD	No
Elm Bark	Antitussive	No
Elm Bark	Demulcent (Oral)	Yes
Ephedrine	Bronchodilator	Yes
Ephedrine	Nasal Decongestant (Oral)	No
Ephedrine Hydrochloride	Brochodilator	Yes
Ephedrine Hydrochloride	Nasal Decongestant (Topical)	Yes
Ephedrine Hydrochloride	Nasal Decongestant (Oral)	No
Ephedrine Hydrochloride	Vasoconstrictor (Eye)	Yes
Ephedrine Sulfate	(Anorectal) Vasoconstrictor (External) (Aqueous Solution)	Yes
Ephedrine Sulfate	Vasoconstrictor (Intrarectal)(Aqueous Solution)	Yes
Ephedrine Sulfate	Bronchodilator	Yes
Ephedrine Sulfate	Nasal Decongestant (Topical/Inhalant)	Yes
Ephedrine Sulfate	Nasal Decongestant (Oral)	No
Epinephrine	(Anorectal) Vasoconstrictor (External)	No
Epinephrine	Vasocontrictor (Intrarectal)	No
Epinephrine	Bronchodilator (Inhalant)	Yes
Epinephrine Bitartrate	Brochodilator (Inhalant)	Yes
Epinephrine Hydrochloride	(Anorectal) Vasoconstrictor (External) (Aqueous Solution)	Yes
Epinephrine Hydrochloride	Vasoconstictor (Intrarectal)	No
Epinephrine Hydrochloride (Racemic)	Bronchodilator (Inhalant)	Yes
Epinephrine Undecylenate	(Anorectal) Vasocontrictor (External)	No
Epinephrine Undecylenate	Vasoconstrictor (Intrarectal)	No
Ergocalciferol	Minor Irritations (Vaginal)	No
Essential Oils	Hair Grower	No
Estradiol	Hair Grower	No
Estradiol	Topical Hormone	No
Estrogens	Aphrodisiac	No

INGREDIENT	USE	SAFE AND EFFECTIVE ❓❗
Estrone	Topical Hormone	No
Estrone	Acne	No
Ether	IPPUAD	No
Ethohexadiol	Dandruff	No
Ethoxylated Alkyl Alcohol	Insect Bite Neutralizer	No
Ethyl Alcohol	Skin Antimicrobial	Yes
Ethyl 4-(Bis(Hydroxypropyl)) Aminobenzoate	Sunscreen	Yes
Ethylhexyl p-Methoxycinnamate	Suncreen	Yes
Ethylmorphine Hydrochloride	Antitussive	No
Ethyl Nitrite	Premenstrual Tension Menstrual Pain	No
Eucalyptol	Antitussive (Lozenge)	No
Eucalyptol	Expectorant (Topical/Inhalant)	No
Eucalyptol	Nasal Decongestant (Topical/Inhalant)	No
Eucalyptol	Antitussive (Mouthwash)	No
Eucalyptol	Expectorant (Lozenge)	No
Eucalyptol	Dandruff	No
Eucalyptol	Antitussive (Topical/Inhalant)	No
Eucalyptol	Nasal Decongestant (Lozenge)	No
Eucalyptol	Nasal Decongestant (Inhalant Room Spray)	No
Eucalyptol	Nasal Decongestant (Mouthwash)	No
Eucalyptol	Antimicrobial (Oral)	No
Eucalyptol	Anesthetic, Analgesic (Oral)	No
Eucalyptus Oil	Antitussive (Lozenge)	No
Eucalyptus Oil	Expectorant (Topical/Inhalant)	No
Eucalyptus Oil	Nasal Decongestant (Topical/Inhalant)	No
Eucalyptus Oil	Antitussive (Mouthwash)	No
Eucalyptus Oil	Expectorant (Lozenge)	No
Eucalyptus Oil	Antitussive (Topical/Inhalant)	No
Eucalyptus Oil	Nasal Decongestant (Mouthwash)	No
Eucalyptus Oil	Counteririrritant (Skin)	No
Eucalyptus Oil	Astringent (External)	No
Eucalyptus Oil	Hair Grower	No
Eucalyptus Oil	Smoking Deterrent	No
Eugenol	Analgesic, Anesthetic, Antipruritic (Skin)	No
Eugenol	Toothache-relief Agent (85 to 87% Concentrations)	Yes
Eugenol	Toothache-relief Agent (1 to 84% Concentrations)	No
Eugenol	Astringent	No
Euphorbia Pilulifera	Bronchodilator	No

INGREDIENT	USE	SAFE AND EFFECTIVE?
Extract Hydrangea	Premenstrual Tension, Menstrual Pain	No
Extract of Cascara	Premenstrual Tension Menstrual Pain	No
Extract of Ergot	Boil	No
Extract Stone Root	Premenstrual Tension Menstrual Pain	No
Extract White Pine Compound	Expectorant	No
Fatty Acids	Hair Grower	No
Fennel Acid	Intestinal Distress	No
Ferric Ammonium Citrate	Weight Control	No
Ferric Chloride	Antimicrobial (Oral)	No
Ferric Chloride	Premenstrual Tension, Menstrual Pain	No
Ferric Chloride	Insect Bite Neutralizer	No
Ferric Chloride	Prevention of Poison Ivy, Oak, and Sumac, Dermatitis	No
Ferric Pyrophosphate	Weight Control	No
Ferric Subsulfate	Astringent (External)	No
Ferrous Fumarate	Weight Control	No
Ferrous Gluconate	Weight Control	No
Ferrous Sulfate	Weight Control	No
Flax Seed	Weight Control	No
Fluid Extract Ergot	Insect Bite Neutralizer	No
Folic Acid	Weight Control	No
Formaldehyde Solution	Tooth Desensitizer	No
Frangula	Stimulant Laxative	No
Fructose	Weight Control	No
Fructose	Alcoholic Intoxication (Prevent)	No
Galega	IPPUAD	No
Gamboge	Stimulant Laxative	No
Garlic, Dehydrated	IPPUAD	No
Garlic, Dehydrated	Intestinal Distress	No
Gastric Mucin	Antacid	No
Gelatin	Demulcent (Oral)	Yes
Gelatin	Demulcent (Eye)	Yes
Gentian, Solic Extract Of	Smoking Deterrent	No
Gentian Violet	Pinworms	No
Gentian Violet	Antimicrobial (Oral)	No
Gentiana Lutea	Menstrual Cramps	—
Ginger	IPPUAD	No
Ginger, Ground	Smoking Deterrent	No
Ginseng	Aphrodisiac	No
Ginseng	Stimulant	No
Ginseng, Korean	Aphrodisiac	No

197

INGREDIENT	USE	SAFE AND EFFECTIVE ?
Glutamic Acid Hydrochloride	IPPUAD	No
Glutamic Acid Hydrochloride	Intestinal Distress	No
Glutamic Acid Hydrochloride	Hypochlorhydria, Achlorhydria	No
Glyercides (Mono- and Di-)	Weight Control	No
Glycerin	(Anorectal) Protectant (External) (Aqueous Solution)	Yes
Glycerin (Suppository)	Hyperosmotic Laxative	Yes
Glycerin	Demulcent (Oral)	Yes
Glycerin	Demulcent (Eye)	Yes
Glycerin	Earwax Softening Agent	No
Glycerin	Skin Protectant	Yes
Glyceryl Aminobenzoate	Sunscreen	Yes
Glyceryl Monostearate	Foot Preparation	No
Glycine	IPPUAD	No
Glycine	Intestinal Distress	No
Glycol Salicylate	Analgesic, Anesthetic, Antipruritic (Skin)	No
Glycyrrhiza	Aphrodisiac	No
Glycyrrhiza	Menstrual Cramps	No
Golden Seal	(Anorectal) Counterirritant (External)	No
Golden Seal	Counterirritant (Intrarectal)	No
Golden Seal	Aphrodisiac	No
Gotu Kola	Aphrodisiac	No
Gramicidin	Skin First Aid Anitbiotic	No
Guaifenesin	Expectorant	No*
Guar Gum	Bulk Laxative	No
Guar Gum	Anorectic (Bulk)	No
Gum Arabic, Powdered	Smoking Deterrent	No
Haloprogin	Antifungal	Yes
Haloprogin	External Feminine Itching	No
Hawthorne, Dry Alcoholic Extract Of	Smoking Deterrent	No
Hectorite	Intestinal Distress	No
Hermicellulase	Intestinal Distress	No
Hermicellulase	Exocrine Pancreatic Insufficiency	No
Hemicellulose of Psyllium	Bulk Laxative	Yes
Hexachlorophene	Antimicrobial (Prescription Use Only)	No
Hexachlorophene	Minor Irritations (Vaginal)	No
Hexachlorophene	Boil	No
Hexylresorcinol	Antimicrobial Soap	No

---

*Guaifenesin. Although no change has been published in the *Federal Register,* the FDA appears to have started the process of reclassifying this ingredient as a safe and effective expectorant. However, we do not recommend that you use it. See p. 51.

INGREDIENT	USE	SAFE AND EFFECTIVE **?**
Hexylresorcinol	Surgical Hand Scrub	No
Hexylresorcinol	Skin Wound Cleanser	Yes
Hexylresorcinol	Skin Antiseptic	No
Hexylresorcinol	Health Care Personnel Handwash	No
Hexylresorcinol	Skin Wound Protectant	No
Hexylresorcinol	Patient Preop. Skin Prep	No
Hexylresorcinol	Analgesic, Anesthetic, Antipruritic (Skin)	No
Hexylresorcinol	Anesthetic, Analgesic (Oral)	Yes
Histamine Dihydrochloride	Counterirritant (Skin)	Yes
Histidine	Weight Control	No
Homatropine Methylbromide	Antidiarrheal	No
Homatropine Methylbromide	IPPUAD	No
Homatropine Methylbromide	Intestinal Distress	No
Homatropine Methylbromide	Premenstrual Tension, Menstrual Pain (Smooth Muscle Relaxant)	No
Homosalate	Sunscreen	Yes
Honey	Astringent (External)	No
Horehound	Antitussive	No
Horehound	Expectorant	No
Horsetail	IPPUAD	No
Huckleberry	IPPUAD	No
Hydrastic Fluid Extract	IPPUAD	No
Hydrastis Canadensis	Weight Control	No
Hydriodic Acid Syrup	IPPUAD	No
Hydrochloric Acid	IPPUAD	No
Hydrochloric Acid Diluted	Hyperchlorhydria, Achlorhydria	No
Hydrocodone Bitartrate	Antitussive	No
Hydrocortisone	Antifungal (Combo with a Category I Antifungal Agent)	Yes
Hydrocortisone	Antipruritic (Skin)	Yes
Hydrocortisone	Dandruff, Seborrheic Dermatitis and Psoriasis	No
Hydrocortisone Acetate	Antifungal (Combo with a Category I Antifungal Agent)	Yes
Hydrocortisone Acetate	Antipruritic (Skin)	Yes
Hydrogen Peroxide	Antimicrobial (Oral)	No
Hydrogen Peroxide	Debriding Agent (Oral)	Yes
Hydrogen Peroxide	Wound-healing Agent in Aqueous Solution (Dental)	No
Hydrogen Peroxide	Wound-cleanser (In Aqueous Solution)	Yes
Hydroquinone	Skin Bleaching	Yes
Hydroxyethylcellulose	Demulcent (Eye)	Yes
Hydroxypropylmethylcellulose	Demulcent (Eye)	Yes

INGREDIENT	USE	SAFE AND EFFECTIVE ?
Hyoscyamine Sulfate	Antidiarrheal	No
Hyoscyamine Sulfate	Anticholerinergic	No
Hyoscyamine Sulfate	Premenstrual Tension Menstrual Pain	No
Ichthammol	Boil	No
Ichthammol	Skin Irritations	No
Ichthammol	Corn and Callus Remover	No
Infusion of Rose Petal	Astringent	No
Inositol	Weight Control	No
Iodine	Corn and Callus Remover	No
Iodine	Weight Contol	No
Iodine	Wart Remover	No
Iodine	Antimicrobial (Oral)	No
Iodine	Toothache Relief Agent	No
Iodine	IPPUAD	No
Iodine Complexed With Phosphate Ester of Alkylaryloxy Polyethylene Glycol	Antimicrobial Soap	No
Iodine Complexed With Phosphate Ester of Alkylaryloxy Polyethylene Glycol	Surgical Hand Scrub	No
Iodine Complexed With Phosphate Ester of Alkylaryloxy Polyetheylene Glycol	Skin Wound Cleanser	No
Iodine Complexed With Phosphate Ester of Alkylaryloxy Polyethylene Glycol	Skin Antiseptic	No
Iodine Complexed With Phosphate Ester of Alkylaryloxy Polyetheylene Glycol	Health Care Personnel Handwash	No
Iodine Complexed With Phosphate Ester of Alkylaryloxy Polyetheylene Glycol	Skin Wound Protectant	No
Iodine Complexed With Phosphate Ester of Alkylaryloxy Polyetheylene Glycol	Patient Preop. Skin Prep.	No
Iodized Botanical Oil	Foot Preparation	No
Iodized Lime	Exectorant	No
Iodoantipyrine	(Internal) Analgesic	No
Iodoantipyrine	Antipyretic	No
Iodontipyrine	Antirheumatic	No
Iodochlorhydroxyquin	Antifungal	Yes
Ipecac Fluid Extract	Expectorant	No
Ipecac Syrup	Emetic (For Acute Toxic Ingestion)	Yes
Ipecac Syrup	Expectorant	No
Ipecac	Emetic	Yes
Ipomea	Stimulant Laxative	No
Iron Ox Bile	Intestinal Distress	No
Isobornyl Thiocyanoacetate	Pediculicide	No
Isobutyl Para-Amino-Benzoate	Boil	No
Isoleucine	Weight Control	No
Isopropyl Alcohol	Astringent (External)	No

INGREDIENT	USE	SAFE AND EFFECTIVE ?
Isopropyl Alcohol	Antiseptic (50-90% V/V)	Yes
Isopropyl Alcohol	Skin Antimicrobial	Yes
Jalap	Stimulant Laxative	No
Java Tea	Diuretic	—
Johnsworth	IPPUAD	No
Johnsworth	Appetite Stimulant	—
Johnsworth	Intestinal Distress	No
Juniper	Intestinal Distress	No
Juniper Potassium Extract	Weight Control	No
Juniper Tar	Dandruff, Seborrheic Dermatitis, Psoriasis	No
Juniper Tar	(Anorectal) Counterirritant (External)	No
Juniper Tar	Counterirritant (Intrarectal)	No
Juniper Tar	Analgesic, Anesthetic, Antipruritic (Skin)	Yes
Juniper Tar	Boil	No
Juniper	Appetite Stimulant	—
Kaolin	Antacid	No
Kaolin	Antidiarrheal	No
Kaolin	(Anorectal) Protectant (External)	Yes
Kaolin	Protectant (Intrarectal)	Yes
Kaolin	Skin Protectant	Yes
Kaolin, Colloidal	IPPUAD	No
Karaya	Bulk Laxative	Yes
Karaya Gum	Anorectic (Bulk)	No
Kerosene	Pediculicide (Less Than 5%)	No
Knotgrass	Appetite Stimulant	—
Knotgrass	Intestinal Distress	No
Knotweed	Diuretic	—
L-Desoxyephedrine	Nasal Decongestant (Topical/Inhalant)	No*
L-Lysine	Weight Control	No
L-Lysine Monohydrochloride	Weight Control	No
Lactic Acid	Alters Vaginal pH	No
Lactic Acid	Lowers Surface Tension and Produces Mucolytic Effects (Vaginal)	No
Lactic Acid	Wart Remover	No
Lactic Acid	IPPUAD	No
Lactobacillus Acidophilus	Antidiarrheal	No

*L-Desoxyephedrine. Although no change has been published in the *Federal Register,* the FDA appears to have started the process of reclassifying this ingredient (alone and in combination with aromatics such as camphor, menthol, methyl salicylate, bornyl acetate, and lavender oil) as safe and effective as a topical nasal decongestant (administered by inhaler). See p. 43. .

INGREDIENT	USE	SAFE AND EFFECTIVE ?
Lactobacillus Acidophilus	For Fever Blister	No
Lactobacillus Bulgaricus	Antidiarrheal	No
Lactobacillus Bulgaricus	For Fever Blister	No
Lactose	Intestinal Distress	No
Lactose	Weight Control	No
Lactose	Smoking Deterrent	No
Lanolin	(Anorectal) Protectant (External)	Yes
Lanolin	Protectant (Intrarectal)	Yes
Lanolin	Hair Grower	No
Lanolin	Emollient (Eye)	Yes
Lanolin	Emollient (Skin)	Yes
Lanolin	Boil	No
Lanolin Anhydrous	Emollient (Eye)	Yes
Lanolin Nonionic Derivatives	Emollient (Eye)	Yes
Lappa Extract	(Anorectal) Miscellaneous (External)	No
Lappa Extract	Miscellaneous (Intrarectal)	No
Lard	Lubricant (Skin)	No
Laurel Isoquinolinium Bromide	Dandruff	No
Laureth 105	Contraceptive	No
Lavender, Compound Tincture	IPPUAD	No
Lawsone With Dihydroxyacetone	Sunscreen	Yes
Lecithin	Weight Control	No
Lemon Oil, Terpene-less	Smoking Deterrent	No
Leptandra Extract	(Anorectal) Miscellaneous (External)	No
Leptandra Extract	Miscellaneous (Intrarectal)	No
Leucine	Weight Control	No
Licorice Root Extract	Smoking Deterrent	No
Licorice	Aphrodisiac	No
Lidocaine	(Anorectal) Anesthetic (External)	No
Lidocaine	Anesthetic (Intrarectal)	No
Lidocaine	Analgesic, Anesthetic, Antipruritic (Skin)	Yes
Lidocaine	Anesthetic, Analgesic (Oral)	No
Lidocaine Hydrochloride	Anesthetic, Analgesic, Antipruritic (Skin)	Yes
Lidocaine Hydrochloride	Anesthetic, Analgesic (Oral)	No
Life Everlasting	Appetite Stimulant	—
Linden	IPPUAD	No
Lipase	Intestinal Distress	No
Live Yeast Cell Derivative	Wound Healing Agent (External)	No
Live Yeast Cell Derivative	Wound Healing Agent (Intrarectal)	No

INGREDIENT	USE	SAFE AND EFFECTIVE ?
Live Yeast Cell Derivative	Wound Healing Aid (Skin)	No
Liver Concentrate	Weight Control	No
Lobeline	Smoking Deterrent	No
Lysine	For Fever Blister	No
Lysine Hydrochloride	Intestinal Distress	No
Magaldrate	Antacid	Yes
Magnesium	Weight Control	No
Magnesium Aluminum-Silicate	Antacid	Yes
Magnesium Aluminum-Silicate	Acne	No
Magnesium Carbonate	Antacid	Yes
Magnesium Carbonate (With Analgesic and/or Caffeine)	Hangover Due to Overindulgence In Alcohol and Food	Yes
Magnesium Carbonate	Analgesic Adjuvant (Antacid or Buffering)	Yes
Magnesium Citrate	Saline Laxative	Yes
Magnesium Hydroxide	Antacid	Yes
Magnesium Hydroxide	IPPUAD	No
Magnesium Hydroxide	Acute Toxic Ingestion	No
Magnesium Hydroxide	Intestinal Distress	No
Magnesium Hydroxide	Saline Laxative	Yes
Magnesium Hydroxide	Analgesic Adjuvant (Antacid or Buffering)	Yes
Magnesium Oxide	Antacid	Yes
Magnesium Oxide	Weight Control	No
Magnesium Salicylate	(Internal) Analgesic	Yes
Magnesium Salicylate	Antipyretic	Yes
Magnesium Salicylate	Antirheumatic	Yes
Magnesium Salicylate	Premenstrual Tension Menstrual Pain	Yes
Magnesium Stearate	Smoking Deterrent	No
Magnesium Sulfate	Acne	No
Magnesium Sulfate	Foot Preparation	No
Mangesium Sulfate	Premenstrual Tension Menstrual Pain	No
Magnesium Sulfate	Saline Laxative	Yes
Magnesium Sulfate	Boils	No
Mangesium Trisilicate	Antacid	Yes
Magnesium Trisilicate	IPPUAD	No
Magnesium Trisilicate (With Analgesic and/or Caffeine)	Hangover Due to Overindulgence In Alcohol	Yes
Malt	Weight Control	No
Malt Soup Extract	Bulk Laxative	Yes
Maltodextrin	Weight Control	No
Manganese Citrate	Weight Control	No

INGREDIENT	USE	SAFE AND EFFECTIVE ❓
Mannitol	IPPUAD	No
Mannitol	Weight Control	No
Meclizine Hydrochloride	Antiemetic (Motion Sickness)	Yes
Menfegol	Contraceptive	No
Menthol	Antifungal	No
Menthol	(Anorectal) Counterirritant (External) (Aqueous Solution)	Yes
Menthol	Counterirritant (Intrarectal)	No
Menthol	Expectorant (Topical/Inhalant)	No
Menthol	Nasal Decongestant (Topical/Inhalant)	No
Menthol	Expectorant (Lozenge)	No
Menthol	Antitussive (Lozenge)	No*
Menthol	Antitussive (Topical/Chestrub)	No*
Menthol	Antitussive (Inhalant Room Spray)	No
Menthol	Nasal Decongestant (Inhalant Room Spray)	No
Menthol	Nasal Decongestant (Lozenge)	No
Menthol	Nasal Decongestant (Mouthwash)	No
Menthol	Dandruff, Seborrheic Dermatitis, Psoriasis	No
Menthol	Counterirritant (Skin) (1.25% to 16%)	Yes
Menthol	Analgesic, Anesthetic Antipruritic (1% or Less) (Skin)	Yes
Menthol	Antimicrobial (Oral)	No
Menthol	Anesthetic, Analgesic (Oral)	Yes
Menthol	Toothache-Relief Agent	No
Menthol	Smoking Deterrent	No
Menthol	Insect Bite Neutralizer	No
Menthol	Wart Remover	No
Menthol	Boil	No
Menthol	Astringent (External)	No
Menthyl Anthranilate	Sunscreen	No
Meralein Sodium	Antimicrobial (Oral)	No
Merbromin	Topical Antimicrobial	No
Mercuric Chloride	Topical Antimicrobial	No
Mercuric Oxide, Yellow	Anti-Infective (Eye)	No
Mercuric Oxide, Yellow	Topical Antimicrobial	No
Mercuric Salicylate	Topical Antimicrobial	No
Mercuric Sulfide	Topical Antimicrobial	No

*Menthol. Although no change has been published in the *Federal Register,* the FDA appears to have started the process of reclassifying this ingredient as a safe and effective antitussive, for use in a lozenge or chest rub. See. p. 53.

INGREDIENT	USE	SAFE AND EFFECTIVE ?
Mercurous Chloride	Boil	No
Mercury	Topical Antimicrobial	No
Mercury Ammoniated	Topical Antimicrobial	No
Mercury Chloride	Topical Antimicrobial	No
Mercury Oleate	Psoriasis	No
Mercury Oleate	Topical Antimicrobial	No
Metaproterenol Sulfate	Bronchodilator (Inhalant)	Yes
Methanol	Skin Prep.	No
Methapyrilene Fumarate	Antihistamine (Withdrawn from Market)	No
Methapyrilene Fumarate	Sedative	No
Methapyrilene Fumarate	Analgesic Adjuvant	No
Methapyrilene Fumarate	Antipyretic Adjuvant	No
Methapyrilene Fumarate	Antirheumatic Adjuvant	No
Methapyrilene Fumarate	Sleep-Aid	No
Methapyrilene Hydrochloride	Antihistamine (Withdrawn from the Market)	No
Methapyrilene Hydrochloride	Sedative	No
Methapyrilene Hydrochloride	Sleep-Aid	No
Methapyrilene Hydrochloride	Smoking Deterrent	No
Methapyrilene Hydrochloride	Premenstrual Tension Menstrual Pain	No
Methapyrilene Hydrochloride	Analgesic, Anesthetic, Antipruritic (Skin)	Yes
Methenamine	Anagesics for Kidney and Bladder Irritation	—
Methenamine	Premenstrual Tension Menstrual Pain	No
Methionine	Weight Control	No
Methoxyphenamine Hydrochloride	Bronchodilator	No
Methoxypolyoxyethylene-Glycol 550 Laurate	Contraceptive	No
Methyl Isobutyl Ketone	Foot Preparation	No
Methyl Nicotinate	Counterirritant	Yes
Methyl Salicylate	Counterirritant	Yes
Methyl Salicylate	Corn and Callus Remover	No
Methyl Salicylate	Antimicrobial (Oral)	No
Methyl Salicylate	Anesthetic, Analgesic (Oral)	No
Methyl Salicylate	Oral Mucosal Analgesic	No
Methyl Salicylate	Toothache-Relief Agent	No
Methyl Salicylate	Smoking Deterrent	No
Methyl Salicylate	Dandruff	No
Methyl Salicylate	Boil	No
Methylbenzethonium Chloride	Antimicrobial Soap	No
Methylbenzethonium Chloride	Surgical Hand Scrub	No
Methylbenzethonium Chloride	Skin Wound Cleanser	Yes
Methylbenzethonium Chloride	Skin Antiseptic	No

INGREDIENT	USE	SAFE AND EFFECTIVE ❓
Methylbenzethonium Chloride	Health Care Personnel Handwash	No
Methylbenzethonium Chloride	Skin Wound Protectant	No
Methylbenzethonium Chloride	Patient Preop. Skin Prep	No
Methylbenzethonium Chloride	Corn and Callus Remover	No
Methylbenzethonium Chloride	Cradle Cap	No
Methylcellulose	Antacid	No
Methylcellulose	Bulk Laxative	Yes
Methylcellulose	Demulcent (Eye)	Yes
Methylcellulose	Anorectic (Bulk)	No
Methylene Blue	Premenstrual Tension Menstrual Pain	No
Methylparaben	Antifungal	No
Methyltestosterone	Aphrodisiac	No
Miconazole Nitrate	Antifungal	Yes
Miconazole Nitrate	External Feminine Itching	No
Milk Solids, Dried	Antacid	Yes
Mineral Oil	(Anorectal) Protectant (External)	Yes
Mineral Oil	Protectant (Intrarectal)	Yes
Mineral Oil	Lubricant Laxative	Yes
Mineral Oil	Emollient (Eye)	Yes
Mineral Oil, Emulsified	Lubricant Laxative	Yes
Mineral Oil, Light	Emollient (Eye)	Yes
Mullein	Miscellaneous (Intrarectal) (Anorectal)	No
Mycozyme	Intestinal Distress	No
Myrrh	Oral Mucosal Protectant	No
Myrrh Fluid Extract Of	IPPUAD	No
Myrrh Tincture Of	Antimicrobial (Oral)	No
Myrrh Tincture Of	Astringent (Oral)	No
Naphazoline Hydrochloride	Nasal Decongestant (Topical)	Yes
Naphazoline Hydrochloride	Vasoconstrictor (Eye)	Yes
Natural Estrogenic Hormone	Topical Hormone	No
Natural Estrogenic Hormone	Premenstrual Tension Menstrual Pain	No
Neomycin Sulfate	Skin First Aid Antibiotic	Yes
Nettle	IPPUAD	No
Niacinamide	Sedative	No
Niacinamide	Hangover	—
Niacinamide	Premenstrual Tension Menstrual Pain	No
Niacinamide	Weight Control	No
Nickel-Pectin	Intestinal Distress	No
Nicotinic Acid	Smoking Deterrent	No
Nitromersol	Topical Antimicrobial	No

INGREDIENT	USE	SAFE AND EFFECTIVE?
Nitromersol Chloride	Antimicrobial (Oral)	No
Nonoxynol 9	Contraceptive	Yes
Nonoxynol 9	Minor Irritations (Vaginal)	No
Nonoxynol 9	Lowers Surface Tension and Produces Mucolytic Effects (Vaginal)	Yes
Nonylphenoxypoly (Ethyleneoxy) Ethanoliodine	Antimicrobial Soap	No
Nonylphenoxypoly (Ethyleneoxy) Ethanoliodine	Surgical Hand Scrub	No
Nonylphenoxypoly (Ethyleneoxy) Ethanoliodine	Skin Wound Cleanser	No
Nonylphenoxypoly (Ethyleneoxy) Ethanoliodine	Skin Antiseptic	No
Nonylphenoxypoly (Ethyleneoxy) Ethanoliodine	Health Care Personnel Handwash	No
Nonylphenoxypoly (Ethyleneoxy) Ethanoliodine	Patient Preop. Skin Prep.	No
Noscapine	Antitussive	No
Noscapine Hydrochloride	Antitussive	No
Nux Vomica	Aphrodisiac	No
Nux Vomica	IPPUAD	No
Nux Vomica	Smoking Deterrent	No
Nystatin	External Feminine Itching	No
Obtundia Surgical Dressing	Insect Bite Neutralizer	No
Octoxynol	Contraceptive	Yes
Octoxynol	Lowers Surface Tension and Produces Mucolytic Effects (Vaginal)	Yes
Octoxynol	Minor Irritations (Vaginal)	No
Oil of Citronella	Insect Repellent	No
Oil of Cloves	Astringent (External)	No
Oil Of Erigeron	Premenstrual Tension Menstrual Pain	No
Oil Of Nutmeg	Premenstrual Tension Menstrual Pain	No
Oil Of Sage	Astringent (External)	No
Oil of Sassafras	Boil	No
Oil of Thyme	Foot Preparation	No
Oil of Turpentine	Insect Bite Neutralizer	No
Oleoresin Capsicium	Premenstrual Tension Menstrual Pain	No
Olive Oil	Hair Grower	No
Opium Powder	Antidiarrheal (When Combined With One Or More Non-Narcotic Medicinal Ingredients)	Yes
Opium, Tincture of	Antidiarrheal (When Combined With One Or More Non-Narcotic Medicinal Ingredients)	Yes

207

INGREDIENT	USE	SAFE AND EFFECTIVE ❓
Organic Vegetables	Weight Control	No
Ortho-Hydroxophenyl Mercuric Chloride	Topical Antimicrobial	No
Orthophosphoric Acid	Intestinal Distress	No
Orthophosphoric Acid	Anticavity Agent (Any Dosage Form)	No
Orthophosphoric Acid	IPPUAD	No
Ox Bile Extract	IPPUAD	No
Ox Bile Extract	Intestinal Distress	No
Ox Bile	Stimulant Laxative	No
Oxybenzone	Sunscreen	Yes
Oxymetazoline Hydrochloride	Nasal Decongestant (Topical)	Yes
Oxyquinoline	Antifungal	No
Oxyquinoline	Skin Preparation	No
Oxyquinoline Citrate	Minor Irritations (Vaginal)	No
Oxyquinoline Sulfate	Antifungal	No
Oxyquinoline Sulfate	Astringent (External)	No
Oxyquinoline Sulfate	Boil	No
Oxyquinoline Sulfate	Antimicrobial (Oral)	No
Oxyquinoline Sulfate	Minor Irritations (Vaginal)	No
Oxytetracycline Hydrochloride	Skin First Aid Antibiotic	Yes
Padimate A	Sunscreen	Yes
Padimate O	Sunscreen	Yes
Pamabrom	Diuretic for Premenstrual and Menstrual Periods	Yes
Pancreatin	IPPUAD	No
Pancreatin	Intestinal Distress	No
Pancreatin	Exocrine Pancreatic Insufficiency	Yes
Pancreatin Enzymes	Weight Control	No
Pancrelipase	IPPUAD	No
Pancrelipase	Intestinal Distress	No
Pancrelipase	Exocrine Pancreatic Insufficiency	Yes
Panthenol	Skin Irritation	No
Panthenol	Corn and Callus Remover	No
Pantothenic Acid	Weight Control	No
Papain	Intestinal Distress	No
Papain	Weight Control	No
Papain	Lowers Surface Tension and Produces Mucolytic Effects (Vaginal)	No
Papaya	Intestinal Distress	No
Papaya Enzymes	Weight Control	No
Paraffin	Emollient (Eye)	Yes
Para-Chlormercuriphenol	Topical Antimicrobial	No
Paregoric	Antidiarrheal (When Combined With One or More Non-Narcotic Medicinal Ingredients)	Yes

INGREDIENT	USE	SAFE AND EFFECTIVE ❓
Parsley	Diuretic	No
Passion Flower Extract	Sleep-Aid	No
Peat	Hangover	No
Pectin	Antacid	No
Pectin	IPPUAD	No
Pectin	Antidiarrheal	No
Pectin	Demulcent (Oral)	Yes
Pega Palo	Aphrodisiac	No
Peppermint	Intestinal Distress	No
Peppermint Oil	Expectorant	No
Peppermint Oil	Nasal Decongestant (Inhalant Room Spray)	No
Peppermint Oil	Expectorant (Lozenge)	No
Peppermint Oil	Insect Bite Neutralizer	No
Peppermint Oil	Antitussive (Topical/Inhalant)	No
Peppermint Oil	Nasal Decongestant (Lozenge)	No
Peppermint Oil	Nasal Decongestant (Mouthwash)	No
Peppermint Oil	IPPUAD	No
Peppermint Oil	Intestinal Distress	No
Peppermint Oil	Foot Preparation	No
Peppermint Oil	Hangover	No
Peppermint Oil	Astringent (External)	No
Peppermint Spirit	IPPUAD	No
Peppermint	Appetite Stimulant	—
Pepsin	IPPUAD	No
Pepsin	Weight Control	No
Pepsin	Intestinal Distress	No
Pepsin	Hypochlorhydria/Achlorhydria In Combination With Bethaine Hydrochloride	No
Peruvian Balsam	(Anorectal) Wound Healing Agent (External)	No
Peruvian Balsam	Wound Healing Agent (Intrarectal)	No
Petrolatum	Boil	No
Petrolatum, White	(Anorectal) Protectant (External)	Yes
Petrolatum, White	Protectant (Intrarectal)	Yes
Petrolatum, White	Emollient (Eye)	Yes
Petrolatum, White	Skin Protectant	Yes
Phenacaine Hydrochloride	(Anorectal) Anesthetic (External)	No
Phenacaine Hydrochloride	Anesthetic (Intrarectal)	No
Phenacetin	Intestinal Distress (Withdrawn From Market)	No
Phenacetin	Weight Control (Withdrawn From Market)	No
Phenacetin	Analgesic (Withdrawn From Market)	No

209

INGREDIENT	USE	SAFE AND EFFECTIVE ❓
Phenacetin	Antipyretic (Withdrawn From Market)	No
Phenacetin	Antirheumatic (Withdrawn From Market)	No
Phenacetin	Premenstrual Tension, Menstrual Pain (Withdrawn From Market)	No
Phenazopyridine Hydrochloride	Kidney and Bladder Irriatation	—
Phenindamine Tartrate	Antihistamine	Yes
Phenindamine Tartrate	Premenstrual Tension, Menstrual Pain	No
Pheniramine Maleate	Antihistamine	Yes
Pheniramine Maleate	Analgesic Adjuvant	No
Pheniramine Maleate	Antipyretic Adjuvant	No
Pheniramine Maleate	Antirheumatic Adjuvant	No
Phenobarbital	Stimulant Corrective (To Correct Ephedrine)	No
Phenol	Antifungal	No
Phenol	Acne	No
Phenol	Antimicrobial Soap (Aqueous Alcoholic)	No
Phenol	Surgical Hand Scrub (Greater Than 1.5% Aqueous Alcoholic)	No
Phenol	Surgical Hand Scrub (1.5% Or Less Aqueous Alcoholic)	No
Phenol	Skin Wound Protectant (Greater Than 1.5% Aqueous Alcoholic)	No
Phenol	Skin Wound Cleanser (1.5% Or Less Aqueous Alcoholic)	No
Phenol	Patient Preop. Skin Prep. (1.5% Or Less Aqueous Alcoholic)	No
Phenol	Patient Preop. Skin Prep. (Greater Than 1.5% Aqueous Alcoholic)	No
Phenol	Boil	No
Phenol	Health Care Personnel Hand Wash (Greater Than 1.5% Aqueous Alcoholic)	No
Phenol	Health Care Personnel Hand Wash (1.5% Or Less Aqueous Alcoholic)	No
Phenol	Skin Wound Protectant (1.5% Or Less Aqueous Alcoholic)	No
Phenol	Skin Antiseptic (Greater Than 1.5% Aqueous Alcoholic)	No
Phenol	Skin Wound Cleanser (Greater Than 1.5% Aqueous Alcoholic)	No
Phenol	Skin Antiseptic (1.5% Or Less Aqueous Alcoholic)	No
Phenol	(Anorectal) Antiseptic (External)	No

INGREDIENT	USE	SAFE AND EFFECTIVE
Phenol	Antiseptic (Intrarectal)	No
Phenol	Analgesic, Anesthetic, Antipruritic (Skin)	Yes
Phenol	Antimicrobial (Oral)	Yes
Phenol	Anesthetic, Analgesic (Oral)	Yes
Phenol	Toothache-Relief Agent	No
Phenol	Oral Mucosal Analgesic	Yes
Phenol	Astringent (External)	No
Phenol	Insect Bite Neutralizer	No
Phenol	Minor Irritations (Vaginal) (Greater Than 1.5% Phenol)	No
Phenol	Seborrheic Derm., Psoriasis	No
Phenolate Sodium	Antifungal	No
Phenolate Sodium	Acne	No
Phenolate Sodium	Analgesic, Anesthetic Antipruritic (Skin)	Yes
Phenolate Sodium	Antimicrobial (Oral)	No
Phenolate Sodium	Seborrheic Derm., Psorasis	No
Phenolate Sodium	Oral Mucosal Analgesic	Yes
Phenolate Sodium	Anesthetic, Analgesic (Oral)	Yes
Phenolate Sodium	Toothache-Relief Agent	No
Phenolate Sodium	Minor Irritations (Greater Than 1.5% Phenol) (Vaginal)	No
Phenolphthalein	Fever Blisters	No
Phenolphthalein, White	Stimulant Laxative	Yes
Phenolphthalein, Yellow	Stimulant Laxative	Yes
Phenoxyacetic Acid	Corn and Callus Remover	No
Phenyl Salicylate	Antidiarrheal	No
Phenyl Salicylate	Acne	No
Phenyl Salicylate	Corn and Callus Remover	No
Phenyl Salicylate	Premenstrual Tension, Menstrual Pain	No
Phenylalanine	Weight Control	No
Phenylephrine Hydrochloride	(Anorectal) Vasoconstrictor (Aqueous Solution; External)	Yes
Phenylephrine Hydrochloride	Vasoconstrictor (Aqueous Solution; (Intrarectal)	Yes
Phenylephrine Hydrochloride	Vasoconstrictor (Intrarectal Suppositories)	No
Phenylephrine Hydrochloride	Nasal Decongestant (Topical/Oral)	Yes
Phenylephrine Hydrochloride	Vasoconstrictor (0.08% To 0.2%) (Eye)	Yes
Phenylephrine Hydrochloride	Fever Blisters	No
Phenylmercuric Acetate	Contraceptive	No
Phenylmercuric Nitrate	Contraceptive	No
Phenylmercuric Nitrate	Topical Antimicrobial	No

211

INGREDIENT	USE	SAFE AND EFFECTIVE ❓
Phenylpropanolamine Hydrochloride	Anorectic	Yes
Phenylpropanolamine Hydrochloride	Nasal Decongestant (Oral)	Yes
Phenylpropanolamine Hydrochloride	Oral Decongestant	No
Phenylpropanolamine Bitartrate	Nasal Decongestant (Oral)	Yes
Phenylpropanolamine Maleate	Nasal Decongestant (Oral)	Yes
Phenyltoloxamine	Analgesic Adjuvant	No
Phenyltoloxamine	Antipyretic Adjuvant	No
Phenyltoloxamine	Antirheumatic Adjuvant	No
Phenyltoloxamine Citrate	Antihistamine	No
Phenyltoloxamine Dihydrogen Citrate	Sedative	No
Phenyltoloxamine Dihydrogen Citrate	Sleep-Aid	No
Phosphate Disodium	Anticavity Agent (Any Dosage Form)	No
Phosphate Disodium	Saline Laxative (In Combination)	Yes
Phosphate Monosodium	Saline Laxative (In Combination)	Yes
Phosphorated Carbohydrate	Antiemetic	No
Phosphorus	Weight Control	No
Phytolacca Berry Juice	Weight Control	No
Picrotoxin	Pediculicide	No
Pineapple Enzymes	Weight Control	No
Pine Needle Oil	Foot Preparation	No
Pine Tar	Expectorant	No
Pine Tar	Boil	No
Pine Tar Preps	Dandruff, Seborrheic Derm., Psorasis	No
Piperazine Citrate	Pinworms	No
Piperocaine Hydrochloride	Anesthetic (Eye)	No
Piperonyl Butoxide With Pyrethrins	Pediculicide	Yes
Piscidia Erythrina	Menstrual Pain	No
Plantago Ovata Husks	Bulk Laxative	Yes
Plantago Seed	Bulk Laxative	Yes
Plantago Seed Husks	Bulk Laxative	Yes
Plantago Seed, Blond	Bulk Laxative	Yes
Podophyllum Resin	Stimulant Laxative	No
Poloxalkol	Stool Softener Laxative	No
Poloxamer 100	Skin Wound Cleanser	Yes
Poloxamer-Iodine Complex	Antimicrobial Soap	No
Poloxamer-Iodine Complex	Surgical Hand Scrub	No
Poloxamer-Iodine Complex	Skin Wound Cleanser	No
Poloxamer-Iodine Complex	Skin Antiseptic	No
Poloxamer-Iodine Complex	Health Care Personnel Handwash	No
Poloxamer-Iodine Complex	Skin Wound Protectant	No
Poloxamer-Iodine Complex	Patient Preop. Skin Prep.	No
Polycarbophil	Antidiarrheal	Yes
Polycarbophil	Bulk Laxative	Yes

INGREDIENT	USE	SAFE AND EFFECTIVE ?
Polyethylene	Acne	No
Polyethylene Glycol 300	Demulcent (Eye)	Yes
Polyethylene Glycol 400	Demulcent (Eye)	Yes
Polymyxin B Sulfate	Skin First Aid Antibiotic (Combined With Bacitracin, Chlortetracycline Hydrochloride, Oxytetracycline Hydrochloride, Tetracycline Hydrochloride Or Neomycin Sulfate)	Yes
Polymyxin B Sulfate	Skin First Aid Antibiotic (Single Ingredient)	No
Polyoxyethylene Monolaurate	Astringent (External)	No
Polysorbate 80	Demulcent (Eye)	Yes
Polyvinyl Alcohol	Demulcent (Eye)	Yes
Potassium Acetate	Premenstrual Tension, Menstrual Pain	No
Potassium Alum	Antifungal	No
Potassium Alum	Antiperspirant	No
Potassium Alum	Astringent (External)	No
Potassium Arsenite	Acute Toxic Ingestion	No
Potassium Bicarbonate	IPPUAD	No
Potassioum Bromide	Sedative	No
Potassium Carbonate	IPPUAD	No
Potassium Carbonate	Antidiarrheal	No
Potassium Chlorate	Antimicrobial (Oral)	No
Potassium Chloride	Replacement of Minerals Lost In Diarrhea	—
Potassium Chloride	Salt Substitute	—
Potassium Citrate	Weight Control	No
Potassium Ferrocyanide	Astringent (External)	No
Potassium Gentian Root	Smoking Deterrent	No
Potassium Guaiacolsulfonate	Expectorant	No
Potassium Iodide	Foot Preparation	No
Potassium Iodide	Expectorant	No
Potassium Iodide	Salt Substiute	—
Potassium Nitrate	Tooth Desensitizer	No
Potassium Nitrate	Premenstrual Tension Menstrual Pain	No
Potassium Nux Vomica	Smoking Deterrent	No
Potassium Sorbate	Minor Irritations (Vaginal)	Yes
Povidone	Demulcent (Eye)	Yes
Povidone-Iodine	Antifungal	No
Povidone-Iodine	Acne	No
Povidone-Iodine	Antimicrobial (Oral)	No
Povidone-Iodine	Minor Irritations (Vaginal)	Yes
Povidone-Iodine	Dandruff, Psoriasis	No
Povidone-Iodine Complex	Antimicrobial Soap	No

INGREDIENT	USE	SAFE AND EFFECTIVE ❓
Povidone-Iodine Complex	Surgical Hand Soap	No
Povidone-Iodine Complex	Skin Wound Cleanser	No
Povidone-Iodine Complex	Skin Antiseptic	No
Povidone-Iodine Complex	Health Care Personnel Handwash	No
Povidone-Iodine Complex	Skin Wound Protectant	No
Povidone-Iodine Complex	Patient Preop. Skin Preparation	No
Pramoxine Hydrochloride	(Anorectal) Anesthetic (External) (Cream Formulation)	Yes
Pramoxine Hydrochloride	(Anorectal) Anesthetic (External) (Jelly Formulation)	Yes
Pramoxine Hydrochloride	Anesthetic (Intrarectal) (Cream Formulation)	No
Pramoxine Hydrochloride	Anesthetic (Intrarectal) (Jelly Formulation)	No
Pramoxine Hydrochloride	Analgesic, Anesthetic, Antipruritic (Skin)	Yes
Progesterone	Breast Developer	No
Progesterone	Topical Hormone	No
Prolase	Intestinal Distress	No
Pormethazine Hydrochloride	Antihistamine	No
Propylene Glycol	Foot Balm & Salve	No
Propylene Glycol	Pediculicide	No
Propylene Glycol	Demulcent (Eye)	Yes
Propylene Glycol	Smoking Deterrent	No
Prophylhexedrine	Nasal Decongestant (Topical, Inhalant)	Yes
Propylparaben	Antifungal	No
Protease	Intestinal Distress	No
Prune Concentrate Dehydrate	Stimulant Laxative	No
Prune Powder	Stimulant Laxative	No
Pseudoephedrine Hydrochloride	Bronchodilator	No
Pseudoephedrine Hydrochloride	Nasal Decongestant (Oral)	Yes
Pseudoephedrine Sulfate	Bronchodilator	No
Pseudoephedrine Sulfate	Nasal Decongestant (Oral)	Yes
Psyllium	Bulk Laxative	Yes
Psyllium	Anorectic (Bulk)	No
Pyrantel Pamoate	Pinworms	Yes
Pyrethrin	Pediculicide	No
Pyrethrins With Piperonyl butoxide	Pediculicide	Yes
Pyridozine Hydrochlorate	Smoking Deterrent	No
Pyridoxine Hydrochloride	Premenstrual Tension, Menstrual Pain	No
Pyridoxine Hydrochloride	Weight Control	No
Pyrilamine Maleate	Acne	No
Pyrilamine Maleate	Antihistamine	Yes
Pyrilamine Maleate	Sedative	No
Pyrilamine Maleate	Analgesic Adjuvant	No

INGREDIENT	USE	SAFE AND EFFECTIVE
Pyrilamine Maleate	Premenstrual Tension	No
Pyrilamine Maleate	Antipyretic Adjuvant	No
Pyrilamine Maleate	Antirheumatic Adjuvant	No
Pyrilamine Maleate (In Combination)	Premenstrual Tension	Yes
Pyrilamine Maleate	Sleep-Aid	No
Pyrilamine Maleate	Insect Bite Neutralizer	No
Pyrilamine Maleate	Anesthetic, Analgesic (Oral)	No
Quinine	(Internal) Analgesic	No
Quinine	Antipyretic	No
Quinine	Antirheumatic	No
Quinine Ascorbate	Smoking Deterrent	No
Quinine Sulfate	Nocturnal Leg Muscle Cramps	No
Racephedrine Hydrochloride	Bronchodilator	Yes
Racephedrine Hydrochloride	Nasal Decongestant (Oral)	No
Racephedrine Hydrochloride	Nasal Decongestant (Topical)	Yes
Red Petrolatum	Sunscreen	Yes
Released Carbon Dioxide	Miscellaneous Laxative	Yes
Resorcinol	Antifungal	No
Resorcinol	Acne	No
Resorcinol	Psoriasis	No
Resorcinol	(Anorectal) Antiseptic (External)	No
Resorcinol	(Anorectal) Keratolytic (External)	Yes
Resorcinol	Antiseptic (Intrarectal)	No
Resorcinol	Analgesic, Anesthetic, Antipruritic (Skin)	Yes
Resorcinol With Sulfur	Acne	Yes
Resorcinol Monoacetate	Acne	No
Resorcinol Monoacetate With Sulfur	Acne	Yes
Rhubarb Fluid Extract	Antidiarrheal	No
Rhubarb Fluid Extract	IPPUAD	No
Rhubarb Chinese	Stimulant Laxative	No
Riboflavin	Premenstrual Tension Menstrual Pain	No
Riboflavin	Weight Loss	No
Rice Polishings	Weight Control	No
Rosin	Boil	No
Rosin Cerate	Boil	No
Saccharin	Weight Loss	No
Salicin	Foot Preparation	No
Salicyl Alcohol	Anesthetic, Analgesic (Oral)	No
Salicylamide	Sedative	No
Salicylamide	Analgesic, Anesthetic, Antipruritic (External)	No
Salicylamide	(Internal) Analgesic	No
Salicylamide	Antipyretic	No
Salicylamide	Antirheumatic	No

INGREDIENT	USE	SAFE AND EFFECTIVE?
Salicylamide	Antirheumatic Adjuvant	No
Salicylamide	Analgesic Adjuvant	No
Salicylamide	Antipyretic Adjuvant	No
Salicylamide	Kidney and Bladder Irritation	—
Salicylamide	Premenstrual Tension Menstrual Pain	No
Salicylamide	Sleep-Aid	No
Salicylic Acid	Antifungal	No
Salicylic Acid	Acne	No
Salicylic Acid	Corn and Callus Remover (12-40%)	Yes
Salicylic Acid	Wart Remover	Yes
Salicylic Acid	Dandruff, Seborrheic Derm. Psoriasis	Yes
Salsalate	(Internal) Analgesic	No
Salsalate	Antipyretic	No
Salsalate	Antirheumatic	No
Sandarac	Toothache-Relief Agent	No
Sarsaparilla	Aphrodisiac	No
Sassafras, Oil of	Foot Preparation	No
Saw Palmetto	Premenstrual Tension, Menstrual Pain	No
Scopolamine Aminoxide Hydrobromide	Sedative	No
Scopolamine Aminoxide Hydrobromide	Sleep-Aid	No
Scopolamine Hydrobromide	Antidiarrheal	No
Scopolamine Hydrobromide	Antiemetic	No
Scopolamine Hydrobromide	Anticholinergic	No
Scopolamine Hydrobromide	Sedative	No
Scopolamine Hydrobromide	Sleep-Aid	No
Sea Minerals	Weight Control	No
Sea Kelp	Anorectic (Bulk)	No
Selenium Sulfide	Dandruff	Yes
Senecio Aureus	Menstrual Cramps	No
Senna	Intestinal Distress	No
Senna Fruit Extract	Stimulant Laxative	Yes
Senna Leaf Extract	Stimulant Laxative	Yes
Senna Pod Concentrate	Stimulant Laxative	Yes
Senna Syrup	Stimulant Laxative	Yes
Sennosides A & B	Stimulant Laxative	Yes
Sesame Seed	Weight Control	No
Shark Liver Oil	(Anorectal) Protectant (External)	Yes
Shark Liver Oil	Protectant (Intrarectal)	Yes
Shark Liver Oil	(Anorectal) Wound Healing Agent (External)	No
Shark Liver Oil	Wound Healing Agent (Intrarectal)	No
Shark Liver Oil	Skin Protectant	Yes

INGREDIENT	USE	SAFE AND EFFECTIVE ❓
Silver Nitrate	Smoking Deterrent	No
Silver Protein, Mild	Anti-Infective (Eye)	No
Silver Acetate	Smoking Deterrent	No
Silver Nitrate	Astringent (External)	No
Simethicone	Antacid	No
Simethicone	Antiflatulent	Yes
Simethicone	IPPUAD	No
Simethicone	Intestinal Distress	No
Sodium	Weight Control	No
Sodium Aluminum Chlorohydroxy Lactate	Antiperspirant (Aerosol)	No
Sodium Aluminum Chlorohydroxy Lactate	Antiperspirant (Non-Aerosol)	No
Sodium Aminobenzoate	Analgesic Adjuvant	No
Sodium Aminobenzoate	Antipyretic Adjuvant	No
Sodium Aminobenzoate	Antirheumatic Adjuvant	No
Sodium Ascorbate	Smoking Deterrent	No
Sodium Benzoate	Premenstrual Tension, Menstrual Pain	No
Sodium Bicarbonate	Antacid	Yes
Sodium Bicarbonate	Anticavity Agent (Any Dosage Form)	No
Sodium Bicarbonate	Intestinal Distress	No
Sodium Bicarbonate	IPPUAD	No
Sodium Bicarbonate	Foot Preparation	No
Sodium Bicarbonate	Analgesic Adjuvant (Antacid or Buffering)	Yes
Sodium Bicarbonate	Debriding Agent (Oral)	Yes
Sodium Bicarbonate	Insect Bite Neutralizer	No
Sodium Bicarbonate	Skin Protectant	Yes
Sodium Bicarbonate	Alters Vaginal pH	No
Sodium Bicarbonate	Anorectic (Bulk) In Combination With Acid Ingredients	No
Sodium Borate	Antifungal	No
Sodium Borate	Acne	No
Sodium Borate	Alters Vaginal pH (Greater Than 1% Boron)	No
Sodium Borate	Minor Irritations (Greater Than 1% Boron) (Vaginal)	No
Sodium Borate	Lowers Surface Tension and Produces Mucolytic Effects (Greater Than 1% Boron) (Vaginal)	No
Sodium Borate	Astringent (Greater Than 1% Boron) (Vaginal)	No
Sodium Borate	Insect Bite Neutralizer	No
Sodium Bromide	Sedative	No
Sodium Bromide	Sleep-Aid	No
Sodium Caprylate	Antifungal	No
Sodium Caprylate	Antimicrobial (Oral)	No

217

INGREDIENT	USE	SAFE AND EFFECTIVE ❓
Sodium Carbonate	Antacid	Yes
Sodium Carbonate	Analgesic Adjuvant (Antacid or Buffering)	Yes
Sodium Carbonate	Alters Vaginal pH	No
Sodium Caseinate	Weight Control	No
Sodium Chloride	Intestinal Distress	No
Sodium Chloride	Foot Balm and Salve	No
Sodium Chloride	Replacement of Minerals Lost In Diarrhea	—
Sodium Chloride	Salt Replacement (Heat Relief)	—
Sodium Chloride	Weight Control	No
Sodium Chloride	(Eye) Hypertonic Agent (2 to 5%)	Yes
Sodium Chloride	Smoking Deterrent	No
Sodium Citrate	Expectorant	No
Sodium Citrate (In Solution)	Overindulgence In Alcohol and Food	Yes
Sodium Citrate	Tooth Densensitizer (In Combination With Citric Acid)	No
Sodium Diacetate	Astringent (External)	No
Sodium Dichromate	Antimicrobial (Oral)	No
Sodium Dihydrogen Phosphate	Anticavity Agent (Any Dosage Form)	No
Sodium Fluoride	Tooth Desensitizer	No
Sodium Fluoride	Anticavity Dental Rinse	Yes
Sodium Fluoride	Anticavity Dentrifice	Yes
Sodium Lactate	Lowers Surface Tension and Produces Mucolytic Effects (Vaginal)	No
Sodium Lauryl Sulfate	Foot Preparation	No
Sodium Lauryl Sulfate	Lowers Surface Tension and Produces Mucolytic Effects (Vaginal)	Yes
Sodium Monofluorophosphate	Anticavity Dental Rinse (6%)	No
Sodium Monofluorophosphate	Anticavity Dentrifice	Yes
Sodium Monofluorophosphate	Tooth Desensitizer	No
Sodium Nitrate	Premenstrual Tension, Menstrual Pain	No
Sodium Oleate	Stimulant Laxative	No
Sodium Perborate Monohydrate	Wound Cleanser (Oral)	No*
Sodium Perborate	Debriding Agent (Oral)	No
Sodium Perborate	Alters Vaginal pH (Greater Than 1% Boron)	No
Sodium Perborate	Lowers Surface Tension and Produces Mucolytic Effects (Vaginal)	No

***Sodium perborate monohydrate.** Although no change has been published in the *Federal Register,* the FDA appears to have started the process of reclassifying this ingredient as a safe and effective skin wound cleanser ingredient.

INGREDIENT	USE	SAFE AND EFFECTIVE ?
Sodium Perborate	Minor Irritations (Greater Than 1% Boron) (Vaginal)	No
Sodium Perborate	Astringent (Greater Than 1% Boron) (Vaginal)	No
Sodium Phosphate	Anticavity Agent (Any Dosage Form)	No
Sodium Phosphate Dibasic Anhydrous Reagent	Anticavity Agent (Any Dosage Form)	No
Sodium Potassium Tartrate	Antacid	Yes
Sodium Propionate	Antifungal	No
Sodium Propionate	Minor Irritations (Vaginal)	Yes
Sodium Salicylate	(Internal) Analgesic	Yes
Sodium Salicylate	Antipyretic	Yes
Sodium Salicylate	Antirheumatic	Yes
Sodium Salicylate	Kidney and Bladder Irritation	—
Sodium Salicylate	Minor Irritations (Vaginal)	No
Sodium Salicylate	Dandruff, Psoriasis	No
Sodium Salicylate	IPPUAD	No
Sodium Salicylic Acid Phenolate	(Anorectal) Antiseptic (External)	No
Sodium Salicylic Acid Phenolate	Antiseptic (Intrarectal)	No
Sodium Salicylic Acid Phenolate	Minor Irritations (Greater Than 1.5% Phenol) (Vaginal)	No
Sodium Sesquicarbonate	Foot Preparation	No
Sodium Sulfate	Foot Preparation	No
Sodium Sulfide	Ingrown Toenail	No
Sodium Thiosulfate	Acne	No
Sodium 3,4-dimethyl-phenyl Glyoxylate	Sunscreen	No
Sorbitol	IPPUAD	No
Sorbitol	Intestinal Distress	No
Sorbitol	Hyperosmotic Laxative	Yes
Soy Bean Protein	Weight Control	No
Soy Meal	Weight Control	No
Spirit of Peppermint	Premenstrual Tension, Menstrual Pain	No
Squill	Expectorant	No
Squill Extract	Expectorant	No
Stannous Fluoride	Anticavity Dental Rinse	Yes
Stannous Fluoride	Anticavity Dentrifice	Yes
Stannous Fluoride	Anticavity Dental Gel	Yes
Stannous Fluoride	Tooth Desensitizer	No
Starch	(Anorectal) Protectant (External)	Yes
Starch	Protectant (Intrarectal)	Yes
Starch	Skin Protectant	Yes
Starch	Astringent (External)	No
Stem Bromelains	Intestinal Distress	No
Stramonium	Anticholinergic (Inhalant)	No
Strawberry	IPPUAD	No

INGREDIENT	USE	SAFE AND EFFECTIVE ❓
Strontium Chloride	Tooth Desensitizer	No
Strychnine	Aphrodisiac	No
Strychnine	IPPUAD	No
Sucrose	Premenstrual Tension, Menstrual Pain	No
Sucrose	Weight Control	No
Sucrose Octaacetate	Nailbiting and Thumbsucking Deterrent	No
Sugar	Smoking Deterrent	No
Sulfacetamide Sodium	(Eye) Anti-Infective	No
Sulferated Oils of Turpentine	Premenstrual Tension, Menstrual Pain	No
Sulfur	Antifungal	No
Sulfur	Acne	Yes
Sulfur	Scabies (5-10%)	Yes
Sulfur	Skin Protectant	No
Sulfur	Dandruff	Yes
Sulfur, Precipitated	(Anorectal) Keratolytic (External)	No
Sulfur, Precipitated	Keratolytic (Intrarectal)	No
Sulfur, Sublimed	(Anorectal) Keratolytic (External)	No
Sulfur, Sublimed	Keratolytic (Intrarectal)	No
Sulisobenzone	Sunscreen	Yes
Sweet Spirits of Nitre	Diaphoretic Diuretic, Intestinal Antispasmodic, Stimulant, Flatulent, Colic	No
Syrup of Pine Tar	Expectorant	No
Talc	Astringent (External)	No
Talc	Smoking Deterrent	No
Tannic Acid	Acute Toxic Ingestion	No
Tannic Acid	Antifungal	No
Tannic Acid	Intestinal Distress	No
Tannic Acid	(Anorectal) Astringent (External)	No
Tannic Acid	Astringent (Intrarectal)	No
Tannic Acid	Ingrown Toenail	No
Tannic Acid	Astringent (External)	No
Tannic Acid	Upset Stomach	No
Tannic Acid	Skin Protectant	No
Tannic Acid	IPPUAD	No
Tannic Acid Glycerite	Astringent (External)	No
Taraxacum Officinale	Menstrual Cramps	No
Tartaric Acid	Antacid	Yes
Tartaric Acid	Saline and Hyperosmotic Laxative	No
Tartaric Acid	Alters Vaginal pH	No
Terpin Hydrate	Expectorant	No
Terpin Hydrate Elixir	Expectorant	No

INGREDIENT	USE	SAFE AND EFFECTIVE ❓∎
Testosterone	Aphrodisiac	No
Tetracaine	(Anorectal) Anesthetic (External)	No
Tetracaine	Anesthetic (Intrarectal)	No
Tetracaine	Analgesic, Anesthetic, Antipruritic (Skin)	Yes
Tetracaine	Anesthetic, Analgesic (Oral)	No
Tetracaine Hydrochloride	Acne	No
Tetracaine Hydrochloride	(Anorectal) Anesthetic (External)	No
Tetracaine Hydrochloride	Anesthetic (Intrarectal)	No
Tetracaine Hydrochloride	Analgesic, Anesthetic, Antipruritic (Skin)	Yes
Tetracaine Hydrochloride	Analgesic, Anesthetic (Oral)	No
Tetracaine Hydrochloride	Hair Grower	No
Tetracycline Hydrochloride	Skin First Aid Antibiotic	Yes
Tetrahydrozoline Hydrochloride	(Eye) Vasoconstrictor	Yes
Thenyldiamine Hydrochloride	Antihistamine	No
Thenyldiamine Hydrochloride	Nasal Decongestant (Topical)	No
Theobromine Sodium Salicylate	Diuretic for Premenstrual And Menstrual Periods	No
Theophylline	Diuretic for Premenstrual And Menstrual Periods	No
Theophylline Anhydrous	Bronchodilator	No
Theophylline Calcium Salicylate	Bronchodilator	No
Theophylline Sodium Glycinate	Bronchodilator	No
Thiamine	Insect Repellent (Internal Use)	No
Thiamine Hydrochloride	Sedative	No
Thiamine Hydrochloride	Weight Control	No
Thiamine Hydrochloride	Sleep-Aid	No
Thiamine Hydrochloride	Premenstrual Tension, Menstrual Pain	No
Thiamine Mononitrate	Weight Control	No
Thiamine Mononitrate	Hangover	No
Thiamine Mononitrate	Smoking Deterrent	No
Thimerosol	Topical Antimicrobial	No
Thiocyanoacetate	Pediculicide	No
Thonzylamine Hydrochloride	Antihistamine	Yes
Threonine	Weight Control	No
Thymol	Antifungal	No
Thymol	Acne	No
Thymol	Antitussive	No
Thymol	Nasal Decongestant (Topical, Inhalant)	No
Thymol	Nasal Decongestant (Lozenge)	No
Thymol	Nasal Decongestant (Inhalant Room Spray)	No

INGREDIENT	USE	SAFE AND EFFECTIVE ?
Thymol	Nasal Decongestant (Mouthwash)	No
Thymol	Analgesic, Anesthetic, Antipruritic (Skin)	No
Thymol	Antimicrobial (Oral)	No
Thymol	Anesthetic, Analgesic (Oral)	No
Thymol	Oral Mucosal Analgesic	No
Thymol	Toothache-Relief Agent	No
Thymol	Dandruff	No
Thymol	Astringent (External)	No
Thymol	Smoking Deterrent	No
Thymol	Boil	No
Thymol	Antipruritic (Skin)	No
Thymol Iodide	Antimicrobial (Oral)	No
Thymol Iodide	Oral Mucosal Analgesic	No
Thymold Iodide	Toothache-Relief Agent	No
Tincture of Green Soap	Antiseptic (Skin)	No
Tincture of Iodine	Antimicrobial Soap	No
Tincture of Iodine	Surgical Hand Scrub	No
Tincture of Iodine	Skin Wound Cleanser	No
Tincture of Iodine	Skin Antiseptic	No
Tincture of Iodine	Health Care Personnel Handwash	No
Tincture of Iodine	Skin Wound Protectant	No
Tincture of Iodine	Patient Preop. Skin Prep.	Yes
Titanium Dioxide	Sunscreen	Yes
Tolindate	Antifungal	No
Tolnaftate	Antifungal	Yes
Tolu	Expectorant	No
Tolu Balsam	Expectorant	No
Tolu Balsam	Antimicrobial (Oral)	No
Tolu Balsam	Expectorant (Oral)	No
Tolu Balsam Tincture	Expectorant	No
Tragacanth Mucilage	Foot Preparation	No
Triacetin	Antifungal	No
Tricalcium Phosphate	Weight Control	No
Triclocarban	Surgical Hand Scrub	No
Triclocarban	Skin Wound Cleanser (For Bar Soap Use Only)	No
Triclocarban	Skin Antiseptic	No
Triclocarban	Health Care Personnel Handwash (For Bar Soap Use Only)	No
Triclocarban	Skin Wound Protectant	No
Triclocarban	Patient Preop. Skin Prep.	No
Triclosan	Antimicrobial Soap	No
Triclosan	Surgical Hand Scrub	No

INGREDIENT	USE	SAFE AND EFFECTIVE **?**
Triclosan	Skin Wound Cleanser	No
Triclosan	Skin Antiseptic	No
Triclosan	Health Care Personnel Handwash	No
Triclosan	Skin Wound Protectant	No
Triclosan	Patient Preop. Skin Prep.	No
Triethanolamine	Insect Bite Neutralizer	No
Triethanolamine Salicylate	Analgesic, Anesthetic, Antipruritic (Skin)	No
Treithanolamine Salicylate	Sunscreen	Yes
Trillium	Intestinal Distress	No
Triple Dye	Antimicrobial Soap	No
Triple Dye	Surgical Hand Scrub	No
Triple Dye	Skin Wound Cleanser	No
Triple Dye	Skin Antiseptic (Use Limited To Neonatal Nursery)	No
Triple Dye	Health Care Personnel Handwash	No
Triple Dye	Skin Wound Protectant	No
Triple Dye	Patient Preop. Skin Prep.	No
Tryptophan	Weight Control	No
Turpentine Oil	Antitussive (Oral)	No
Turpentine Oil	Expectorant (Topical, Inhalant)	No
Turpentine Oil	Nasal Decongestant (Topical, Inhalant)	No
Turpentine Oil	Antitussive (Topical, Inhalant)	No
Turpentine Oil	Expectorant (Oral)	No
Turpentine Oil	Nasal Decongestant (Oral)	No
Turpentine Oil	Counterirritant (Skin)	Yes
Turpentine Oil, Rectified	Counterirritant (Intrarectal)	No
Turpentine Oil, Rectified	(Anorectal) Counterirritant (External)	No
Tyrosine	Weight Control	No
Undecoylium Chloride-Iodine Complex	Antimicrobial Soap	No
Undecoylium Chloride-Iodine Complex	Surgical Hand Scrub	No
Undecoylium Chloride-Iodine Complex	Skin Wound Cleanser	No
Undecoylium Chloride-Iodine Complex	Skin Antiseptic	No
Undecoylium Chloride-Iodine Complex	Health Care Personnel Handwash	No
Undecoylium Chloride-Iodine Complex	Skin Wound Protectant	No
Undecoylium Chloride-Iodine Complex	Patient Preop. Skin Prep.	No
Undecylenate Preps	Dandruff, Seborrheic Derm. Psoriasis	No
Urea	Premenstrual Tension, Menstrual Pain	No
Urea	Antipruritic (2-10%, Skin)	Yes
Uva Ursi	Weight Control	No
Uva Ursi Potassium Extract	Weight Control	No

INGREDIENT	USE	SAFE AND EFFECTIVE ?
Valine	Weight Control	No
Venice Turpentine	Premenstrual Tension, Menstrual Pain	No
Vitamin A	(Anorectal) Wound Healing Agent (External)	No
Vitamin A	Wound Healing Agent (Intrarectal)	No
Vitamin A	Weight Control	No
Vitamin A	Minor Irritations (Vaginal)	No
Vitamin A	Corn and Callus Remover	No
Vitamin A Acetate	Weight Control	No
Vitamin A Acid	Corn and Callus Remover	No
Vitamin A Palmitate	Weight Control	No
Vitamin D	(Anorectal) Wound Healing Agent (External)	No
Vitamin D	Wound Healing Agent (Intrarectal)	No
Vitamin D	Weight Control	No
Vitamin E	Weight Control	No
Vitamin E	Acne	No
Vitamin E	Stimulant	No
Vitromersol	Topical Antimicrobial	No
Wheat Germ	Weight Control	No
Wheat Germ Oil	Hair Grower	No
White Ointment	Emollient (Eye)	Yes
White Pine	Expectorant	No
White Wax	Emollient (Eye)	Yes
Wintergreen Oil	Astringent (External)	No
Witch Hazel	Foot Preparation	No
Witch Hazel Water	(Anorectal) Astringent (External)	Yes
Woodruff	Intestinal Distress	No
Wool Alcohols	(Anorectal) Protectant (External)	Yes
Wool Alcohols	Protectant (Intrarectal)	Yes
Xanthan Gum	Anorectic (Bulk)	No
Xylometazoline Hydrochloride	Nasal Decongestant (Topical)	Yes
Xylem	Hangover	No
Yeast	Weight Control	No
Yohimbine	Aphrodisiac	No
Zinc Acetate	Skin Protectant	Yes
Zinc Acetate	Wound Healing Aid	No
Zinc Caprylate	Antifungal	No
Zinc Carbonate	Skin Protectant	Yes
Zinc Chloride	Astringent (External)	No
Zinc Chloride	Corn and Callus Remover	No
Zinc Chloride	Astringent (Oral)	Yes

INGREDIENT	USE	SAFE AND EFFECTIVE ❓∎
Zinc Oxide	Acne	No
Zinc Oxide	(Anorectal) Protectant (External)	Yes
Zinc Oxide	Protectant (Intrarectal)	Yes
Zinc Oxide	(Anorectal) Astringent (External)	Yes
Zinc Oxide	Astringent (Intrarectal)	Yes
Zinc Oxide	Antiseptic (Skin)	No
Zinc Oxide	Skin Protectant	Yes
Zinc Oxide	Astringent (External)	No
Zinc Oxide	Insect Bite Neutralizer	No
Zinc Oxide	Boil	No
Zinc Phenolsulfonate	Antidiarrheal	No
Zinc Phenolsulfonate	Antiemetic	No
Zinc Phenolsulfonate	Astringent (External)	No
Zinc Propionate	Antifungal	No
Zinc Pyrithione	Dandruff, Seborrheic Derm.	Yes
Zinc Stearate	Acne	No
Zinc Stearate	Astringent (External)	No
Zinc Sulfate	Foot Preparation	No
Zinc Sulfate	Astringent (Eye)	Yes
Zinc Sulfate	Astringent (Vaginal)	No
Zinc Sulfate	Astringent (External)	No
Zinc Sulfide	Acne	No
Zinc Thiosulfate	Acne	—
Zinc Undecylenate	Antifungal	Yes
Zirconium Oxide	Insect Bite Neutralizer	No
Zyloxin	Topical Antimicrobial	No
2-Amino-2-Methyl-2-Propanol-8-Bromo-Theophyllinate	Premenstrual Tension, Menstrual Pain	Yes
2-Ethylhexyl Salicylate	Sunscreen	Yes
2-Ethylhexyl 2-Cyano-3, 3-Diphenacrylate	Sunscreen	Yes
2-Ethylhexyl 4-Phenyl-Benzophenone-2 Carboxylic Acid	Sunscreen	No
2-Phenylbenzimidazole-5-Sulfonic Acid	Sunscreen	Yes
3-(4-Methylbenzylidene)-Camphor	Sunscreen	No

NB The following ingredients were inadvertantly omitted from the Status of Ingredients list, when the updated compilation was prepared. All of these ingredients *lack evidence of safety, effectiveness, or both,* when used as OTC *menstrual or diuretic* drug products: Barosma, Cnicus benedictus (blessed thistle), Corn Silk, Couch grass, Dog grass extract, Extract buchu, Extract uva ursi, Hydrastis canadensis (golden seal), Oil of juniper, Pipsissewa and Triticum.

BRAND NAME INDEX

Safe and Effective: **FDA** — "YES" means that the FDA, in a Panel Report or other Federal Register Notice, found all active ingredients in the product safe and effective for that use. "NO" means at least one ingredient, the combination of ingredients, or the dosage form lacks evidence of safety or effectiveness.

                 HRG — "YES" and "NO" is Health Research Group's opinion of the same product. In addition, N/E means that we have not fully evaluated the drug or category of drugs.

Problem: "S(Ingredient)" or "E(Ingredient)" means the particular ingredient lacks evidence of safety or effectiveness.

                 $ means that HRG believes the product is not a good buy because a less expensive effective treatment, often a single-ingredient generic, is available.

PROBLEM	ALTERNATIVE	PAGE	PRODUCT
$	Generic Petroleum Jelly	—	**A and D Ointment**
S(Phenacetin), E(Caffeine), $	Generic Aspirin	7,28	**A.S.A. COMPOUND**
SE(Chloroxylenol), E(Thymol), N/E (Acetone, Wormwood), $	Moist Heat; Generic Aspirin or Aceta- minophen, If Necessary	7,18	**ABSORBINE, JR. (Lotion)**
E(Dosage form — suppositories)	Generic Acetaminophen	7,27	**ACEPHEN (Suppositories)**
$	Frequent Soap and Water Rinsing Will Allow Most Minor Wounds to Heal	—	**ACHROMYCIN Ointment**
E(Triprolidine, Colds) S(Pseudoephedrine), $	Allergy: Generic Chlorphe- niramine; Cold: Treat Individual Symptoms	33,61	**ACTIFED Tablets and Syrup**
Not For Allergies	Generic Oxymetazoline or Phenylephrine Spray	33,43	**AFRIN Nasal Spray and Drops**
S(Pseudoephedrine), $	Allergy: Generic Chlor- pheniramine Pills Cold: Generic Oxymetazoline or Phenylephrine Spray	33,43	**AFRINOL REPETABS**
	Cotton Socks, Keep Feet Very Dry	—	**AFTATE**
S(Mineral Oil), $	High Liquid, High Fiber Diet	87,99	**AGORAL Plain**
S(Mineral Oil, Phenolphthalein), $	High Liquid, High Fiber Diet	87,99	**AGORAL Raspberry & Marshmallow**
$	See Chart p. 113 For Best Buy	101,115	**ALUDROX (Liquid and Tablets)**
Occasional Use Only, $	Baking Soda	101,114	**ALKA-2 Chewable ANTACID**

PRODUCT	USE	INGREDIENTS	SAFE AND EFFECTIVE? FDA	HRG
ALKA SELTZER Effervescent Antacid (Gold)	Antacid	Sodium Bicarbonate, Citric Acid	YES	YES
ALKA SELTZER Pain Reliever and Effervescent Antacid (Blue)	Antacid / Painkiller	Aspirin, Sodium Bicarbonate, Citric Acid	YES / YES	NO / YES
ALKA SELTZER PLUS Cold Medicine	Cold	Phenylpropanolamine Bitartrate, Chlorpheniramine Maleate	*	NO
ALLEREST Tablets and Children's Chewables	Allergy	Phenylpropanolamine HCl., Chlorpheniramine Maleate	YES	NO
ALLEREST Nasal Spray	Nasal	Phenylephrine HCl.	YES	YES
ALLEREST Time-Release Capsules	Allergy	Phenylpropanolamine HCl. Chlorpheniramine Maleate	NO	NO
ALLIMIN Tablets	Anti-Flatulent	Dried Garlic Powder (Allium Savitum)	NO	NO
ALTERNAGEL	Antacid	Aluminum Hydroxide	YES	YES
AMERICAINE	Hemorrhoids	Benzocaine, Benzethonium, Chloride, Polyethylene Glycol base	N/E	NO
AMPHOJEL	Antacid	Aluminum Hydroxide gel	YES	YES
ANACIN, ANACIN MAXIMUM STRENGTH	Painkiller	Aspirin, Caffeine	NO	NO
ANACIN-3, ANACIN-3 MAXIMUM STRENGTH	Painkiller	Acetaminophen	YES	YES

Safe and Effective: **FDA** — "YES" means that the FDA, in a Panel Report or other Federal Register Notice, found all active ingredients in the product safe and effective for that use. "NO" means at least one ingredient, the combination of ingredients, or the dosage form lacks evidence of safety or effectiveness.

HRG — "YES" and "NO" is Health Research Group's opinion of the same product. In addition, N/E means that we have not fully evaluated the drug or category of drugs.

Problem: "S(Ingredient)" or "E(Ingredient)" means the particular ingredient lacks evidence of safety or effectiveness.

$ means that HRG believes the product is not a good buy because a less expensive effective treatment, often a single-ingredient generic, is available.

228

PROBLEM	ALTERNATIVE	PAGE	PRODUCT
Occasional Use Only, $	Baking Soda	101,114	**ALKA SELTZER Effervescent Antacid (Gold)**
As Antacid: S(Aspirin), $	Antacid: See Chart p. 113	7,24 101,114	**ALKA SELTZER Pain Reliever & Effervescent**
As Painkiller: $	For Best Buy Painkiller: Generic Aspirin		**Antacid (Blue)**
FDA: E(Chlorpheniramine);* HRG: also S(Phenylpropanloamine), $	Treat Individual Symptoms	33,44	**ALKA SELTZER PLUS Cold Medicine**
SE(Phenylpropanolamine), $	Generic Chlorpheniramine, If Needed	33, 61	**ALLEREST Tablets and Children's Chewables**
Not for Allergy	Generic Phenylephrine or Oxymetazoline Spray	33,43	**ALLEREST Nasal Spray**
FDA: E(Timed-Release Form) HRG: also S(Phenylpropanolamine), $	Generic Chlorpheniramine, If Needed	33,61	**ALLEREST Time-Release Capsules**
E(Garlic Powder)	None	101,115	**ALLIMIN Tablets**
$	See Chart p. 113 For Best Buy	101,114	**ALTERNAGEL**
FDA: N/E (Benzethonium) HRG: Also S(Benzocaine), $	Keep Clean & Dry; Petroleum Jelly or Zinc Oxide, If Necessary	131,142	**AMERICAINE**
$	See Chart p. 113 For Best Buy	101,114	**AMPHOJEL**
E(Caffeine), $	Generic Aspirin	7,29	**ANACIN, A.M.S.**
$	Generic Acetaminopher	7,27	**ANACIN-3, A.M.S.**

---

*Antihistamines, including the ingredient in this product, lack evidence of effectiveness in treating the symptoms of a cold, in the judgment of the FDA Advisory Panel. The FDA's review of prescription drugs also found drugs containing antihistamines to be INEFFECTIVE in treatment of a cold. The FDA's Director of OTC Drug Evaluation has indicated that the FDA has started the process of reclassifying antihistamines as effective in OTC products for treating a cold. We disagree with this change, and believe that this drug should not be used to treat colds.

PRODUCT	USE	INGREDIENTS	SAFE AND EFFECTIVE? FDA	HRG
ANALGESIC BALM	External Painkiller	Methyl Salicylate, Menthol	YES	N/E
ANOREXIN	Weight Loss	Phenylpropanolamine HCl., Caffeine	YES	NO
ANUSOL Ointment	Hemorrhoids	Zinc Oxide Pramoxine, Peruvian Balsam	NO	NO
ANUSOL Suppositories	Hemorrhoids	Peruvian Balsam, Bismuth Subgallate, Bismuth Resorcinol Compound	NO	NO
APPEDRINE, MAXIMUM STRENGTH	Weight Loss	Phenylpropanolamine HCl., Vitamins	NO	NO
AQUA-BAN	Menstrual	Ammonium Chloride, Caffeine	YES	NO
ARTHRITIS PAIN FORMULA	Painkiller	Aspirin, Aluminum Hydroxide, Magnesium Hydroxide	YES	NO
A.R.M. Allergy Relief Medicine	Allergy	Phenylpropanolamine Chlorpheniramine Maleate	YES	NO
ARTHRITIS PAIN FORMULA, Aspirin Free	Painkiller	Acetaminophen	YES	YES
ASCRIPTIN, ASCRIPTIN A/D	Painkiller	Aspirin, Aluminum Hydroxide, Magnesium Hydroxide	YES	NO
ASPERCREME (Lotion and Cream)	External Painkiller	Triethanolamine Salicylate	NO	NO
ASPERGUM	Painkiller, Sore Throat	Aspirin	YES	NO
ASPIRIN Suppositories	Painkiller	Aspirin	NO	NO

Safe and Effective: FDA — "YES" means that the FDA, in a Panel Report or other Federal Register Notice, found all active ingredients in the product safe and effective for that use. "NO" means at least one ingredient, the combination of ingredients, or the dosage form lacks evidence of safety or effectiveness.

HRG — "YES" and "NO" is Health Research Group's opinion of the same product. In addition, N/E means that we have not fully evaluated the drug or category of drugs.

Problem: "S (Ingredient)" or "E (Ingredient)" means the particular ingredient lacks evidence of safety or effectiveness.

$ means that HRG believes the product is not a good buy because a less expensive effective treatment, often a single-ingredient generic, is available.

PROBLEM	ALTERNATIVE	PAGE	PRODUCT
$	Moist Heat; Generic Aspirin or Acetaminophen If Necessary	7,18	**ANALGESIC BALM**
SE(Phenylpropanolamine HCl.)	Eat A Bit Less, Exercise More: Lose a Pound a Week	67,81	**ANOREXIN**
E(Peruvian Balsam), $	Keep Clean & Dry; Petroleum Jelly, If Necessary	131,141	**ANUSOL Ointment**
E(Peruvian Balsam, Bismuth Subgallate), $	Keep Clean & Dry; Petroleum Jelly, If Necessary	131,141	**ANUSOL Suppositories**
FDA: E(Vitamins); HRG: SE(Phenylpropanolamine), $	Eat A Bit Less, Exercise More: Lose a Pound a Week	67,81	**APPEDRINE, MAXIMUM STRENGTH**
Inappropriate Therapy, $	Generic Aspirin or Acetaminophen, Eat Less Salt	7,30	**AQUA-BAN**
E(Buffers), $	Generic Aspirin	7,24	**ARTHRITIS PAIN FORMULA**
S(Phenylpropanolamine), $	Generic Chlorpheniramine		**A.R.M. Allergy Relief Medicine**
Not Anti-Inflammatory, $	Generic Acetaminophen	7,27	**ARTHRITIS PAIN FORMULA, Aspirin Free**
E(Buffers), $	Generic Aspirin	7,24	**ASCRIPTIN ASCRIPTIN A/D**
E(Triethanolamine Salicylate) $	Moist Heat; Generic Aspirin or Acetaminophen, If Necessary	7,18	**ASPERCREME (Lotion and Cream)**
E(Dosage Form), $	Generic Aspirin Tablets	7,25	**ASPERGUM**
E(Dosage Form), $	Generic Aspirin Tablets	7,26	**ASPIRIN Suppositories**

PRODUCT	USE	INGREDIENTS	SAFE AND EFFECTIVE? FDA	HRG
ASTHMAHALER	Asthma	Epinephrine as Bitartrate	YES	YES
AUREOMYCIN Ointment	Skin Anti-Biotic	Chlortetracycline	YES	N/E
AYDS Appetite Suppressant	Weight Loss	Benzocaine	YES	NO
BC Tablet & Powder	Painkiller	Aspirin, Salicylamide, Caffeine	NO	NO
BACTINE First Aid Spray	Skin Wound	Benzalkonium Chloride, Lidocaine	YES	N/E
BANTRON	Smoking Deterrent	Lobeline Sulfate, Tribasic Calcium Phosphate, Magnesium Carbonate	NO	NO
BASALJEL, EXTRA STRENGTH BASALJEL	Antacid	Aluminium Hydroxide	YES	YES
BAYER ASPIRIN, BAYER CHILD-REN'S ASPIRIN	Painkiller	Aspirin	YES	YES
BAYER CHILDREN'S COLD TABLETS	Cold	Aspirin, Phenylpropano-lamine HCl.	YES	NO
BAYER COUGH SYRUP FOR CHILDREN	Cough, Cold	Phenylpropanolamine HCl., Dextromethorphan	YES	NO
BAYER TIME-RELEASE ASPIRIN	Painkiller	Aspirin	NO	NO
BENADRYL Antihistamine Cream	Skin Itching	Diphenhydramine	YES	N/E

Safe and Effective: **FDA** — "YES" means that the FDA, in a Panel Report or other Federal Register Notice, found all active ingredients in the product safe and effective for that use. "NO" means at least one ingredient, the combination of ingredients, or the dosage form lacks evidence of safety or effectiveness.

HRG — "YES" and "NO" is Health Research Group's opinion of the same product. In addition, N/E means that we have not fully evaluated the drug or category of drugs.

Problem: "S(Ingredient)" or "E(Ingredient)" means the particular ingredient lacks evidence of safety or effectiveness.

$ means that HRG believes the product is not a good buy because a less expensive effective treatment, often a single-ingredient generic, is available.

PROBLEM	ALTERNATIVE	PAGE	PRODUCT
See a Health Care Professional for Diagnosis and Treatment		33,64	ASTHMAHALER
$	Frequent Soap and Water Rinsing Will Allow Most Minor Wounds to Heal.	—	AUREOMYCIN Ointment
E(Benzocaine)	Eat a Bit Less, Exercise More: Lose a Pound a Week	67,83	AYDS Appetite Suppressant
SE(Salicylamide) E(Caffeine), $	Generic Aspirin	7,29	BC Tablet & Powder
$	Frequent Soap and Water Rinsing Will Allow Most Minor Wounds to Heal	—	BACTINE First Aid Spray
E(Lobeline Sulfate)	Slowly Taper Down	—	BANTRON
$	See Chart p. 113 For Best Buy	101,114	BASALJEL, EXTRA STRENGTH BASALJEL
$	Generic Aspirin	7,21	BAYER ASPIRIN, BAYER CHILDREN'S ASPIRIN
S(Phenylpropanolamine), $	Treat Individual Symptoms	33,44	BAYER CHILDREN'S COLD TABLETS
S(Phenylpropanolamine), $	Productive Cough: Drink Warm Liquids; Dry Cough: Generic Dextromethorphan	33,54	BAYER COUGH SYRUP FOR CHILDREN
E(Timed-Release Dosage), $	Generic Aspirin	7,26	BAYER TIME-RELEASE ASPIRIN
$	Generic Antihistamine Pills, If Necessary	—	BENADRYL Antihistamine Cream

PRODUCT	USE	INGREDIENTS	SAFE AND EFFECTIVE?	
			FDA	HRG
BEN-GAY External Analgesic Products	External Painkiller	Methyl Salicylate, Menthol	YES	N/E
BENOXYL	Acne	Benzoyl Peroxide	YES	YES
BENYLIN	Cough	Diphenhydramine HCl.	YES	NO
BENYLIN DM	Cough	Dextromethorphan Hydrobromide, Ammonium Chloride, Sodium Citrate	NO	NO
BENZEDREX Inhaler	Nasal Decongestant	Propylhexedrine, Menthol, Aromatics	NO	NO
BETADINE Ointment, Skin Cleanser, Solution	Skin Cleanser, Skin Wound Cleanser	Povidone Iodine	NO	NO
BISACODYL	Laxative	Bisacodyl	YES	NO
BISODOL Powder	Antacid	Sodium Bicarbonate, Magnesium Carbonate	YES	YES
BISODOL Antacid Tablets	Antacid	Calcium Carbonate, Magnesium Hydroxide	YES	YES
BLACK DRAUGHT SYRUP	Laxative	Casanthranol	YES	NO
BLISTEX Ointment	Chapped Lips, Cold Sore, Fever Blister	Camphor, Phenol, Lanolin, Petroleum base	YES	N/E
BONINE	Motion Sickness	Meclizine HCl.	YES	YES
BOROFAX	Chapped Skin Abrasions Diaper Rash	Boric Acid, Lanolin	NO	NO
BRIOSCHI	Antacid	Sodium Bicarbonate	YES	YES
BROMO-SELTZER	Painkiller, Antacid	Acetaminophen, Sodium Bicarbonate, Citric Acid	YES	NO

Safe and Effective: **FDA** — "YES" means that the FDA, in a Panel Report or other Federal Register Notice, found all active ingredients in the product safe and effective for that use. "NO" means at least one ingredient, the combination of ingredients, or the dosage form lacks evidence of safety or effectiveness.

HRG — "YES" and "NO" is Health Research Group's opinion of the same product. In addition, N/E means that we have not fully evaluated the drug or category of drugs.

Problem: "S (Ingredient)" or "E (Ingredient)" means the particular ingredient lacks evidence of safety or effectiveness.

$ means that HRG believes the product is not a good buy because a less expensive effective treatment, often a single-ingredient generic, is available.

234

PROBLEM	ALTERNATIVE	PAGE	PRODUCT
$	Moist Heat, Generic Aspirin or Acetamino- phen, If Necessary	7,18	**BEN-GAY External Analgesic Products**
$	Generic Benzoyl Peroxide	—	**BENOXYL**
S(Diphenhydramine), $	Productive Cough: Drink Warm Liquids; Dry Cough: Generic Dextromethorphan	33,53	**BENYLIN**
E(Ammonium Chloride & Sodium Citrate), $	Productive Cough: Drink Warm Liquids; Dry Cough: Generic Dextromethorphan	33,52	**BENYLIN DM**
E(Menthol), $	Allergies: Generic Chlor- pheniramine Pills, Colds: Generic Oxymetazoline or Phenylephrine Spray	33,40	**BENZEDREX Inhaler**
SE(Povidone Iodine), $	Frequent Soap and Water Rinsing Will Allow Most Minor Bites and Wounds To Heal	—	**BETADINE Ointment, Skin Cleanser, Solution**
S(Bisacodyl), $	High Liquid, High Fiber Diet	87,98	**BISACODYL**
Occasional Use Only, $	Baking Soda	101,114	**BISODOL Powder**
Occasional Use Only, $	Baking Soda	101,114	**BISODOL Antacid Tablets**
S(Casanthranol), $	High Liquid, High Fiber, Diet	87,98	**BLACK DRAUGHT SYRUP**
$	Generic Petroleum Jelly	—	**BLISTEX Ointment**
$	Generic Meclizine	117,130	**BONINE**
SE(Boric Acid), $	Generic Petroleum Jelly	—	**BOROFAX**
Occasional Use Only, $	Generic Baking Soda	101,114	**BRIOSCHI**
Unnecessary	Generic Acetaminophen or Baking Soda	7,27 101,114	**BROMO-SELTZER**

235

PRODUCT	USE	INGREDIENTS	SAFE AND EFFECTIVE? FDA	HRG
BRONITIN Asthma Pills	Bronchial Asthma	Ephedrine, Theophylline, Guaifenesin, Pyrilamine Maleate	NO	NO
BRONKAID Tablets	Bronchial Asthma	Ephedrine, Theophylline, Guaifenesin, Magnesium Trisilicate	NO	NO
BRONKAID Mist and Mist Suspension	Bronchial Asthma	Epinephrine (Mist) Epinephrine Bitartrate (Mist Suspension)	YES	YES
BRONKOTABS	Bronchial Asthma	Ephedrine Sulfate, Theophylline, Guaifenesin, Phenobarbital	NO	NO
BUF Acne Cleansing Bar	Acne	Salicylic Acid and Sulfur In Soap	NO	NO
BUFFERIN, BUFFERIN EXTRA STRENGTH	Painkiller	Aspirin, Magnesium Carbonate, Aluminum Glycinate	YES	NO
BUFFERIN, Arthritis Painkiller Strength	Painkiller	Aspirin, Magnesium Carbonate, Aluminium Glycinate	YES	NO
C3 Cold Cough Capsules	Cold, Cough	Dextromethorphan HBr., Phenylpropanolamine HCl. Chlorpheniramine Maleate	NO	NO
CALADRYL Lotion and Cream	Skin Itching	Diphenhydramine HCl. Calamine, Camphor Alcohol	YES	N/E
CALDECORT Rectal	Itch Ointment	0.5% Hydrocortisone	YES	NO
CAMALOX	Antacid	Aluminum Hydroxide, Magnesium Hydroxide, Calcium Carbonate	YES	YES
CAMPHO-PHENIQUE	First Aid	Camphor, Phenol	YES	N/E
CARTER'S LITTLE PILLS	Laxative	Bisacodyl	YES	NO

Safe and Effective: **FDA** — "YES" means that the FDA, in a Panel Report or other Federal Register Notice, found all active ingredients in the product safe and effective for that use. "NO" means at least one ingredient, the combination of ingredients, or the dosage form lacks evidence of safety or effectiveness.

HRG — "YES" and "NO" is Health Research Group's opinion of the same product. In addition, N/E means that we have not fully evaluated the drug or category of drugs.

Problem: "S(Ingredient)" or "E(Ingredient)" means the particular ingredient lacks evidence of safety or effectiveness.

$ means that HRG believes the product is not a good buy because a less expensive effective treatment, often a single-ingredient generic, is available.

PROBLEM	ALTERNATIVE	PAGE	PRODUCT
SE(Theophylline) , E(Pyrilamine, Guaifenesin*)	Consult a Health Care Professional	33,65	**BRONITIN Asthma Pills**
E(Guaifenesin),* SE(Theophylline)	Consult a Health Care Professional	33,65	**BRONKAID Tablets**
See A Health Care Professional For Diagnosis and Treatment		33,64	**BRONKAID Mist and Mist Suspension**
SE(Theophylline), E(Phenobarbital)	Consult a Health Care Professional	33,65	**BRONKOTABS**
E(Salicylic Acid), $	Generic Benzoyl Peroxide	—	**BUF Acne Cleansing Bar**
E(Buffers), $	Generic Aspirin	7,24	**BUFFERIN, BUFFERIN EXTRA STRENGTH**
E(Buffers), $	Generic Aspirin	7,24	**BUFFERIN, Arthritis Painkiller Strength**
E(Time-Release Form), $	Treat Individual Symptoms	33,49	**C3 Cold Cough Capsules**
$	Generic Antihistamine Pills, If Necessary	—	**CALADRYL Lotion and Cream**
E(Hydrocortisone), $	Keep Clean & Dry; Petroleum Jelly, If Necessary	131,145	**CALDECORT Rectal**
$	See Chart p. 113 For Best Buy	101,115	**CAMALOX**
$	Frequent Soap and Water Rinsing Will Allow Most Minor Bites and Wounds To Heal	—	**CAMPHO-PHENIQUE**
S(Bisacodyl), $	High Liquid, High Fiber Diet	87,98	**CARTER'S LITTLE PILLS**

---

*Guaifenesin lacks evidence of effectiveness as an expectorant, in the judgment of the FDA Advisory Panel. The FDA's Director of OTC Drug Evaluation has indicated that they have started the process of reclassifying guaifenesin as effective as an expectorant. We disagree with this change, and believe that this ingredient is a waste of money.

PRODUCT	USE	INGREDIENTS	SAFE AND EFFECTIVE? FDA	HRG
CEPACOL Mouthwash/Gargle	Mouthwash/ Gargle	Cetylpyridinium Chloride Alcohol, Phosphate Buffers, Aromatics	NO	NO
CEPACOL Throat Lozenges	Sore Throat	Cetylpyridinium Chloride Benzyl Alcohol, Sucrose	NO	NO
CEPACOL Anesthetic Troches	Sore Throat	Cetylpyridinium Chloride Benzocaine, Sucrose	NO	NO
CEPASTAT Spray/Gargle	Sore Throat	Phenol, Glycerin	YES	YES
CEPASTAT Lozenges, Regular and Children's	Sore Throat	Phenol, Menthol	YES	YES
CEROSE Compound Capsules	Cold	Acetaminophen, Phenyl- ephrine HCl., Chlorpheni- ramine Maleate	YES	NO
CHARCOCAPS	Bloating, Fullness, Cramps	Activated Charcoal	NO	NO
CHERACOL	Cough	Codeine Phosphate Guaifenesin, Alcohol	*	NO
CHERACOL D	Cough	Dextromethorphan Hbr. Guaifenesin, Alcohol	*	NO
CHLORASEPTIC Cough Control Lozenges	Cough Sore Throat	Dextromethorphan, Sodium Phenolate, Phenol	YES	NO
CHLORASEPTIC Liquid, Lozenges (Menthol, Cherry), and Spray	Sore Throat	Phenol, Sodium Phenolate	YES	YES

Safe and Effective: **FDA** — "YES" means that the FDA, in a Panel Report or other Federal Register Notice, found all active ingredients in the product safe and effective for that use. "NO" means at least one ingredient, the combination of ingredients, or the dosage form lacks evidence of safety or effectiveness.

HRG — "YES" and "NO" is Health Research Group's opinion of the same product. In addition, N/E means that we have not fully evaluated the drug or category of drugs.

Problem: "S(Ingredient)" or "E(Ingredient)" means the particular ingredient lacks evidence of safety or effectiveness.

$ means that HRG believes the product is not a good buy because a less expensive effective treatment, often a single-ingredient generic, is available.

PROBLEM	ALTERNATIVE	PAGE	PRODUCT
SE(Cetylpyridinium as Antimicrobial), $	Generic Aspirin or Acetaminophen (See Text on Strep Throat)	33,55	**CEPACOL Mouthwash/Gargle**
SE(Cetylpyridinium as Antimicrobial), $	Generic Aspirin or Acetaminophen (See Text on Strep Throat)	33,57	**CEPACOL Throat Lozenges**
SE(Cetylpyridinium as Antimicrobial), $	Generic Aspirin or Acetaminophen (See Text on Strep Throat)	33,57	**CEPACOL Anesthetic Troches**
$	Generic Aspirin or Acetaminophen (See Text on Strep Throat)	33,56	**CEPASTAT Spray/Gargle**
$	Generic Aspirin or Acetaminophen; (See Text on Strep Throat)	33,56	**CEPASTAT Lozenges, Regular and Children's**
S(Phenylephrine), $	Treat Individual Symptoms	33,48	**CEROSE Compound Capsules**
E(Activated Charcoal)	None Needed	101,115	**CHARCOCAPS**
E(Guaifenesin), * $	Productive Cough: Drink Warm Liquids; Dry Cough: Generic Dextromethorphan	33,51	**CHERACOL**
E(Guaifenesin), * $	Productive Cough: Drink Warm Liquids; Dry Cough: Generic Dextromethorphan	33,52	**CHERACOL D**
Irrational Fixed Combination, $	Treat Individual Symptoms	33,54	**CHLORASEPTIC Cough Control Lozenges**
$	Generic Aspirin or Acetaminophen (See Text on Strep Throat)	33,56	**CHLORASEPTIC Liquid Lozenges (Menthol, Cherry) and Spray**

---

*Guaifenesin lacks evidence of effectiveness as an expectorant, in the judgment of the FDA Advisory Panel. The FDA's Director of OTC Drug Evaluation has indicated that they have started the process of reclassifying guaifenesin as effective as an expectorant. We disagree with this change, and believe that this ingredient is a waste of money.

PRODUCT	USE	INGREDIENTS	SAFE AND EFFECTIVE?	
			FDA	HRG
CHLOR-TRIMETON Allergy Syrup, Tablets, Repetabs	Allergy	Chlorpheniramine Maleate	YES	YES
CHLOR-TRIMETON DECONGESTANT Tablets, Long Acting Repetabs	Allergy	Pseudoephedrine Sulfate, Chlorpheniramine Maleate	YES	NO
CHOOZ	Antacid	Calcium Carbonate	YES	YES
CLEAR EYES	Eye Drops	Naphazoline HCl.	YES	N/E
CLEARASIL, CLEARASIL SUPER STRENGTH	Acne	Benzoyl Peroxide	YES	YES
CODEXIN Extra Strength Capsules	Weight Loss	Phenylpropanolamine HCl., Caffeine	YES	NO
COLACE	Laxative	Docusate Sodium	YES	NO
COMFOLAX	Laxative	Docusate Sodium	YES	NO
COMFOLAX PLUS	Laxative	Docusate Sodium, Casanthranol	YES	NO
COMPOZ	Sleep Aid	Pyrilamine Maleate	NO	NO
COMTREX Multi-Symptom Cold Reliever, Liquid, Capsules, Tablets	Cold	Acetaminophen, Phenyl-propanolamine HCl., Chlorpheniramine Maleate Dextromethorphan HBr.	*,**	NO
CONAR Expectorant	Cough	Noscapine, Phenylephrine HCl., Guaifenesin	NO	NO

Safe and Effective: **FDA** — "YES" means that the FDA, in a Panel Report or other Federal Register Notice, found all active ingredients in the product safe and effective for that use. "NO" means at least one ingredient, the combination of ingredients, or the dosage form lacks evidence of safety or effectiveness.

HRG — "YES" and "NO" is Health Research Group's opinion of the same product. In addition, N/E means that we have not fully evaluated the drug or category of drugs.

Problem: "S (Ingredient)" or "E (Ingredient)" means the particular ingredient lacks evidence of safety or effectiveness.

$ means that HRG believes the product is not a good buy because a less expensive effective treatment, often a single-ingredient generic, is available.

PROBLEM	ALTERNATIVE	PAGE	PRODUCT
$	Generic Chlorpheni-ramine, If Needed	33,60	**CHLOR-TRIMETON Allergy Syrup, Tablets, Repetabs**
S(Pseudoephedrine), $	Generic Chlorpheni-ramine, If Needed	33,60	**CHLOR-TRIMETON DECONGESTANT Tablets, Long Acting Repetabs**
Occasional Use Only, $	Baking Soda	101,114	**CHOOZ**
	OTC Eye Drops Not Needed	—	**CLEAR EYES**
$	Generic Benzoyl Peroxide	—	**CLEARASIL CLEARASIL SUPER STRENGTH**
SE(Phenylpropano-lamine)	Eat a Bit Less, Exercise More: Lose a Pound a Week	67,75	**CODEXIN Extra Strength Capsules**
S(Docusate Sodium), $	High Liquid, High Fiber Diet	87,99	**COLACE**
S(Docusate Sodium), $	High Liquid, High Fiber Diet	87,99	**COMFOLAX**
S(Docusate Sodium, Casanthranol), $	High Liquid, High Fiber Diet	87,99	**COMFOLAX PLUS**
SE(Pyrilamine Maleate)	Use Non Drug Remedies	147,160	**COMPOZ**
Irrational Combi-nation **, E(Antihis-amine)*	Treat Individual Symptoms	33,47	**COMTREX Multi-Symptom Cold Reliever, Liquid, Capsules, Tablets**
FDA: E(Noscapine, Guaifenesin***); HRG: Also S(Phenyl-ephrine), $	Productive Cough: Drink Warm Liquids; Dry Cough: Generic Dextromethorphan	33,54	**CONAR Syrup**

*Antihistamines, including the ingredient in this product, lack evidence of effectiveness in treating the symptoms of a cold, in the judgment of the FDA Advisory Panel. The FDA's review of prescription drugs also found drugs containing antihistamines to be INEFFEC-TIVE in treatment of a cold. The FDA's Director of OTC Drug Evaluation has indicated that the FDA has started the process of reclassifying antihistamines as effective in OTC pro-ducts for treating a cold. We disagree with this change, and believe that this drug should not be used to treat colds.

**Combination drugs containing ingredients from four categories (analgesic/antipyretic, antihistamine, antitussive, and nasal decongestant) lack evidence of effectiveness, in the judgment of the FDA Advisory Panel. The FDA's Director of OTC Drug Evaluation has indicated that the FDA has started the process of reclassifying this particular combination as effective. We disagree with this charge, and believe that this kind of combination is an unwise "shotgun" approach.

***Guaifenesin lacks evidence of effectiveness as an expectorant, in the judgment of the FDA Advisory Panel. The FDA's Director of OTC Drug Evaluation has indicated that they have started the process of reclassifying guaifenesin as effective as an expectorant. We disagree with this change, and believe that this ingredient is a waste of money.

PRODUCT	USE	INGREDIENTS	SAFE AND EFFECTIVE? FDA	HRG
CONCEPTROL	Contraceptive	Nonoxynol	YES	YES
CONGESPIRIN Chewable Cold Tablets for Children	Cold	Aspirin, Phenylephrine HCl.	YES	NO
CONGESPIRIN for Children Cough Syrup	Cough	Dextromethorphan HBr.	YES	YES
CONGESPIRIN Liquid Cold Medicine	Cold	Acetaminophen, Phenyl-propolamine HCl., Alcohol 10%	YES	NO
CONTAC Time Capsules	Cold, Sinus, Allergy	Phenylpropanolamine HCl. Chlorpheniramine Maleate	YES	NO
CONTAC JR. Liquid	Cough, Cold	Acetaminophen, Alcohol 10%, Phenylpropanolamine HCl., Dextromethorphan HBr.	YES	NO
CONTAC SEVERE Cold Formula	Cold	Acetaminophen, Pseudo-ephedrine HCl., Chlor-pheiramine Maleate, Dex-tromethorphan HBr.	* **	NO
CONTROL Capsules	Weight Loss	Phenylpropanolamine HCl.	YES	NO
COPE	Painkiller	Aspirin, Caffeine, Magnesium Hydroxide, Aluminum Hydroxide	NO	NO
CORICIDIN Cough Syrup	Cough	Dextromethorphan Phenylpropanolamine HCl., Guaifenesin	***	NO
CORICIDIN "D" Decongestant Tablets	Cold, Sinus	Aspirin, Phenylpropano-lamine HCl., Chlorpheni-ramine Maleate	**	NO

Safe and Effective: **FDA** — "YES" means that the FDA, in a Panel Report or other Federal Register Notice, found all active ingredients in the product safe and effective for that use. "NO" means at least one ingredient, the combination of ingredients, or the dosage form lacks evidence of safety or effectiveness.

HRG — "YES" and "NO" is Health Research Group's opinion of the same product. In addition, N/E means that we have not fully evaluated the drug or category of drugs.

Problem: "S(Ingredient)" or "E(Ingredient)" means the particular ingredient lacks evidence of safety or effectiveness.

$ means that HRG believes the product is not a good buy because a less expensive effective treatment, often a single-ingredient generic, is available.

PROBLEM	ALTERNATIVE	PAGE	PRODUCT
Shop for least expensive nonoxynol or octoxynol contraceptive		—	CONCEPTROL
S(Phenylephrine), $	Treat Individual Symptoms	33,48	CONGESPIRIN Chewable Cold Tablets for Children
$	Generic Dextromethorphan	33,52	CONGESPIRIN for Children Cough Syrup
S(Phenylpropano-lamine)	Treat Individual Symptoms	33,44	CONGESPIRIN Liquid Cold Medicine
S(Phenylpropano-lamine), $	Treat Individual Symptoms	33,48	CONTAC Time Capsules
S(Phenylpropano-lamine), $	Treat Individual Symptoms	33,48	CONTAC JR. Liquid
FDA: E(Chlorpheni-ramine,** Irrational Combination*) HRG: Also S(Pseudoephe-drine), $	Treat Individual Symptoms	33,48	CONTAC SEVERE Cold Formula
SE(Phenylpropano-lamine)	Eat a Bit Less, Exercise More: Lose a Pound a Week	67,81	CONTROL Capsules
FDA: E(Caffeine) HRG: Also E(Buf-fers), $	Generic Aspirin	7,29	COPE
FDA: E(Guaifenesin)*** HRG: Also S(Phenyl-propanolamine), $	Treat Individual Symptoms	33,52	CORICIDIN Cough Syrup
E(Chlorpheniramine Maleate), **$	Treat Individual Symptoms	33,48	CORICIDIN "D" Decongestant Tablets

*Combination drugs containing ingredients from four categories (analgesic/antipyretic, antihistamine, antitussive, and nasal decongestant) lack evidence of effectiveness, in the judgment of the FDA Advisory Panel. The FDA's Director of OTC Drug Evaluation has indicated that the FDA has started the process of reclassifying this particular combination as effective. We disagree with this charge, and believe that this kind of combination is an unwise "shotgun" approach.

**Antihistamines, including the ingredient in this product, lack evidence of effectiveness in treating the symptoms of a cold, in the judgment of the FDA Advisory Panel. The FDA's review of prescription drugs also found drugs containing antihistamines to be INEFFECTIVE in treatment of a cold. The FDA's Director of OTC Drug Evaluation has indicated that the FDA has started the process of reclassifying antihistamines as effective in OTC products for treating a cold. We disagree with this change, and believe that this drug should not be used to treat colds.

***Guaifenesin lacks evidence of effectiveness as an expectorant, in the judgment of the FDA Advisory Panel. The FDA's Director of OTC Drug Evaluation has indicated that they have started the process of reclassifying guaifenesin as effective as an expectorant. We disagree with this change, and believe that this ingredient is a waste of money.

			SAFE AND EFFECTIVE?	
PRODUCT	USE	INGREDIENTS	FDA	HRG
CORICIDIN Extra Strength Sinus Headache Tablets	Allergy, Sinus	Acetamaminophen, Phenylpropanolamine, HCl., Chlorpheniramine Maleate	YES	NO
CORICIDIN Tablets	Cold	Aspirin, Chlorpheniramine Maleate	*	NO
CORRECTOL	Laxative	Docusate Sodium, Phenolphthalein	YES	NO
CORTEF Rectal Itch Ointment	Rectal Itch	Hydrocortisone (0.5%)	YES	NO
CORYBAN-D Cough Syrup	Cough, Cold	Dextromethorphan HBr. Guaifenesin, Phenylephrine, HCl., Acetaminophen, Alcohol 7.5%	NO	NO
CO-TYLENOL Cold Formula, Tablets, Capsules and Liquid	Cold, Cough	Acetaminophen, Pseudoephedrine HCl., Chlorpheniramine Maleate Dextromethorphan HBr., Alcohol 7.5% (liquid only)	***	NO
CO-TYLENOL Liquid Cold Formula, Children's	Cold	Acetaminophen, Phenylpropanolamine, HCl., Chlorpheniramine Maleate	*	NO
CREOMULSION	Cough	Beechwood Creosote, Cascara, Ipecac, Menthol, White Pine, Cherry	NO	NO
CUTICURA Antibacterial Medicated Soap	Antimicrobial Soap	Triclocarban	NO	NO
CYSTEX	Painkiller	Salicylamide, Methenamine, Sodium Salicylate, Benzoic Acid	NO	NO
DATRIL, DATRIL 500	Painkiller	Acetaminophen	YES	YES

Safe and Effective: **FDA** — "YES" means that the FDA, in a Panel Report or other Federal Register Notice, found all active ingredients in the product safe and effective for that use. "NO" means at least one ingredient, the combination of ingredients, or the dosage form lacks evidence of safety or effectiveness.

HRG — "YES" and "NO" is Health Research Group's opinion of the same product. In addition, N/E means that we have not fully evaluated the drug or category of drugs.

Problem: "S(Ingredient)" or "E(Ingredient)" means the particular ingredient lacks evidence of safety or effectiveness.

$ means that HRG believes the product is not a good buy because a less expensive effective treatment, often a single-ingredient generic, is available.

PROBLEM	ALTERNATIVE	PAGE	PRODUCT
S(Phenylpropano-lamine), $	Treat Individual Symptoms	33,44	**CORICIDIN Extra Strength Sinus Headache Tablets**
E(Chlorpheniramine)*, $	Treat Individual Symptoms	33,47	**CORICIDIN Tablets**
S(Docusate Sodium, Phenolphthalein), $	High Liquid, High Fiber Diet	87,98	**CORRECTOL**
E(Hydrocortisone), $	Keep Clean & Dry; Petroleum Jelly or Zinc Oxide, If Necessary	131,145	**CORTEF Rectal Itch Ointment**
FDA: E(Guaifenesin),** Irrational Combination HRG: Also S (Phenylephrine), $	Treat Individual Symptoms	33,48	**CORYBAN-D Syrup**
FDA: E(Irrational Combination)*** HRG: Also S(Pseudoephdrine), $	Treat Individual Symptoms	33,47	**CO-TYLENOL Cold Formula, Tablets, Capsules and Liquid**
FDA: E(Chlorpheniramine)* HRG: Also S(Phenylpropanolamine), $	Treat Individual Symptoms	33,47	**CO-TYLENOL Liquid Cold Formula, Children's**
E(Beechwood Creosote, Ipecac), N/E (Menthol, Cascara), $	Productive Cough-Drink Warm Liquids; Dry Cough, Generic Dextromethorphan	33,51	**CREOMULSION**
SE(Triclocarban), $	Plain Soap and Water	—	**CUTICURA Antibacterial Medicated Soap**
SE(Salicylamide), $	Generic Aspirin	7,28	**CYSTEX**
$	Generic Acetaminophen	7,27	**DATRIL, DATRIL 500**

*Antihistamines, including the ingredient in this product, lack evidence of effectiveness in treating the symptoms of a cold, in the judgment of the FDA Advisory Panel. The FDA's review of prescription drugs also found drugs containing antihistamines to be INEFFECTIVE in treatment of a cold. The FDA's Director of OTC Drug Evaluation has indicated that the FDA has started the process of reclassifying antihistamines as effective in OTC products for treating a cold. We disagree with this change, and believe that this drug should not be used to treat colds.

**Guaifenesin lacks evidence of effectiveness as an expectorant, in the judgment of the FDA Advisory Panel. The FDA's Director of OTC Drug Evaluation has indicated that they have started the process of reclassifying guaifenesin as effective as an expectorant. We disagree with this change, and believe that this ingredient is a waste of money.

***Combination drugs containing ingredients from four categories (analgesic/antipyretic, antihistamine, antitussive, and nasal decongestant) lack evidence of effectiveness, in the judgment of the FDA Advisory Panel. The FDA's Director of OTC Drug Evaluation has indicated that the FDA has started the process of reclassifying this particular combination as effective. We disagree with this charge, and believe that this kind of combination is an unwise "shotgun" approach.

PRODUCT	USE	INGREDIENTS	SAFE AND EFFECTIVE? FDA	HRG
DAYCARE Liquid, Capsules	Cold, Cough	Acetaminophen, Phenyl-propanolamine, HCl., Dextro-methorphan HBr., Alcohol 10% (liquid only)	YES	NO
DEBROX Drops	Ear Wax Remover	Carbamide Peroxide in Anhydrous Glycerin	YES	N/E
DEEP-DOWN PAIN RELIEF RUB	External Painkiller	Methyl Salicylate, Methyl Nicotinate, Camphor, Menthol	YES	N/E
DELCID	Antacid	Aluminum Hydroxide, Magnesium Hydroxide	YES	YES
DELFEN FOAM	Contra-ceptive	Nonoxynol	YES	YES
DEMAZIN Repetabs	Cold, Allergy, Sinus	Phenylephrine HCl. Chlorpheniramine Maleate	NO	NO
DEMAZIN Syrup	Cold, Allergy, Sinus	Phenylephrine HCl. Chlorpheniramine Maleate, Alcohol 7.5%	YES	NO
DERMA MEDICONE Ointment	Skin Irritation	Benzocaine, 8-Hydroxy-quinoline sulfate, Menthol, Ichthammol, Zinc Oxide	NO	NO
DERMOLATE Anal-Itch Ointment	Anal Itch	Hydrocortisone (0.5%)	YES	NO
DESENEX Antifungal Powder, Foam, Ointment, Soap Liquid	Athlete's Foot	Undecylenic Acid, Zinc Undecylenate (Powder and and Ointment)	YES	N/E
DESITIN Ointment	Skin	Zinc Oxide, Cod Liver Oil, Talc, Petrolatum, Lanolin Base	YES	N/E
DEWITT'S PILLS for Backache and Joint Pains	Painkiller	Salicylamide, Potassium Nitrate, Uva Ursi, Buchu, Caffeine	NO	NO

Safe and Effective: **FDA** — "YES" means that the FDA, in a Panel Report or other Federal Register Notice, found all active ingredients in the product safe and effective for that use. "NO" means at least one ingredient, the combination of ingredients, or the dosage form lacks evidence of safety or effectiveness.

HRG — "YES" and "NO" is Health Research Group's opinion of the same product. In addition, N/E means that we have not fully evaluated the drug or category of drugs.

Problem: "S(Ingredient)" or "E(Ingredient)" means the particular ingredient lacks evidence of safety or effectiveness.

$ means that HRG believes the product is not a good buy because a less expensive effective treatment, often a single-ingredient generic, is available.

PROBLEM	ALTERNATIVE	PAGE	PRODUCT
S(Phenylpropano-lamine)	Treat Individual Symptoms	33,48	DAYCARE Liquid, Capsules
		—	DEBROX Drops
$	Moist Heat; Generic Aspirin or Acetamino-phen, If Necessary	7,18	DEEP-DOWN PAIN RELIEF RUB
	See Chart p. 113 For Best Buy	101,112	DELCID
Shop for Least Expensive Nonoxynol or Octoxynol Contraceptive		—	DELFEN FOAM
FDA:(Timed-Release Form) HRG: Also S (Phenylephrine), $	Treat Individual Symptoms	33,48	DEMAZIN Repetabs
S(Phenylephrine), $	Treat Individual Symptoms	33,48	DEMAZIN Syrup
E(Ichthammol), $	Generic Petroleum Jelly	—	DERMA MEDICONE Ointment
E(Hydrocortisone), $	Keep Clean & Dry; Pe-troleum Jelly or Zinc Oxide, If Necessary	131,145	DERMOLATE Anal-Itch Ointment
	Cotton Socks, Keep Feet Very Dry	—	DESENEX Antifungal Powder, Foam, Ointment, Soap Liquid
N/E (Talc), $	Generic Petroleum Jelly	—	DESITIN Ointment
S(Salicylamide), E(Sali-cylamide, Caffeine), N/E (Potassium Nitrate, Uva Ursi, Buchu), $	Generic Aspirin	7,28	DEWITT'S PILLS for Backache and Joint Pains

PRODUCT	USE	INGREDIENTS	SAFE AND EFFECTIVE? FDA	HRG
DEXATRIM and DEXATRIM Extra-Strength Capsules	Weight Loss	Phenylpropanolamine HCl., Caffeine	YES	NO
DEXATRIM, Caffeine Free	Weight Loss	Phenylpropanolamine HCl.,	YES	NO
DIALOSE	Laxative	Docusate Potassium	YES	NO
DIALOSE PLUS	Laxative	Docusate Potassium, Casanthranol	YES	NO
DIETAC Maximum Strength Once a Day Diet Capsules, and Pre Meal Diet Aid Capsules	Weight Loss	Phenylpropanolamine HCl.	YES	NO
DIETAC Once a Day Diet Capsules	Weight Loss	Phenylpropanolamine HCl., Caffeine	YES	NO
DI-GEL Tablets, Liquid	Antacid	Aluminum Hydroxide, Magnesium Hydroxide, Simethicone	YES	YES
DIMACOL Liquid, Capsules	Cough, Cold	Dextromethorphan HBr, Guaifenesin, Pseudoephedrine HCl.	*	NO
DIMETANE Tablets, Liquid	Allergy	Brompheniramine Maleate	YES	YES
DIMETANE Decongestant Elixir/Tablets	Cold	Phenylephrine HCl., Brompheniramine Maleate Alcohol 2.3% (in Elixir)	YES	NO
DIOTHANE	Hemorrhoids	Diperodon, 8-Quinolinol Benzoate	NO	NO
DIUREX	Menstrual	Potassium Salicylate, Uva Ursi, Buchu, Salicylamide, Juniper Berries, Methylene Blue, Magnesium Trisilicate	NO	NO
DOAN'S PILLS	Painkiller	Magnesium Salicylate	YES	YES

Safe and Effective: **FDA** — "YES" means that the FDA, in a Panel Report or other Federal Register Notice, found all active ingredients in the product safe and effective for that use. "NO" means at least one ingredient, the combination of ingredients, or the dosage form lacks evidence of safety or effectiveness.

HRG — "YES" and "NO" is Health Research Group's opinion of the same product. In addition, N/E means that we have not fully evaluated the drug or category of drugs.

Problem: "S(Ingredient)" or "E(Ingredient)" means the particular ingredient lacks evidence of safety or effectiveness.

$ means that HRG believes the product is not a good buy because a less expensive effective treatment, often a single-ingredient generic, is available.

PROBLEM	ALTERNATIVE	PAGE	PRODUCT
SE(Phenylpropano-lamine)	Eat a Bit Less, Exercise More; Lose a Pound a Week	67,81	**DEXATRIM and DEXATRIM Extra-Strength Capsules**
SE(Phenylpropano-lamine)	Eat a Bit Less, Exercise More; Lose a Pound a Week	67,81	**DEXATRIM, Caffeine Free**
S(Docusate Potassium), $	High Liquid, High Fiber Diet	87,99	**DIALOSE**
S(Docusate Potassium, Casanthranol , $	High Liquid, High Fiber Diet	87,99	**DIALOSE PLUS**
SE(Phenylpropano-lamine), $	Eat a Bit Less, Exercise More; Lose a Pound a Week	67,81	**DIETAC Maximum Strength Once a Day Diet Cap-sules, and Pre Meal Diet Aid Capsules**
SE(Phenylpropano-lamine), $	Eat A Bit Less; Exercise More: Lose a Pound a Week	67,81	**DIETAC Once a Day Diet Capsules**
E(Simethicone), $	See Chart p. 113 For Best Buy	101,111	**DI-GEL Tablets, Liquid**
FDA: E(Guaifenesin)* HRG: Also S(Pseudo-ephedrine), $	Treat Individual Symptoms	33,48	**DIMACOL Liquid, Capsules**
$	Generic Bromphenir-amine, If Needed	33,60	**DIMETANE Tablets, Liquid**
S(Phenylephrine), $	Treat Individual Symptoms	33,47	**DIMETANE Decongestant Elixir/Tablets**
SE(Diperodon, Intra-rectal Use), E(Dipero-don, External Use), $	Keep Clean & Dry; Pe-roleum Jelly or Zinc Oxide, If Necessary	131,142	**DIOTHANE**
SE(Salicylamide), $	Eat Less Salt; Generic Aspirin or Acetamino-phen If Necessary	7,30	**DIUREX**
$	Generic Aspirin	7,27	**DOAN'S PILLS**

---

*Guaifenesin lacks evidence of effectiveness as an expectorant, in the judgment of the FDA Advisory Panel. The FDA's Director of OTC Drug Evaluation has indicated that they have started the process of reclassifying guaifenesin as effective as an expectorant. We disagree with this change, and believe that this ingredient is a waste of money.

PRODUCT	USE	INGREDIENTS	SAFE AND EFFECTIVE? FDA	HRG
DOAN'S RUB	External Painkiller	Methyl Salicylate, Menthol	YES	N/E
DR. SCHOLL'S Athlete's Foot Gel, Spray, Powder, Spray Powder	Athlete's Foot	Tolnaftate	YES	N/E
DR. SCHOLL'S 2 Drop Corn-Callus Remover	Corn-Callus Remover	Salicylic Acid, Ether, Alcohol	YES	N/E
DONNAGEL	Diarrhea	Kaolin, Pectin, Hyoscyamine Sulfate, Atropine Sulfate, Hyoscine HBr.	NO	NO
DONNAGEL PG	Diarrhea	Kaolin, Pectin, Hyoscyamine Sulfate, Atropine Sulfate, Hyoscine HBr., Powdered Opium	NO	NO
DORCOL Pediatric Cough Syrup	Cough, Cold	Phenylpropanolamine HCl., Dextromethorphan HBr., Guaifenesin, Alcohol 5%	*	NO
DOXIDAN	Laxative	Danthron, Docusate Calcium	YES	NO
DRAMAMINE Liquid, Tablets	Motion Sickness	Dimenhydrinate	YES	YES
DRISTAN-AF Tablets	Cold, Allergy, Sinus	Acetaminophen, Phenylephrine HCl., Chlorpheniramine Maleate, Caffeine	NO	NO
DRISTAN 12-HOUR Nasal Decongestant Capsules	Nasal Decongestant	Phenylephrine HCl., Chlorpheniramine Maleate	NO	NO
DRISTAN Decongestant, Antihistamine, Analgesic Capsules	Cold, Allergy, Sinus	Aspirin, Phenylpropanolamine HCl., Chlorpheniramine Maleate, Caffeine	NO	NO

Safe and Effective: **FDA** — "YES" means that the FDA, in a Panel Report or other Federal Register Notice, found all active ingredients in the product safe and effective for that use. "NO" means at least one ingredient, the combination of ingredients, or the dosage form lacks evidence of safety or effectiveness.

HRG — "YES" and "NO" is Health Research Group's opinion of the same product. In addition, N/E means that we have not fully evaluated the drug or category of drugs.

Problem: "S(Ingredient)" or "E(Ingredient)" means the particular ingredient lacks evidence of safety or effectiveness.

$ means that HRG believes the product is not a good buy because a less expensive effective treatment, often a single-ingredient generic, is available.

PROBLEM	ALTERNATIVE	PAGE	PRODUCT
N/E Methyl Salicylate	Moist Heat; Generic Aspirin or Acetaminophen If Necessary	7,18	DOAN'S RUB
	Cotton Socks, Keep Feet Very Dry	—	DR. SCHOLL'S Athlete's Foot Gel, Spray, Powder, Spray Powder
		—	DR. SCHOLL'S 2 Drop Corn-Callus Remover
SE(Hyoscyamine Sulfate, Atropine Sulfate), E(Kaolin, Pectin), $	Avoid Irritating Foods, Drink 1-2 Quarts Clear Liquids Daily	117,127	DONNAGEL
SE(Atropine, Hyoscyamine) E(Kaolin Pectin)	Avoid Irritating Foods, Drink 1-2 Quarts Clear Liquids Daily	117,127	DONNAGEL PG
FDA: E(Guaifenesin)* HRG: Also S(Phenylpropanolamine), $	Treat Individual Symptoms	33,54	DORCOL Pediatric Cough Syrup
S(Danthron, Docusate Calcium), $	High Liquid, High Fiber Diet	87,98	DOXIDAN
$	Buy Generic Dimenhydrate or Meclizine	117,130	DRAMAMINE Liquid, Tablets
FDA: E(Caffeine) HRG: Also S(Phenylephrine), $	Treat Individual Symptoms	33,48	DRISTAN-AF Tablets
FDA: E(Timed-Release Form) HRG: Also S (Phenylephrine), $	Treat Individual Symptoms	33,43	DRISTAN 12-Hour Nasal Decongestant Capsules
FDA: E(Caffeine) HRG: Also S(Phenylpropanolamine), $	Treat Individual Symptoms	33,49	DRISTAN Decongestant, Antihistamine, Analgesic Capsules

*Guaifenesin lacks evidence of effectiveness as an expectorant, in the judgment of the FDA Advisory Panel. The FDA's Director of OTC Drug Evaluation has indicated that they have started the process of reclassifying guaifenesin as effective as an expectorant. We disagree with this change, and believe that this ingredient is a waste of money.

251

PRODUCT	USE	INGREDIENTS	SAFE AND EFFECTIVE? FDA	HRG
DRISTAN ULTRA COLDS Formula Capsules and Tablets and Nighttime Liquid	Cough, Cold	Acetaminophen, Pseudoephedrine HCl., Dextromethorphan HBr., Chlorpheniramine Maleate, Alcohol 25% (Liquid)	*	NO
DRISTAN LONG LASTING Nasal Mist	Nasal Decongestant	Oxymetazoline HCl.	YES	YES
DRISTAN NASAL MIST	Nasal Decongestant	Phenylephrine HCl., Pheniramine Maleate	NO	NO
DRIXORAL	Allergy	Pseudoephedrine, Dexbrompheniramine	YES	NO
DRY & CLEAR Acne Medication	Acne	Benzoyl Peroxide	YES	YES
DULCOLAX	Laxative	Bisacodyl	YES	NO
DURADYNE	Painkiller	Aspirin, Acetaminophen, Phenacetin, Caffeine	NO	NO
DURAGESIC	Painkiller	Aspirin, Salicylsalicylic Acid (Salsalate)	NO	NO
DURATION Long Acting Topical Nasal Decongestant	Cold, Sinus, Allergy	Oxymetazoline, Menthol, Camphor, Eucalyptol	YES	YES
ECOTRIN	Painkiller	Aspirin	NO	NO
EFFERSYLLIUM	Laxative	Psyllium	YES	YES
EMETROL	Nausea and Vomiting	Invert Sugar, Phosphoric Acid	NO	NO
EMKO BECAUSE Contraceptor/ Contraceptive Foam and Pre-Fil	Contraceptive	Nonoxynol	YES	YES
EMPIRIN	Painkiller	Aspirin	YES	YES
ENCARE	Contraceptive	Nonoxynol	YES	YES
EVAC-U-GEN	Laxative	Yellow Phenolphthalein	YES	NO

Safe and Effective: FDA — "YES" means that the FDA, in a Panel Report or other Federal Register Notice, found all active ingredients in the product safe and effective for that use. "NO" means at least one ingredient, the combination of ingredients, or the dosage form lacks evidence of safety or effectiveness.

HRG — "YES" and "NO" is Health Research Group's opinion of the same product. In addition, N/E means that we have not fully evaluated the drug or category of drugs.

Problem: "S(Ingredient)" or "E(Ingredient)" means the particular ingredient lacks evidence of safety or effectiveness.

$ means that HRG believes the product is not a good buy because a less expensive effective treatment, often a single-ingredient generic, is available.

PROBLEM	ALTERNATIVE	PAGE	PRODUCT
FDA: E(Irrational Combination)* HRG: Also S(Pseudoephedrine), $	Treat Individual Symptoms	33,49	DRISTAN ULTRA COLDS Formula Capsules and Tablets and Nighttime Liquid
Not For Allergies	Generic Oxymetazoline or Phenylephrine Spray	33,43	DRISTAN LONG LASTING Nasal Mist
N/E(Pheniramine for Colds), $	Generic Phenylephrine or Oxymetazoline Spray	33,43	DRISTAN NASAL MIST
S(Pseudoephedrine), $	Treat Individual Symptoms	33,61	DRIXORAL
$	Generic Benzoyl Peroxide	—	DRY & CLEAR Acne Medication
S(Bisacodyl)	High Liquid, High Fiber Diet	87,98	DULCOLAX
S(Phenacetin), E(Caffeine), $	Generic Aspirin	7,28	DURADYNE
SE(Salsalate), $	Generic Aspirin	7,22	DURAGESIC
Not for Allergies, $	Generic Oxymetazoline or Phenylephrine Spray	33,43	DURATION Long Acting Topical Nasal Decongestant
E(Enteric Coating), $	Generic Aspirin	7,26	ECOTRIN
$	High Liquid, High Fiber Diet	87,97	EFFERSYLLIUM
E(Phosphorated Carbohydrate), $	Avoid Solid Foods; Drink 1-2 Quarts Clear Liquids Per Day	117,129	EMETROL
Shop for Least Expensive Octoxynol Contraceptive	Nonoxynol or	—	EMKO BECAUSE Contraceptor/ Contraceptive Foam Pre-Fil
$	Generic Aspirin	7,22	EMPIRIN
Shop for Least Expensive Octoxynol Contraceptive	Nonoxynol or	—	ENCARE
S(Phenolphthalein), $	High Liquid, High Fiber Diet	87,98	EVAC-U-GEN

*Combination drugs containing ingredients from four categories (analgesic/antipyretic, antihistamine, antitussive, and nasal decongestant) lack evidence of effectiveness, in the judgment of the FDA Advisory Panel. The FDA's Director of OTC Drug Evaluation has indicated that the FDA has started the process of reclassifying this particular combination as effective. We disagree with this charge, and believe that this kind of combination is an unwise "shotgun" approach.

PRODUCT	USE	INGREDIENTS	SAFE AND EFFECTIVE?	
			FDA	HRG
EXCEDRIN, EXCEDRIN EXTRA STRENGTH	Painkiller	Aspirin, Acetaminophen, Caffeine	NO	NO
EXCEDRIN P.M.	Sleeping Pill Painkiller	Pyrilamine Maleate, Aspirin, Acetaminophen	NO	NO
EX-LAX Chocolated Laxative and Pills	Laxative	Yellow Phenolphthalein	YES	NO
EX-LAX EXTRA GENTLE	Laxative	Yellow Phenolphthalein and Docusate Sodium	YES	NO
E-Z TRIM	Weight Loss	Phenylpropanolamine HCl.	YES	NO
FEEN-A-MINT	Laxative	Yellow Phenolphthalein	YES	NO
FLEET ENEMA	Laxative	Sodium Bicarbonate, Sodium Phosphate	YES	NO
FLUIDEX	Menstrual	Buchu, Couch Grass, Corn Silk, Hydrangea	NO	NO
FORMULA 44 Cough Mixture	Cough	Dextromethorphan HBr., Doxylamine Succinate, Alcohol 10%	YES	NO
FORMULA 44 Cough Control Disks	Cough, Sore Throat	Dextromethorphan HBr., Benzocaine, Menthol, Anethole, Peppermint Oil	NO	NO
FORMULA 44-D Syrup	Cough, Cold	Dextromethorphan HBr., Phenylpropanolamine HCl. Guaifenesin, Alcohol 10%	*	NO
FOSTEX 5% Peroxide Gel	Acne	Benzoyl Peroxide	YES	YES
FOSTEX Cleanser Bar and Cream	Acne	Sulfur, Salicylic Acid	NO	NO
4 WAY NASAL SPRAY	Cold, Sinus, Allergy	Naphazoline HCl., Phenylephrine HCl., Pyrilamine Maleate	NO	NO

PROBLEM	ALTERNATIVE	PAGE	PRODUCT
E(Caffeine), $	Generic Aspirin	7,29	**EXCEDRIN, EXCEDRIN EXTRA STRENGTH**
SE(Pyrilamine Maleate), $	Non Drug Remedy or Generic Aspirin	147,160 7,29	**EXCEDRIN P.M.**
S(Phenolphthalein), $	High Liquid, High Fiber Diet	87,98	**EX-LAX Chocolated Laxative and Pills**
S(Phenolphthalein, Docusate Sodium), $	High Liquid, High Fiber Diet	87,98	**EX-LAX EXTRA GENTLE**
SE(Phenylpropanolamine)	Eat a Bit Less, Exercise More; Lose a Pound a Week	67,81	**E-Z TRIM**
S(Phenolphthalein), $	High Liquid, High Fiber Diet	87,98	**FEEN-A-MINT**
S(Enema), $	High Liquid, High Fiber Diet	87,100	**FLEET ENEMA**
N/E(Buchu, Couch Grass, Corn Silk, Hydrangea), $	Eat Less Salt; Generic Aspirin or Acetaminophen, If Needed	7,30	**FLUIDEX**
E(Doxylamine), $	Productive Cough: Drink Warm Liquids; Dry Cough: Generic Dextromethorphan	33,54	**FORMULA 44 Cough Mixture**
FDA: E(Menthol, Anethole, Peppermint Oil) HRG: Also Irrational Fixed Combination, $	Treat Individual Symptoms	33,53	**FORMULA 44 Cough Control Disks**
FDA: E(Guaifenesin)* HRG: Also S(Phenylpropanolamine), $	Treat Individual Symptoms	33,44	**FORMULA 44-D Syrup**
$	Generic Benzoyl Peroxide	—	**FOSTEX 5% Peroxide Gel**
E(Salicylic Acid)	Plain Soap and Water; Generic Benzoyl Peroxide	—	**FOSTEX Cleanser Bar and Cream**
FDA: N/E(Pyrilamine Maleate as Nasal Spray) & Irrational Combination HRG: Also S(Naphazoline)	Generic Phenylephrine or Oxymetazoline	33,42	**4 WAY NASAL SPRAY**

---

*Guaifenesin lacks evidence of effectiveness as an expectorant, in the judgment of the FDA Advisory Panel. The FDA's Director of OTC Drug Evaluation has indicated that they have started the process of reclassifying guaifenesin as effective as an expectorant. We disagree with this change, and believe that this ingredient is a waste of money.

PRODUCT	USE	INGREDIENTS	SAFE AND EFFECTIVE? FDA	HRG
4 WAY LONG ACTING Nasal Spray	Decongestant	Xylometazoline HCl.	YES	YES
FREEZONE Corn & Callus Remover	Corn/Callus	Zinc Chloride, Salicylic Acid	NO	NO
GAS X	Anti-Flatulent	Simethicone	YES	NO
	Bloating, Fullness, Cramps	Simethicone	NO	NO
GAVISCON Antacid Tablets/ Suspension	Antacid	Aluminum Hydroxide, Magnesium Trisilicate, Alginic Acid	YES	YES
GELUSIL, GELUSIL-M	Antacid	Aluminium Hydroxide, Magnesium Hydroxide, Simethicone	YES	YES
GELUSIL II	Antacid	Aluminum Hydroxide, Magnesium Hydroxide, Simethicone	YES	YES
GLYCERIN Suppositories	Laxative	Glycerin	YES	NO
GOODY'S Headache Powders	Painkiller	Aspirin, Acetaminophen, Caffeine	NO	NO
HALEY'S MO	Laxative	Mineral Oil, Magnesium Hydroxide	YES	NO
HALLS Mentho-lyptus Cough Drops	Cough	Menthol, Eucalyptus Oil	NO	NO
HALLS Decongestant Cough Formula	Cough	Phenylpropanolamine HCl., Dextromethorphan HBr., Menthol, Eucalyptus Oil	NO	NO
HEAD AND CHEST	Cough, Cold	Phenylpropanolamine HCl., Guaifenesin	*	NO
HEAD AND SHOULDERS Antidandruff Shampoo	Dandruff	Zinc Pyrethione	YES	N/E

Safe and Effective: **FDA** — "YES" means that the FDA, in a Panel Report or other Federal Register Notice, found all active ingredients in the product safe and effective for that use. "NO" means at least one ingredient, the combination of ingredients, or the dosage form lacks evidence of safety or effectiveness.

HRG — "YES" and "NO" is Health Research Group's opinion of the same product. In addition, N/E means that we have not fully evaluated the drug or category of drugs.

Problem: "S(Ingredient)" or "E(Ingredient)" means the particular ingredient lacks evidence of safety or effectiveness.

$ means that HRG believes the product is not a good buy because a less expensive effective treatment, often a single-ingredient generic, is available.

256

PROBLEM	ALTERNATIVE	PAGE	PRODUCT
Not for Allergies	Generic Xylometazoline or Phenylephrine Spray	33,43	4 WAY LONG ACTING Nasal Spray
E(Zinc Chloride)		—	FREEZONE
E(Simethicone)	None Needed	101,115	GAS X
E(Simethicone)	None Needed		
	See Chart p. 113 For Best Buy	101,107, 115	GAVISCON Antacid Tablets/ Suspension
E(Simethicone), $	See Chart p. 113 For Best Buy	101,111 113	GELUSIL, GELUSIL-M
E(Simethicone)	See Chart p. 113 For Best Buy	101,111 113	GELUSIL II
S(Glycerin), $	High Liquid, High Fiber Diet	87,99	GLYCERIN Suppositories
E(Caffeine), $	Generic Aspirin	7,29	GOODY'S Headache Powders
S(Mineral Oil, Magnesium Hydroxide), $	High Liquid, High Fiber Diet	87,99	HALEY'S MO
E(Eucalyptus Oil), $	Productive Cough: Drink Warm Liquids: Dry Cough: Generic Dextromethorphan	33,53	HALLS Mentholyptus Cough Drops
FDA: E(Eucalyptus Oil) HRG: Also S(Phenylpropanolamine), $	Productive Cough: Drink Warm Liquids; Dry Cough: Generic Dextromethorphan	33,54	HALLS Decongestant Cough Formula
E(Guaifenesin), * $	Productive Cough: Drink Warm Liquids; Dry Cough: Generic Dextromethorphan; Cold: Treat Individual Symptoms	33,45	HEAD AND CHEST
		—	HEAD AND SHOULDERS Antidandruff Shampoo

---

*Guaifenesin lacks evidence of effectiveness as an expectorant, in the judgment of the FDA Advisory Panel. The FDA's Director of OTC Drug Evaluation has indicated that they have started the process of reclassifying guaifenesin as effective as an expectorant. We disagree with this change, and believe that this ingredient is a waste of money.

PRODUCT	USE	INGREDIENTS	SAFE AND EFFECTIVE?	
			FDA	HRG
HEADWAY	Cold, Sinus, Allergy	Acetaminophen, Phenyl-propanolamine HCl., Chlorpheniramine Maleate	YES	NO
HEET	External Painkiller	Methyl Salicylate, Capsicum, Camphor, Menthol, Methyl Nicotinate, Alcohol	YES	N/E
HEMORRIN	Hemorrhoids	Bismuth Subgallate, Bismuth Resorcin Compound, Peruvian Balsam, Zinc Oxide	NO	NO
HOLD 4 HOUR Cough Suppressant Lozenges	Cough	Dextromethorphan	YES	YES
HYDROCIL Instant	Laxative	Psyllium	YES	YES
ICY HOT BALM and Rub	External Analgesic	Methyl Salicylate Menthol	YES	N/E
INTERCEPT Contraceptive Inserts	Contraceptive	Nonoxynol	YES	YES
JOHNSON AND JOHNSON First Aid Cream	Skin Wound Protectant	Cetyl Alcohol, Glycerol Stearate, Isopropyl Palmitate Stearyl Alcohol, Synthetic Beeswax	NO	NO
KAODENE	Diarrhea	Kaolin, Pectin	NO	NO
KAODENE with Paregoric	Diarrhea	Kaolin, Pectin Paregoric	NO	NO
KAOPECTATE, Kaopectate Concentrate	Diarrhea	Kaolin, Pectin	NO	NO
KASOF	Laxative	Docusate Potassium	YES	NO
KONSYL	Laxative	Psyllium	YES	YES
L.A. FORMULA	Laxative	Psyllium	YES	YES

PROBLEM	ALTERNATIVE	PAGE	PRODUCT
S(Phenylpropano-lamine), $	Treat Individual Symptoms	33,48	**HEADWAY**
$	Moist Heat; Generic Aspirin or Acetamino-phen, If Necessary	7,18	**HEET**
E(Bismuth Subgallate, Peruvian Balsam), $	Keep Clean & Dry; Pe-troleum Jelly or Zinc Oxide, If Necessary	131,144	**HEMORRIN**
$	Productive Cough: Drink Warm Liquids; Dry Cough: Generic Dextromethorphan	33,52	**HOLD 4 HOUR Cough Suppres-sant Lozenges**
$	High Liquid, High Fiber Diet	87,97	**HYDROCIL Instant**
$	Moist Heat; Generic Aspirin or Acetamino-phen If Necessary	7,18	**ICY HOT BALM and Rub**
Shop For Least Expensive	Nonoxynol or Octoxynol Contraceptive	—	**INTERCEPT Contraceptive Inserts**
E(Cetyl Alcohol), $	Frequent Soap and Water Rinsing Will Allow Most Bites and Wounds to Heal	—	**JOHNSON AND JOHNSON First Aid Cream**
E(Kaolin, Pectin), $	Avoid Irritating Foods, Drink 1-2 Quarts Clear Liquids Daily	117,127	**KAODENE**
E(Kaolin, Pectin), $	Avoid Irritating Foods, Drink 1-2 Quarts Clear Liquids Daily	117,127	**KAODENE with Paregoric**
E(Kaolin, Pectin), $	Avoid Irritating Foods, Drink 1-2 Quarts Clear Liquids Daily	117,127	**KAOPECTATE, Kaopectate Concentrate**
S(Docusate Potas-sium), $	High Liquid, High Fiber Diet	87,99	**KASOF**
$	High Liquid, High Fiber Diet	87,97	**KONSYL**
$	High Liquid, High Fiber Diet	87,97	**L.A. FORMULA**

PRODUCT	USE	INGREDIENTS	SAFE AND EFFECTIVE?	
			FDA	HRG
LIQUIPRIN	Painkiller	Acetaminophen	YES	YES
LISTERINE Antiseptic	Mouth-wash, Antiseptic	Thymol, Eucalyptol, Methyl Salicylate, Menthol	NO	NO
LYDIA E. PINKHAM Tablets	Menstrual	Jamaica Dogwood, Pleurisy Root, Licor-ice, Ferrous Sulfate	NO	NO
MAALOX #1, #2, Tablets, TC, Suspension	Antacid	Aluminum Hydrox-ide, Magnesium Hy-droxide	YES	YES
MAALOX PLUS Tablets, Suspension	Antacid	Aluminum Hydroxide, Magnesium Hydroxide, Simethicone	YES	YES
MALTSUPEX	Laxative	Malt Soup Extract	YES	YES
MAREZINE	Motion Sickness	Cyclizine	YES	YES
MEASURIN	Painkiller	Aspirin	YES	YES
MEDI-QUIK Anti-septic Anesthetic First Aid Spray	First Aid Spray	Lidocaine, Benzalkonium Chloride, Camphor	YES	N/E
MENTHOLATUM Deep Heating Rub and Lotion	External Painkiller	Methyl Salicylate, Menthol	YES	N/E
MERCURO-CHROME II Antiseptic/Double Anesthetic First Aid Spray/Liquid	Skin Wound Cleanser	Lidocaine, Benzalkonium Chloride, Menthol, Isopropyl Alcohol	YES	N/E
METAMUCIL	Laxative	Psyllium	YES	YES
MIDOL	Menstrual	Aspirin, Cinnamedrine, Caffeine	NO	NO
MILK OF MAGNESIA	Laxative	Magnesium Hydroxide	YES	NO

Safe and Effective: **FDA** — "YES" means that the FDA, in a Panel Report or other Federal Register Notice, found all active ingredients in the product safe and effective for that use. "NO" means at least one ingredient, the combination of ingredients, or the dosage form lacks evidence of safety or effectiveness.

HRG — "YES" and "NO" is Health Research Group's opinion of the same product. In addition, N/E means that we have not fully evaluated the drug or category of drugs.

Problem: "S (Ingredient)" or "E (Ingredient)" means the particular ingredient lacks evidence of safe-ty or effectiveness.

$ means that HRG believes the product is not a good buy because a less expensive effective treatment, often a single-ingredient generic, is available.

PROBLEM	ALTERNATIVE	PAGE	PRODUCT
$	Generic Acetaminophen	7,27	**LIQUIPRIN**
E(Thymol, Eucalyptol Methyl Salicylate, Menthol As Anti-microbials), $	No Medicine Necessary	33,55	**LISTERINE**
E(Jamaica Dog-wood, Pleurisy Root, Licorice), $	Generic Aspirin or Acetaminophen, Eat Less Salt	7,30	**LYDIA E. PINKHAM Tablets**
	See Chart p. 113 For Best Buy	101,112	**MAALOX #1, #2 Tablets, TC, Suspension**
E(Simethicone), $	See Chart p. 113 For Best Buy	101,111	**MAALOX PLUS Tablets, Suspension**
$	High Liquid, High Fiber Diet	87,97	**MALTSUPEX**
$	Generic cyclizine, meclizine	117,130	**MAREZINE**
$	Generic Aspirin	7,22	**MEASURIN**
$	Frequent Soap and Water Rinsing Will Allow Most Minor Bites and Wounds To Heal	7,18	**MEDI-QUIK Anti-septic Anesthetic First Aid Spray**
$	Moist Heat; Generic Aspirin or Acetamino-phen, If Necessary	7,18	**MENTHOLATUM Deep Heating Rub and Lotion**
$	Frequent Soap and Water Rinsing Will Allow Most Minor Bites and Wounds To Heal	—	**MERCURO-CHROME II Antiseptic/Double Anesthetic First Aid Spray/Liquid**
$	High Liquid, High Fiber Diet	87,97	**METAMUCIL**
E(Cinnamedrine), $	Generic Aspirin or Acetaminophen, Eat Less Salt	7,30	**MIDOL**
S(Magnesium Hydroxide), $	High Liquid, High Fiber Diet	87,98	**MILK OF MAGNESIA,**

PRODUCT	USE	INGREDIENTS	SAFE AND EFFECTIVE? FDA	HRG
MINIT-RUB	External Painkiller	Methyl Salicylate, Menthol, Camphor	YES	N/E
MITROLAN	Laxative	Calcium Polycarbophil	YES	YES
MOBIGESIC	Painkiller	Magnesium Salicylate, Phenyltoloxamine Citrate	NO	NO
MOBISYL	External Painkiller	Triethanolamine Salicylate	NO	NO
MODANE	Laxative	Danthron	YES	NO
MODANE BULK	Laxative	Psyllium	YES	YES
MODANE SOFT	Laxative	Docusate Sodium	YES	NO
MOMENTUM Muscular Backache Formula	Painkiller	Aspirin, Salicylsalicylic Acid (Salsalate), Phenyltoloxamine Citrate	NO	NO
MURINE Regular Formula	Eyedrops	Glycerin, Potassium Chloride, Sodium Chloride, Sodium Phosphate	YES	N/E
MURINE PLUS	Eye Drops	Tetrahydrozoline	YES	N/E
MYCIGUENT	Skin Antibiotic	Neomycin Sulfate	YES	NO
MYCITRACIN	Skin Antibiotic	Bacitracin, Polymyxin B, Neomycin Sulfate	YES	NO
MYLANTA, MYLANTA II Tablets and Suspension	Antacid	Aluminum Hydroxide, Magnesium Hydroxide, Simethicone	YES	YES
MYLICON-80, MYLICON Tablets and Drops	Antiflatulent Bloating, Fullness, Cramps	Simethicone Simethicone	YES NO	NO NO

Safe and Effective: FDA — "YES" means that the FDA, in a Panel Report or other Federal Register Notice, found all active ingredients in the product safe and effective for that use. "NO" means at least one ingredient, the combination of ingredients, or the dosage form lacks evidence of safety or effectiveness.

HRG — "YES" and "NO" is Health Research Group's opinion of the same product. In addition, N/E means that we have not fully evaluated the drug or category of drugs.

Problem: "S(Ingredient)" or "E(Ingredient)" means the particular ingredient lacks evidence of safety or effectiveness.

$ means that HRG believes the product is not a good buy because a less expensive effective treatment, often a single-ingredient generic, is available.

PROBLEM	ALTERNATIVE	PAGE	PRODUCT
$	Moist Heat; Generic Aspirin or Acetaminophen If Necessary	7,18	**MINIT-RUB**
$	High Liquid, High Fiber Diet	87,97	**MITROLAN**
E(Phenyltoloxamine Citrate), $	Generic Aspirin	7,29	**MOBIGESIC**
E(Triethanolamine Salicylate), $	Moist Heat; Generic Aspirin or Acetaminophen If Necessary	7,18	**MOBISYL**
S(Danthron), $	High Liquid, High Fiber Diet	87,98	**MODANE**
$	High Liquid, High Fiber Diet	87,97	**MODANE BULK**
S(Docusate Sodium), $	High Liquid, High Fiber Diet	87,99	**MODANE SOFT**
SE(Salsalate), E(Phenyltoloxamine Citrate), $	Generic Aspirin	7,29	**MOMENTUM Muscular Backache Formula**
	No OTC Eye Drops Needed	—	**MURINE Regular Formula**
	No OTC Eye Drops Needed	—	**MURINE PLUS**
S(Neomycin Sulfate), $	Frequent Soap and Water Rinsing Will Allow Most Minor Bites and Wounds To Heal	—	**MYCIGUENT**
S(Neomycin Sulfate), $	Frequent Soap and Water Rinsing Will Allow Most Minor Bites and Wounds To Heal	—	**MYCITRACIN**
E(Simethicone)	See Chart p. 113 For Best Buy	101,112	**MYLANTA, MYLANTA II Tablets and Suspension**
E(Simethicone), $	None Needed	101,115	**MYLICON-80,**
E(Simethicone), $	None Needed		**MYLICON Tablets and Drops**

PRODUCT	USE	INGREDIENTS	SAFE AND EFFECTIVE? FDA	HRG
MYOFLEX CREME	External Analgesic	Triethanolamine Salicylate	NO	NO
NATURE'S REMEDY	Laxative	Aloe, Cascara Sagrada	YES	NO
NEOLOID Castor Oil	Laxative	Castor Oil	YES	NO
NEOSPORIN Ointment	Skin Anti-biotic	Neomycin Sulfate, Bacitracin Zinc, Polymyxin B Sulfate, White Petrolatum	YES	NO
NEO-SYNEPHRINE Nasal Spray, Drops, Jelly	Nasal Decongestant	Phenylephrine HCl.	YES	YES
NEO-SYNEPHRINE 12 Hour Nasal Spray	Nasal Decongestant	Oxymetazoline HCl.	YES	YES
NEO-SYNEPHRINE II Long Acting Nasal Spray, Nose Drops	Nasal Decongestant	Oxymetazoline HCl.	YES	YES
NEO-SYNEPHRI-NOL DAY RELIEF Capsules	Decongestant	Pseudoephedrine HCl.	NO	NO
NERVINE	Sleeping Pill	Pyrilamine Maleate	NO	NO
NOVAHISTINE Cold Tablets and Elixir	Cold, Sinus, Allergy	Phenylpropanolamine HCl., Chlorpheniramine Maleate, Alcohol 5% (Elixir)	YES	NO
NOVAHISTINE Cough Formula	Cough	Dextromethorphan HBr., Guaifenesin, Alcohol 7.5%	*	NO

Safe and Effective: **FDA** — "YES" means that the FDA, in a Panel Report or other Federal Register Notice, found all active ingredients in the product safe and effective for that use. "NO" means at least one ingredient, the combination of ingredients, or the dosage form lacks evidence of safety or effectiveness.

HRG — "YES" and "NO" is Health Research Group's opinion of the same product. In addition, N/E means that we have not fully evaluated the drug or category of drugs.

Problem: "S(Ingredient)" or "E(Ingredient)" means the particular ingredient lacks evidence of safety or effectiveness.

$ means that HRG believes the product is not a good buy because a less expensive effective treatment, often a single-ingredient generic, is available.

264

PROBLEM	ALTERNATIVE	PAGE	PRODUCT
E(Triethanolamine Salicylate), $	Moist Heat; Generic Aspirin or Acetaminophen, If Necessary	7,18	**MYOFLEX CREME**
S(Aloe, Cascara Sagrada), $	High Liquid, High Fiber Diet	87,98	**NATURE'S REMEDY**
S(Castor Oil), $	High Liquid, High Fiber Diet	87,98	**NEOLOID** Castor Oil
S(Neomycin Sulfate), $	Frequent Soap and Water Rinsing Will Allow Most Minor Bites and Wounds To Heal. *Disregard* Current Neosporin Ad: "If it needs a bandage, it needs Neosporin"	—	**NEOSPORIN Ointment**
Not For Allergy	Generic Phenylephrine or Oxymetazoline Spray	33,43	**NEO-SYNEPHRINE Nasal Spray, Drops, Jelly**
Not For Allergy	Generic Oxymetazoline or Phenylephrine Spray	33,43	**NEO-SYNEPHRINE 12 Hour Nasal Spray**
Not For Allergy	Generic Oxymetazoline or Phenylephrine Spray	33,43	**NEO-SYNEPHRINE II Long Acting Nasal Spray, Nose Drops**
E(Timed Release Form)	Generic Oxymetazoline or Phenylephrine Spray	33,44, 49	**NEO-SYNEPHRI-NOL DAY RELIEF Capsules**
SE(Pyrilamine Maleate), $	Use Non-Drug Remedies	147,160	**NERVINE**
S(Phenylpropanolamine), E(Chlorpheniramine), $	Treat Individual Symptoms	33,47	**NOVAHISTINE Cold Tablets and Elixir**
E(Guaifenesin), * $	Productive Cough: Drink Warm Liquids; Dry Cough: Generic Dextromethorphan	33,52	**NOVAHISTINE Cough Formula**

---

*Guaifenesin lacks evidence of effectiveness as an expectorant, in the judgment of the FDA Advisory Panel. The FDA's Director of OTC Drug Evaluation has indicated that they have started the process of reclassifying guaifenesin as effective as an expectorant. We disagree with this change, and believe that this ingredient is a waste of money.

PRODUCT	USE	INGREDIENTS	SAFE AND EFFECTIVE?	
			FDA	HRG
NOVAHISTINE Cough and Cold Formula	Cough, Cold, Allergy	Dextromethorphan HBr., Pseudoephedrine HCl., Chlorphenramine Maleate, Alcohol 5%	YES	NO
NOVAHISTINE Sinus Tablets	Cold, Sinus Allergy	Acetaminophen, Pseudo-ephedrine HCl., Chlor-pheniramine Maleate	YES	NO
NUPERCAINAL Ointment	Hemorrhoids	Dibucaine	NO	NO
NUPERCAINAL Suppositories	Hemorrhoids	Dibucaine, Zinc Oxide, Cocoa Butter, Bismuth Subgallate	NO	NO
NYQUIL	Cold	Acetaminophen, Dextro-methorphan HBr., Ephe-drine Sulfate, Doxylamine Succinate, Alcohol 25%	NO	NO
NYTOL DPH	Sleeping Pill	Diphenhydramine	YES	NO
ODRINIL	Menstrual, Premenstrual	Buchu, Uva Ursi, Corn Silk, Juniper, Caffeine	NO	NO
ORNEX Deconges-tant Analgesic Capsules - No Drowsiness Formula	Cold	Acetaminophen, Phenyl-propanolamine	YES	NO
ORTHO-CREME	Contraceptive	Nonoxynol	YES	YES
ORTHO-GYNOL	Contraceptive	P-Diisobutyl-phenoxypoly-ethoxyethanol	YES	YES
OTRIVIN	Nasal Decongestant	Xylometazoline HCl.	YES	YES
OXY-5 and OXY-10 Lotion and OXY-WASH	Acne	Benzoyl Peroxide	YES	YES
OXY SCRUB	Acne	Sodium Tetraborate Decahydrate	NO	NO

Safe and Effective: **FDA** — "YES" means that the FDA, in a Panel Report or other Federal Register Notice, found all active ingredients in the product safe and effective for that use. "NO" means at least one ingredient, the combination of ingredients, or the dosage form lacks evidence of safety or effectiveness.

HRG — "YES" and "NO" is Health Research Group's opinion of the same product. In addition, N/E means that we have not fully evaluated the drug or category of drugs.

Problem: "S(Ingredient)" or "E(Ingredient)" means the particular ingredient lacks evidence of safe-ty or effectiveness.

$ means that HRG believes the product is not a good buy because a less expensive effective treatment, often a single-ingredient generic, is available.

266

PROBLEM	ALTERNATIVE	PAGE	PRODUCT
S(Pseudoephedrine), E(Chlorpheniramine), $	Treat Individual Symptoms	33,48	**NOVAHISTINE Cough and Cold Formula**
S(Pseudoephedrine), E(Chlorpheniramine), $	Treat Individual Symptoms	33,47	**NOVAHISTINE Sinus Tablets**
SE(Dibucaine), $	Keep Clean & Dry; Petroleum Jelly or Zinc Oxide If Necessary	131,142	**NUPERCAINAL Ointment**
SE(Dibucaine), E(Bismuth Subgallate), $	Keep Clean & Dry; Petroleum Jelly or Zinc Oxide If Necessary	131,142	**NUPERCAINAL Suppositories**
FDA: E(Ephedrine Sulfate), Irrational Combination* HRG: S(Ephedrine), E(Doxylamine), $	Treat Individual Symptoms	33,48	**NYQUIL**
SE(Diphenhydramine)	Use Non-Drug Remedies	147,159	**NYTOL DPH**
E(Buchu, Uva Ursi, Corn Silk, Juniper)	Generic Aspirin or Acetaminophen, Eat Less Salt	7,30	**ODRINIL**
S(Phenylpropanolamine), $	Treat Individual Symptoms	33,44	**ORNEX Decongestant Analgesic Capsules - No Drowsiness Formula**
Shop For Least Expensive Octoxynol Contraceptive	Nonoxynol or	—	**ORTHO-CREME**
Shop For Least Expensive Octoxynol Contraceptive	Nonoxynol or	—	**ORTHO-GYNOL**
Not For Allergy	Generic Xylometazoline or Phenylephrine Spray	33,43	**OTRIVIN**
$	Generic Benzoyl Peroxide	—	**OXY-5 and OXY-10 Lotion and OXY-WASH**
E(Abrasive Materials)	Generic Benzoyl Peroxide	—	**OXY-SCRUB**

---

*Combination drugs containing ingredients from four categories (analgesic/antipyretic, antihistamine, antitussive, and nasal decongestant) lack evidence of effectiveness, in the judgment of the FDA Advisory Panel. The FDA's Director of OTC Drug Evaluation has indicated that FDA has started the process of reclassifying this particular combination as effective. We disagree with this charge, and believe that this kind of combination is an unwise "shotgun" approach.

PRODUCT	USE	INGREDIENTS	SAFE AND EFFECTIVE?	
			FDA	HRG
PAMPRIN	Menstrual	Acetaminophen, Pyrilamine Maleate, Pamabrom	YES	NO
PARAPECTOLIN	Anti-Diarrheal	Paregoric, Kaolin, Pectin	NO	NO
PAZO Ointment	Hemorrhoids	Benzocaine, Ephedrine Sulfate, Camphor, Zinc Oxide, Petrolatum, Lanolin	NO	NO
PAZO Suppositories	Hemorrhoids	Benzocaine, Ephedrine Sulfate, Camphor, Zinc Oxide, Hydrogenated Vegetable Oil	NO	NO
PEPTO BISMOL	Diarrhea	Bismuth Subsalicylate	*	NO
	Nausea and Vomiting	Bismuth Subsalicylate	NO	NO
	Upset Stomach (Over-Indulgence)	Bismuth Subsalicylate	YES	NO
PERCOGESIC	Painkiller	Acetaminophen, Phenyltoloxamine	NO	NO
PERDIEM	Laxative	Psyllium, Senna	YES	NO
PERI-COLACE	Laxative	Casanthranol, Docusate Sodium	YES	NO
PERTUSSIN 8-Hour Cough Formula	Cough	Dextromethorphan HBr. 9.5% Alcohol	YES	YES
PERTUSSIN Cough Syrup for Children	Cough	Dextromethorphan, Guaifenesin	**	NO

PROBLEM	ALTERNATIVE	PAGE	PRODUCT
E(Pyrilamine Maleate), $	Generic Aspirin or Acetaminophen, Eat Less Salt	7,18	**PAMPRIN**
E(Kaolin, Pectin), $	Avoid Irritating Foods, Drink 1-2 Quarts Clear Liquids Daily	117,125	**PARAPECTOLIN**
SE(Camphor), $	Keep Clean & Dry; Petroleum Jelly or Zinc Oxide, If Necessary	131,142	**PAZO Ointment**
SE(Camphor), $ E(Benzocaine)	Keep Clean & Dry; Petroleum Jelly or Zinc Oxide If Necessary	131,142	**PAZO Suppositories**
E(Bismuth Subsalicylate), * $	Avoid Irritating Foods, Drink 1-2 Quarts Clear Liquids Daily	117,125	**PEPTO-BISMOL**
E(Bismuth Subsalicylate), $	Avoid Solid Foods; Drink 1-2 Quarts Clear Liquids Daily	117,129	**PEPTO-BISMOL**
E(Bismuth Subsalicylate), $	None	101,110	**PEPTO-BISMOL**
E(Phenyltoloxamine), $	Generic Acetaminophen	7,29	**PERCOGESIC**
S(Senna), $	High Liquid, High Fiber Diet	87,98	**PERDIEM**
S(Casanthranol, Docusate Sodium), $	High Liquid, High Fiber Diet	87,99	**PERI-COLACE**
$	Productive Cough: Drink Warm Liquids; Dry Cough: Generic Dextromethorphan	33,52	**PERTUSSIN 8-Hour Cough Formula**
E(Guaifenesin)** $	Productive Cough: Drink Warm Liquids; Dry Cough: Generic Dextromethorphan	33,52	**PERTUSSIN Cough Syrup for Children**

---

*Bismuth subsalicylate lacks evidence of effectiveness as an antidiarrheal ingredient, in the judgment of the FDA Advisory Panel. The FDA's Director of OTC Drug Evaluation has indicated that the FDA has started the process of reclassifying it as effective in treating some symptoms of diarrhea. We disagree with this charge, and believe this drug is unnecessary.

**Guaifenesin lacks evidence of effectiveness as an expectorant, in the judgment of the FDA Advisory Panel. The FDA's Director of OTC Drug Evaluation has indicated that they have started the process of reclassifying guaifenesin as effective as an expectorant. We disagree with this change, and believe that this ingredient is a waste of money.

PRODUCT	USE	INGREDIENTS	SAFE AND EFFECTIVE? FDA	HRG
PHILLIPS MILK OF MAGNESIA	Antacid	Magnesium Hydroxide	YES	YES
	Laxative		YES	NO
PHOSPHALJEL	Antacid	Aluminum Phosphate Gel	YES	YES
POLYSPORIN Ointment	Skin Antibiotic	Polymyxin B. Bacitracin, Zinc, White Petrolatum	YES	N/E
PONTOCAINE Ointment	Hemorrhoids	Tetracaine HCl., Menthol, White Petrolatum, White Wax	NO	NO
PONTOCAINE Cream	Hemorrhoids	Tetracaine HCl., Methylparaben, Sodium Bisulfite	NO	NO
PREPARATION H Ointment, Suppositories	Hemorrhoids	Shark Liver Oil Live Yeast Cell Derivative	NO	NO
PRETTS	Weight Loss	Alginic Acid Sodium Carboxymethylcellulose	NO	NO
PRIMATENE TABLETS ("M" or "P")	Asthma	Phenobarbital, Theophylline Ephedrine HCl, Pyrilamine Maleate (M) or Phenobarital (P)	NO	NO
PRIMATENE MIST Suspension	Asthma	Epinephrine, Alcohol	YES	YES
PROCTODON	Hemorrhoids	Diperodon HCl	NO	NO
PROLAMINE Super Strength	Weight Loss	Phenylpropanolamine	YES	NO
PYRROXATE Capsules	Cold, Allergy, Sinus	Acetaminophen, Phenylpropanolamine HCL, Chlorpheniramine Maleate	YES	NO

Safe and Effective: FDA — "YES" means that the FDA, in a Panel Report or other Federal Register Notice, found all active ingredients in the product safe and effective for that use. "NO" means at least one ingredient, the combination of ingredients, or the dosage form lacks evidence of safety or effectiveness.

HRG — "YES" and "NO" is Health Research Group's opinion of the same product. In addition, N/E means that we have not fully evaluated the drug or category of drugs.

Problem: "S(Ingredient)" or "E(Ingredient)" means the particular ingredient lacks evidence of safety or effectiveness.

$ means that HRG believes the product is not a good buy because a less expensive effective treatment, often a single-ingredient generic, is available.

PROBLEM	ALTERNATIVE	PAGE	PRODUCT
May Cause Diarrhea S(Magnesium Hydroxide), $ $	See Chart, p. 113 For Best Buy High Liquid, High Fiber Diet	101,115 87,98	**PHILLIPS MILK OF MAGNESIA**
$	See Chart p. 113 For Best Buy	101,114	**PHOSPHALJEL**
$	Frequent Soap and Water Rinsing Will Allow Most Minor Bites and Wounds To Heal	—	**POLYSPORIN** Ointment
E(Tetracaine HCl), $	Keep Clean and Dry; Petroleum Jelly or Zinc Oxide, If Necessary	131,142	**PONTOCAINE** Ointment
E(Tetracaine HCl), $	Keep Clean and Dry; Petroleum Jelly or Zinc Oxide, If Necessary	131,142	**PONTOCAINE** Cream
E(Live Yeast Cell Derivative, Shark Liver Oil in Amount Provided), $	Keep Clean and Dry; Petroleum Jelly or Zinc Oxide, If Necessary	131,144	**PREPARATION H** Ointment, Suppositories
E(Alginic Acid, Sodium Carboxymethylcellulose), $	Eat a Bit Less, Exercise More; Lose a Pound a Week	67,83	**PRETTS**
E(Pyrilamine Maleate, M; Phenobarbital, P); SE(Theophylline)	Consult a Health Care Professional	33,66	**PRIMATENE TABLETS** ("M" or "P")
See a Health Care Professional for Diagnosis and Treatment		33,64	**PRIMATENE MIST** Suspension
S(Diperodon for Intrarectal Use), E(Diperodon for External Use), $	Keep Clean and Dry; Petroleum Jelly or Zinc Oxide, If Necessary	131,142	**PROCTODON**
SE (Phenylpropanolamine)	Eat a Bit Less, Exercise More; Lose a Pound a Week	67,81	**PROLAMINE** Super Strength
S (Phenylpropanolamine), $	Treat Individual Symptoms	33,36	**PYRROXATE** Capsules

PRODUCT	USE	INGREDIENTS	SAFE AND EFFECTIVE? FDA	HRG
QUIET WORLD	Sleeping Pill	Aspirin, Acetaminophen, Pyrilamine Maleate	NO	NO
Q-VEL Muscle Relaxant and Pain Relief	Nocturnal Leg Muscle Cramps	Quinine Sulfate	NO	NO
RECTAL MEDICONE Unguent and Suppositories	Hemorrhoids	Benzocaine, Menthol, Zinc Oxide, Peruvian Balsam, Petrolatum, Lanolin (unguent), 8 Hydroxyquinoline, Cocoa Butter (Supp.) Veg. Oil (Supp.)	NO	NO
REGUTOL	Laxative	Docusate Sodium	YES	NO
RHEABAN	Diarrhea	Activated Attapulgite	**	NO
RID	Lice	Pyrethrins, Piperonyl Butoxide Technical 3%, Equivalent to 2.4% (Butoylcarbityl) (6 Propylpiperonyl) Ether and to 0.6 Related Compounds	YES	N/E
RIOPAN Tablet/ Chewable Tablet/ Suspension	Antacid	Magaldrate	YES	YES
RIOPAN PLUS	Antacid	Magaldrate, Simethicone	YES	YES
ROBITUSSIN Syrup	Cough	Guaifenesin, Alcohol 3.5%	*	NO
ROBITUSSIN CF Syrup	Cough, Nasal Decongestant	Dextromethorphan HBr., Phenylpropanolamine HCl. Guaifenesin, Alcohol 4.75%	*	NO

Safe and Effective: FDA — "YES" means that the FDA, in a Panel Report or other Federal Register Notice, found all active ingredients in the product safe and effective for that use. "NO" means at least one ingredient, the combination of ingredients, or the dosage form lacks evidence of safety or effectiveness.

HRG — "YES" and "NO" is Health Research Group's opinion of the same product. In addition, N/E means that we have not fully evaluated the drug or category of drugs.

Problem: "S(Ingredient)" or "E(Ingredient)" means the particular ingredient lacks evidence of safety or effectiveness.

$ means that HRG believes the product is not a good buy because a less expensive effective treatment, often a single-ingredient generic, is available.

PROBLEM	ALTERNATIVE	PAGE	PRODUCT
SE (Pyrilamine Maleate) $	Use Non Drug Remedies	147,160	**QUIET WORLD**
SE (Quinine Sulfate)	If Severe, Seek Medical Help	147,153	**Q-VEL Muscle Relaxant and Pain Relief**
E (Benzocaine and Menthol for Intrarectal Use, Peruvian Balsam), $	Keep Clean and Dry; Petroleum Jelly or Zinc Oxide, If Necessary	131,144	**RECTAL MEDICONE Unguent and Suppositories**
S (Docusate Sodium), $	High Liquid, High Fiber Diet	87,99	**REGUTOL**
E (Attapulgite),**$	Avoid Irritating Foods, Drink 1-2 Quarts Clear Liquids Daily	117,126	**RHEABAN**
—	—	—	**RID**
—	See Chart p. 113 For Best Buy	101,115 113	**RIOPAN Tablet/ Chewable Tablet/ Suspension**
E(Simethicone)	See Chart p. 113 For Best Buy	101,111	**RIOPAN PLUS**
E(Guaifenesin),* $	Productive Cough: Drink Warm Liquids; Dry Cough: Generic Dextromethorphan	33,51	**ROBITUSSIN Syrup**
FDA: E(Guaifenesin)* HRG: Also S(Phenylpropanolamine), $	Treat Individual Symptoms	33,54	**ROBITUSSIN CF**

---

*Guaifenesin lacks evidence of effectiveness as an expectorant, in the judgment of the FDA Advisory Panel. The FDA's Director of OTC Drug Evaluation has indicated that they have started the process of reclassifying guaifenesin as effective as an expectorant. We disagree with this change, and believe that this ingredient is a waste of money.

**Attapulgite lacks evidence of effectiveness as an antidiarrheal ingredient, in the judgment of the FDA Advisory Panel. The FDA's Director of OTC Drug Evaluation has indicated that the FDA has started the process of reclassifying it as effective in treating some symptoms of diarrhea. We disagree with this change, and believe this drug is unnecessary.

PRODUCT	USE	INGREDIENTS	SAFE AND EFFECTIVE?	
			FDA	HRG
ROBITUSSIN-DM	Cough	Dextromethorphan HBr., Guaifenesin	*	NO
ROBITUSSIN-DM COUGH CALMERS Lozenges	Cough	Dextromethorphan HBr., Guaifenesin	*	NO
ROBITUSSIN-PE Syrup	Cough, Nasal Decongestant	Guaifenesin, Pseudoephedrine HCl, Alcohol 1.4%	*	NO
ROLAIDS	Antacid	Dihydroxy Aluminum, Sodium Carbonate	YES	YES
ST. JOSEPH ASPIRIN For Children	Painkiller	Aspirin	YES	YES
ST. JOSEPH COLD TABLETS For Children	Cold	Aspirin, Phenylpropanolamine HCL	YES	NO
ST. JOSEPH COUGH SYRUP For Children	Cough	Dextromethorphan	YES	YES
SCOPE	Mouthwash	Cetylpyridinium Chloride, Domiphen Bromide, Glycerin, Sodium Saccharine, Benzoic Acid, Alcohol 18.5%	NO	NO
SELSUN BLUE	Dandruff	Selenium Sulfide	YES	N/E
SEMICID Vaginal Contraceptive Suppositories	Contraceptive	Nonoxynol	YES	YES
SENOKOT	Laxative	Senna	YES	NO
SENOKOT-S	Laxative	Senna, Docusate Sodium	YES	NO
SENSODYNE Toothpaste	Tooth Desensitizing	Strontium Chloride Hexahydrate	NO	NO

Safe and Effective: **FDA** — "YES" means that the FDA, in a Panel Report or other Federal Register Notice, found all active ingredients in the product safe and effective for that use. "NO" means at least one ingredient, the combination of ingredients, or the dosage form lacks evidence of safety or effectiveness.

HRG — "YES" and "NO" is Health Research Group's opinion of the same product. In addition, N/E means that we have not fully evaluated the drug or category of drugs.

Problem: "S(Ingredient)" or "E(Ingredient)" means the particular ingredient lacks evidence of safety or effectiveness.

$ means that HRG believes the product is not a good buy because a less expensive effective treatment, often a single-ingredient generic, is available.

PROBLEM	ALTERNATIVE	PAGE	PRODUCT
E(Guaifenesin), * $	Productive Cough: Drink Warm Liquids; Dry Cough: Generic Dextromethorphan	33,52	**ROBITUSSIN-DM**
E(Guaifenesin), * $	Productive Cough: Drink Warm Liquids; Dry Cough: Generic Dextromethorphan	33,52	**ROBITUSSIN-DM COUGH CALMERS Lozenges**
FDA: E(Guaifenesin)* HRG: Also, S(Pseudoephedrine), $	Productive Cough: Drink Warm Liquids; Dry Cough: Generic Dextromethorphan	33,54	**ROBITUSSIN-PE Syrup**
Occasional Use Only, $	See Chart p. 113 For Best Buy	101,114 113	**ROLAIDS**
$	Generic Aspirin	7,25	**ST. JOSEPH ASPIRIN for Children**
S(Phenylpropanolamine), $	Treat Individual Symptoms	33,44	**ST.JOSEPH COLD TABLETS for Children**
$	Productive Cough: Drink Warm Liquids; Dry Cough: Generic Dextromethorphan	33,52	**ST. JOSEPH COUGH SYRUP for children**
SE(Cetylpyridinium Chloride and Domiphen Bromide as Antimicrobials), $	No Medical Need for Mouthwash	33,55	**SCOPE**
		—	**SELSUN BLUE**
Shop for Least Expensive Nonoxynol or Octoxynol Contraceptive		—	**SEMICID Vaginal Contraceptive Suppositories**
S(Senna), $	High Liquid, High Fiber Diet	87,98	**SENOKOT**
S(Senna, Docusate Sodium), $	High Liquid, High Fiber Diet	87,98	**SENOKOT-S**
E(Strontium Chloride Hexahydrate), $		—	**SENSODYNE Toothpaste**

*Guaifenesin lacks evidence of effectiveness as an expectorant, in the judgment of the FDA Advisory Panel. The FDA's Director of OTC Drug Evaluation has indicated that they have started the process of reclassifying guaifenesin as effective as an expectorant. We disagree with this change, and believe that this ingredient is a waste of money.

PRODUCT	USE	INGREDIENTS	SAFE AND EFFECTIVE? FDA	HRG
SERUTAN	Laxative	Vegetable Hemicellulose Derived from Plantago Ovata	YES	YES
SIMECO	Antacid	Aluminum Hydroxide Magnesium Hydroxide Simethicone	YES	YES
SINAREST Tablets and SINAREST Extra Strength	Sinus	Acetaminophen, Phenyl-propanolamine HCl., Chlorpheniramine Maleate	YES	NO
SINE AID	Sinus	Acetaminophen, Phenyl-propanolamine HCl.	YES	NO
SINE-OFF Tablets	Sinus	Aspirin, Phenylpropano-lamine HCl., Chlorphen-aramine Maleate	YES	NO
SINE-OFF Extra Strength No Drowsiness Formula	Sinus	Acetaminophen, Phenyl-propanolamine HCl.	YES	NO
SINEX Decongestant Nasal Spray	Nasal Decongestant	Phenylephrine HCl., Cetyl-pryridinium HCl.	YES	N/E
SINEX Long Acting Decongest-tant Nasal Spray	Nasal Decongestant	Oxymetazoline HCl.	YES	YES
SINUTAB and SINUTAB Extra Strength Tablets	Sinus	Acetaminophen, Phenyl-propanolamine HCl., Phenyltoloxamine Citrate	NO	NO
666 Cold Preparation	Cough, Cold	Sodium Salicylate Phenylpropanolamine HCl., Ammonium Chlor-ide, Sodium Citrate, Mag-nesium Sulfate	NO	NO
SLEEP-EZE	Sleeping Pill	Pyrilamine Maleate	NO	NO
SLIM LINE Candy	Weight Loss	Benzocaine	YES	NO
SLOAN'S Liniment	External Analgesic	Turpentine, Kerosene, Pine Oil, Camphor, Methyl Salicylate, Capsicum Oleoresin	NO	NO

Safe and Effective: FDA — "YES" means that the FDA, in a Panel Report or other Federal Register Notice, found all active ingredients in the product safe and effective for that use. "NO" means at least one ingredient, the combination of ingredients, or the dosage form lacks evidence of safety or effectiveness.

HRG — "YES" and "NO" is Health Research Group's opinion of the same product. In addition, N/E means that we have not fully evaluated the drug or category of drugs.

Problem: "S(Ingredient)" or "E(Ingredient)" means the particular ingredient lacks evidence of safe-ty or effectiveness.

$ means that HRG believes the product is not a good buy because a less expensive effective treatment, often a single-ingredient generic, is available.

PROBLEM	ALTERNATIVE	PAGE	PRODUCT
$	High Liquid, High Fiber Diet	87,97	SERUTAN
E(Simethicone)	See Chart p. 113 For Best Buy	101,111 113	SIMECO
S(Phenylpropano- lamine), Irrational Combination, $	Treat Individual Symptoms	33,47	SINAREST Tablets and SINAREST Extra Strength
S(Phenylpropano- lamine), $	Generic Aspirin or Acetaminophen	33,44	SINE AID
S(Phenylpropano- lamine), $	Treat Individual Symptoms	33,45	SINE-OFF Tablets
S(Phenylpropano- lamine, Irrational Combination), $	Treat Individual Symptoms	33,45	SINE-OFF Extra Strength No Drowsiness Formula
N/E(Cetylpyridinium), Not for Allergies, $	Generic Phenylephrine or or Oxymetazoline Spray	33,43	SINEX Decongestant Nasal Spray
Not for Allergies	Generic Oxymetazoline or Phenylphrine Spray	33,43	SINEX Long Acting Deconges- tant Nasal Spray
FDA: E(Phenyl- toloxamine Citrate) HRG: Also S(Phenyl- propanolamine), $	Treat Individual Symptoms	33,49	SINUTAB and SINUTAB Extra Strength
FDA: E(Ammonium Chloride, Sodium Citrate) HRG: Also S(Phenylpropano- lamine), $	Treat Individual Symptoms	33,51	666 Cold Preparation
SE(Pyrilamine Maleate)	Use Non Drug Remedies	147,160	SLEEP-EZE
E(Benzocaine)	Eat a Bit Less, Exercise More; Lose a Pound a Week	67,83	SLIM LINE Candy
E(Methyl Salicylate, Dose)	Moist Heat; Generic Aspirin or Acetamino- phen If Necessary	7,18	SLOAN'S Liniment

PRODUCT	USE	INGREDIENTS	SAFE AND EFFECTIVE?	
			FDA	**HRG**
SOLARCAINE Lotion, Cream, Spray	Skin First Aid	Benzocaine, Triclosan	NO	NO
SOMINEX Formula 2	Sleeping Pill	Diphenhydramine	YES	NO
STANBACK Powder	Painkiller	Aspirin, Salicylamide Caffeine	NO	NO
STRI-DEX B.P.	Acne	Benzoyl Peroxide	YES	YES
STRI-DEX Medicated Pads	Acne	Salicylic Acid, Alcohol	NO	NO
SUCRETS Sore Throat Lozenges	Sore Throat	Hexylresorcinol	YES	NO
SUCRETS Cold Decongestant Formula Lozenges	Nasal Decongestant	Phenylpropanolamine HCl.	YES	NO
SUCRETS Cough Control Formula Lozenges	Cough	Dextromethorphan	YES	YES
SUDAFED Cough Syrup	Cough	Dextromethorphan HBr., Guainfenesin, Pseudo-ephedrine HCl. Alcohol 2.4%	*	NO
SUDAFED Tablets and Liquid	Nasal Decongestant	Pseudoephedrine	YES	NO
SUDAFED Plus Tablets and Liquid	Nasal Decongestant	Pseudoephedrine HCl. Chlorpheniramine Maleate	YES	NO
SURFAK	Laxative	Docusate Calcium	YES	NO

Safe and Effective: FDA — "YES" means that the FDA, in a Panel Report or other Federal Register Notice, found all active ingredients in the product safe and effective for that use. "NO" means at least one ingredient, the combination of ingredients, or the dosage form lacks evidence of safety or effectiveness.

HRG — "YES" and "NO" is Health Research Group's opinion of the same product. In addition, N/E means that we have not fully evaluated the drug or category of drugs.

Problem: "S(Ingredient)" or "E(Ingredient)" means the particular ingredient lacks evidence of safety or effectiveness.

$ means that HRG believes the product is not a good buy because a less expensive effective treatment, often a single-ingredient generic, is available.

278

PROBLEM	ALTERNATIVE	PAGE	PRODUCT
SE(Triclosan)	Soap and Water for Small Wounds; Generic Aspirin or Acetaminophen If Needed for Sunburn Pain	—	SOLARCAINE Lotion, Creme, Spray
SE(Diphenhydramine)	Use Non-Drug Remedies	147,159	SOMINEX Formula 2
SE(Salicylamide), E(Caffeine), $	Generic Aspirin	7,28	STANBACK Powder
$	Generic Benzoyl Peroxide	—	STRI-DEX B.P.
E(Salicylic Acid), $	Soap and Water	—	STRI-DEX Medicated Pads
$	Aspirin or Acetaminophen, If Necessary; See Text On Strep Throat	33,56	SUCRETS Sore Throat Lozenges
S(Phenylpropanolamine), $	Allergies: Generic Chlorpheniramine Pills; Decongestant: Generic Oxymetazoline or Phenylephrine Spray	33,57	SUCRETS Cold Decongestant Formula
$	Productive Cough: Drink Warm Liquids; Dry Cough: Generic Dextromethorphan	33,54	SUCRETS Cough Control Formula Lozenges
FDA: E(Guaifenesin)* HRG: Also S(Pseudoephedrine), $	Productive Cough-Drink Warm Liquids; Dry Cough: Generic Dextromethorphan	33,54	SUDAFED Cough Syrup
S(Pseudoephedrine), $	Allergies: Generic Chlorpheniramine Pills; Colds: Generic Oxymetazoline or Phenylephrine Spray	33,44	SUDAFED Tablets and Liquid
S(Pseudoephedrine), $	Allergies: Generic Chlorpheniramine Pills; Colds: Generic Oxymetazoline or Phenylephrine Spray	33,48	SUDAFED Plus
S(Docusate Calcium), $	High Liquid, High Fiber Diet	87,99	SURFAK

---

*Guaifenesin lacks evidence of effectiveness as an expectorant, in the judgment of the FDA Advisory Panel. The FDA's Director of OTC Drug Evaluation has indicated that they have started the process of reclassifying guaifenesin as effective as an expectorant. We disagree with this change, and believe that this ingredient is a waste of money.

PRODUCT	USE	INGREDIENTS	SAFE AND EFFECTIVE?	
			FDA	HRG
SUNRIL Premenstrual Capsules	Premenstrual	Acetaminophen, Pamabrom, Pyrilamine Maleate	YES	NO
TEDRAL Tablets, Elixir, Suspension	Asthma	Ephedrine, Theophylline, Phenobarbital	NO	NO
TEGRIN Medicated Shampoo	Dandruff	Coal Tar Extract	YES	N/E
TELDRIN Multi-symptom Allergy Reliever	Allergy	Acetaminophen Pseudo-ephedrine HCl. Chlorphen-aramine Maleate	YES	NO
TELDRIN Timed Release Allergy Capsules	Allergy	Chlorpheniramine Maleate	YES	YES
TEMPRA	Painkiller	Acetaminophen	YES	YES
THINZ-SPAN	Weight Loss	Phenylpropanolamine Caffeine, Vitamins and Minerals	NO	NO
TINACTIN Cream, Solution, Powder and Aerosol Powder	Athlete's Foot	Tolnaftate	YES	N/E
TITRALAC	Antacid	Calcium Carbonate	YES	YES
TRENDAR Premenstrual Tablets	Menstrual	Acetaminophen, Pamabrom	YES	NO
TRIAMINIC Expectorant	Cough, Cold	Guaifenesin, Phenyl-propanolamine HCl, Alcohol 5%	*	NO
TRIAMINIC-DM	Cough	Dextromethorphan, HBr. Phenylpropanolamine HCl.	YES	NO
TRIAMINIC Syrup	Cold, Sinus, Allergy	Phenylpropanolamine HCl., Chlorpheniramine Maleate	YES	NO
TRIAMINICIN Tablets	Cold, Sinus Allergy	Aspirin, Phenyl-propanolamine HCl., Chlorpheniramine Maleate Caffeine	NO	NO

Safe and Effective: **FDA** — "YES" means that the FDA, in a Panel Report or other Federal Register Notice, found all active ingredients in the product safe and effective for that use. "NO" means at least one ingredient, the combination of ingredients, or the dosage form lacks evidence of safety or effectiveness.

HRG — "YES" and "NO" is Health Research Group's opinion of the same product. In addition, N/E means that we have not fully evaluated the drug or category of drugs.

Problem: "S(Ingredient)" or "E(Ingredient)" means the particular ingredient lacks evidence of safety or effectiveness.

$ means that HRG believes the product is not a good buy because a less expensive effective treatment, often a single-ingredient generic, is available.

PROBLEM	ALTERNATIVE	PAGE	PRODUCT
E(Pyrilamine), $	Eat Less Salt; Generic Aspirin or Acetamino-phen, If Necessary	7,30	SUNRIL Premen-strual Capsules
SE(Theophylline) E(Phenobarbital)	Consult a Health Care Professional	33,66	TEDRAL Tablets, Elixir, Suspension
		—	TEGRIN Medicated Shampoo
S(Pseudoephedrine), $	Generic Chlorpheniramine	33,61	TELDRIN Multi-symptom Allergy Reliever
$	Generic Chlorpheniramine	33,60	TELDRIN Timed Release Allergy Capsules
$	Generic Acetaminophen	7,27	TEMPRA
FDA: E(Vitamins & Minerals) HRG: Also SE(Phenylpropano-lamine)	Eat a Bit Less, Exercise More; Lose a Pound a Week	67,81	THINZ-SPAN
$	Keep Area Dry, Cotton Socks For Athlete's Foot	—	TINACTIN Cream, Solution, Powder and Aerosol Powder
Occasional Use Only	See Chart p. For Best Buy	101,114	TITRALAC
Innappropriate Treatment, $	Eat Less Salt; Generic Aspirin or Acetaminophen	7,30	TRENDAR Pre-menstrual Tablets
FDA: E(Guaifenesin)* HRG: Also S(Phenyl-propanolamine)	Treat Individual Symptoms	33,54	TRIAMINIC Expectorant
S(Phenylpropano-lamine), $	Productive Cough: Drink Warm Liquids; Dry Cough: Generic Dextromethorphan	33,54	TRIAMINIC-DM
S(Phenylpropano-lamine), $	Treat Individual Symptoms	33,48	TRIAMINIC Syrup
FDA: E(Caffeine) HRG: Also S(Phenyl-propanolamine), $	Treat Individual Symptoms	33,48	TRIAMINICIN Tablets

---

*Guaifenesin lacks evidence of effectiveness as an expectorant, in the judgment of the FDA Advisory Panel. The FDA's Director of OTC Drug Evaluation has indicated that they have started the process of reclassifying guaifenesin as effective as an expectorant. We disagree with this change, and believe that this ingredient is a waste of money.

PRODUCT	USE	INGREDIENTS	SAFE AND EFFECTIVE?	
			FDA	HRG
TRONOLANE Cream	Hemorrhoids	Pramoxine HCl.	YES	NO
TRONOLANE Suppositories	Hemorrhoids	Pramoxine HCl.	NO	NO
TUMS	Antacid	Calcium Carbonate	YES	YES
TUSSAGESIC Tablets and Suspension	Cough, Cold	Acetaminophen, Dextromethorphan HBr., Phenylpropanolamine HCl., Pheniramine Maleate, Pyrilamine Maleate, Terpin Hydrate	NO	NO
TYLENOL Tablets, Capsules, Chewable Tablets, Drops, Elixir, Extra Strength Tablets and Capsules	Painkiller	Acetaminophen	YES	YES
UNISOM	Sleeping Pill	Doxylamine Succinate	YES	NO
VANQUISH	Painkiller	Aspirin, Acetaminophen, Caffeine, Aluminum Hydroxide, Magnesium Hydroxide	NO	NO
VASELINE Pure Petroleum Jelly	Skin Protectant	White Petrolatum	YES	YES
VASELINE First-Aid Carbolated Petroleum Jelly	Skin Protectant	Chloroxylenol, Phenol, Lanolin, Petroleum Jelly	NO	NO
VICKS Cough Syrup	Cough	Dextromethorphan HBr., Guaifenesin, Sodium Citrate, Alcohol 5%	NO	NO
VICKS VAPORUB	Nasal Decongestant Cough, External Analgesic	Menthol, Spirits of Turpentine, Eucalytus Oil, Camphor, Cedar Leaf Oil, Nutmeg Oil, Petroleum Base	NO	NO

Safe and Effective: **FDA** — "YES" means that the FDA, in a Panel Report or other Federal Register Notice, found all active ingredients in the product safe and effective for that use. "NO" means at least one ingredient, the combination of ingredients, or the dosage form lacks evidence of safety or effectiveness.

HRG — "YES" and "NO" is Health Research Group's opinion of the same product. In addition, N/E means that we have not fully evaluated the drug or category of drugs.

Problem: "S(Ingredient)" or "E(Ingredient)" means the particular ingredient lacks evidence of safety or effectiveness.

$ means that HRG believes the product is not a good buy because a less expensive effective treatment, often a single-ingredient generic, is available.

282

PROBLEM	ALTERNATIVE	PAGE	PRODUCT
Inappropriate Treatment, $	Keep Clean & Dry; Petroleum Jelly or Zinc Oxide, If Necessary	131,142	**TRONOLANE Cream**
E(Intrarectal Use of Pramoxine)	Keep Clean & Dry; Petroleum Jelly or Zinc Oxide, If Necessary	131,142	**TRONOLANE Suppositories**
Occasional Use Only	Baking Soda	101,114	**TUMS**
FDA: E(Terpin Hydrate), Irrational Combination HRG: Also S(Phenylpropanolamine), $	Treat Individual Symptoms	33,48	**TUSSAGESIC Tablets and Suspension**
$	Generic Acetaminophen	7,27	**TYLENOL Tablets, Capsules, Chewable Tablets, Drops, Elixir, Extra Strength Tablets and Capsules**
SE(Doxylamine Succinate)	Use Non-Drug Remedies	147,160	**UNISOM**
FDA: E(Caffeine) HRG: Also E(Buffers) $	Generic Aspirin	7,29	**VANQUISH**
$	Generic Petroleum Jelly	131,141	**VASELINE Pure Petroleum Jelly**
SE(Chloroxylenol), $	Soap and Water Rinsing Will Allow Most Minor Bites and Wounds To Heal	—	**VASELINE First-Aid Carbolated Petroleum Jelly**
E(Guafenesin,* Sodium Citrate), $	Productive Cough: Drink Warm Liquids; Dry Cough: Generic Dextromethorphan	33,52	**VICKS Cough Syrup**
E(Turpentine Oil)	Treat Individual Symptoms	33,53	**VICKS VAPORUB**

*Guaifenesin lacks evidence of effectiveness as an expectorant, in the judgment of the FDA Advisory Panel. The FDA's Director of OTC Drug Evaluation has indicated that they have started the process of reclassifying guaifenesin as effective as an expectorant. We disagree with this change, and believe that this ingredient is a waste of money.

PRODUCT	USE	INGREDIENTS	SAFE AND EFFECTIVE? FDA	HRG
VICTORS Cough Lozenges	Cough	Menthol, Eucalyptus Oil	NO	NO
VIROMED Liquid	Cough, Cold	Acetaminophen, Pseudoephedrine, Dextromethorphan HBr., Sodium Citrate, Alcohol 16.63%	NO	NO
VIROMED Tablets	Cough, Cold	Aspirin, Pseudoephedrine HCl., Chlorpheniramine Maleate, Dextromethorphan HBr., Guaifenesin	NO	NO
VISINE Eye Drops	Eye Drops	Tetrahydrozoline HCl.	YES	N/E
VISINE A.D. Eye Drops	Eye Drops	Tetrahydrozoline HCl., Zinc Sulfate	YES	N/E
WYANOID Ointment	Hemorrhoids	Benzocaine, Boric Acid, Zinc Oxide, Peruvian Balsam, Castor Oil, Petrolatum, Ephedrine Sulfate	NO	NO
WYANOID Suppositories	Hemorrhoids	Belladonna Extract, Ephedrine Sulfate, Zinc Oxide, Boric Acid, Bismuth Oxyiodide, Bismuth Subcarbonate, Peruvian Balsam, Cocoa Butter	NO	NO

Safe and Effective: **FDA** — "YES" means that the FDA, in a Panel Report or other Federal Register Notice, found all active ingredients in the product safe and effective for that use. "NO" means at least one ingredient, the combination of ingredients, or the dosage form lacks evidence of safety or effectiveness.

HRG — "YES" and "NO" is Health Research Group's opinion of the same product. In addition, N/E means that we have not fully evaluated the drug or category of drugs.

Problem: "S(Ingredient)" or "E(Ingredient)" means the particular ingredient lacks evidence of safety or effectiveness.

$ means that HRG believes the product is not a good buy because a less expensive effective treatment, often a single-ingredient generic, is available.

284

PROBLEM	ALTERNATIVE	PAGE	PRODUCT
E(Eucalyptus Oil)	Productive Cough: Drink Warm Liquids; Dry Cough: Generic Dextromethorphan		**VICTORS Cough Lozenges**
FDA: E(Sodium Citrate), Irrational Combination HRG: Also S(Pseudo-ephedrine), $	Treat Individual Symptoms	33,48	**VIROMED Liquid**
FDA: E(Guaifenesin)* Irrational Combination HRG: Also S(Pseudo-ephedrine) $	Treat Individual Symptoms	33,48	**VIROMED Tablets**
	No OTC Eye Drops Needed	—	**VISINE Eye Drops**
	No OTC Eye Drops Needed	—	**VISINE A.D. Eye Drops**
SE(Boric Acid), E(Peruvian Balsam), $	Keep Clean & Dry Petroleum Jelly or Zinc Oxide, If Necessary	131,143	**WYANOID Ointment**
SE(Boric Acid, Bella-donna Extract) E(Bis-muth Subcarbonate, Peruvian Balsam), $	Keep Clean & Dry; Petroleum Jelly or Zinc Oxide, If Necessary	131,143	**WYANOID Suppositories**

*Guaifenesin lacks evidence of effectiveness as an expectorant, in the judgment of the FDA Advisory Panel. The FDA's Director of OTC Drug Evaluation has indicated that they have started the process of reclassifying guaifenesin as effective as an expectorant. We disagree with this change, and believe that this ingredient is a waste of money.

285

GLOSSARY

ACID: One of a group of chemicals which characteristically have a sour taste. Acid in the stomach helps to digest food.

ACUTE ILLNESS: An illness that occurs suddenly and runs a short course.

ADJUVANT: A substance added to medication to increase the effect of the drug's main active ingredient(s).

ADSORBENT: A substance that attracts or holds on to other chemicals.

AEROPHAGIA: Swallowing air.

ALLERGIC RHINITIS: Itchy runny nose, itchy watery eyes, and itchy throat caused by allergy to substances in the air such as pollen, mold and animal hair.

ALLERGY: Hypersensitivity (over-reaction) to substances such as drugs, food and pollen.

AMPHETAMINE: "Uppers" or speed. One of a group of chemicals which stimulate the central nervous system. Amphetamines may also increase blood pressure, reduce appetite and cause jitteriness and inability to sleep.

ANAL: Relating to the anus.

ANAL CRYPT: Small pockets found between the anus and the rectum.

ANALGESIC: A pain-reliever. Internal analgesics are pain-relieving drugs that are taken internally, usually by mouth; topical or local analgesics are applied to the skin.

ANAPHYLAXIS: A serious allergic reaction requiring immediate medical attention. It may include difficulty in breathing, drop in blood pressure and sometimes death.

ANESTHETIC: A drug which deadens pain by producing a local or general (body-wide) loss of sensation.

ANEURYSM: A weak-walled sac which protrudes from the wall of a blood vessel; or an abnormally diluted, thin-walled area in a blood vessel.

ANORECTAL: Related to the rectum and anus.

ANORECTIC: A substance that suppresses the appetite.

ANTACID: A drug that neutralizes acid in the stomach.

ANTI-ASTHMATIC: A drug used to treat asthma.

ANTI-ANXIETY DRUG: A drug used to treat the symptoms of anxiety or nervousness.

ANTIBIOTIC: A drug (made from mold or bacteria) used to treat infections by killing or stopping the growth of the bacteria or other microorganisms that cause them.

ANTICHOLINERGIC: A drug that (by blocking certain impulses) blocks bodily secretions. These drugs are used in cough, cold and also diarrheal medicines, and although ineffective for this use, are also contained in some medicines for the treatment of hemorrhoids.

ANTICOAGULANT: A drug which slows the clotting of blood.

ANTIDEPRESSANT: A drug used to treat depression.

ANTIDIARRHEAL: A drug used to treat diarrhea.

ANTIEMETIC: A drug which prevents or treats nausea and vomiting.

ANTIFLATULENT: A drug used to treat "gas."

ANTIHISTAMINE: Drugs which counteract the effects of histamine, a chemical produced by the body during an allergic reaction. Antihistamines are used to treat allergies. Because they often cause drowsiness, they are also sold as nighttime sleep-aids.

ANTI-INFLAMMATORY: A drug used to reduce inflammation, such as the joint inflammation associated with rheumatoid arthritis.

ANTIMICROBIAL: A drug that kills or inhibits the growth of microorganisms that cause infections, such as viruses or bacteria.

ANTIPYRETIC: A drug for reducing fever.

ANTIRHEUMATIC: A drug used to treat arthritis (see ANTI-INFLAMMATORY).

ANTISEPTIC: A substance that prevents infection by destroying microorganisms (such as bacteria).

ANTITUSSIVE: A drug used to suppress coughing.

ARTHRITIS: Inflammation of one or more joints, with joint swelling, redness and/or pain during movement. (See OSTEO-ARTHRITIS, RHEUMATOID ARTHRITIS, INFECTIOUS ARTHRITIS, and GOUT.)

ASTHMA: A disease causing intermittent narrowing of the airways. Symptoms include wheezing and difficulty in breathing.

ASTRINGENT: A substance which makes the skin and mucous membranes shrink or "pucker."

BACTERIA: Microscopic creatures, many of which cause infections (such as strep throat, pneumonia and urinary infections).

BETA-CAROTENE: A chemical found in carrots, sweet potatoes and leafy vegetables that is converted into Vitamin A in the body.

BILATERAL SYMMETRY: The distribution of a physical condition in the same areas on the right and left side of the body.

BULK-FORMING LAXATIVES: Products which relieve constipation by increasing the amount of fiber passing through the digestive tract, thus making the stool softer and easier to pass.

BRONCHODILATOR: A drug used to treat asthma which opens the airways in the lung, making breathing easier.

BYSSINOSIS: A lung disease found in textile workers after long-term exposure to cotton dust. Symptoms include wheezing, tightness in the chest and difficulty in breathing.

CALORIE: A unit of food energy.

CARBOHYDRATE: A substance found in food; starches and sugars are both carbohydrates. Vegetables, fruit, bread and grains are all rich in carbohydrates. The body breaks carbohydrates down into simple sugars such as glucose, which are used for energy.

> **Simple carbohydrate:** Sugar found in sweet foods, including fruit and honey.

> **Complex carbohydrate** (starch): Carbohydrate which must be broken down by the body, and is found in vegetables, grains, potatoes and bread.

CARCINOGEN: A cancer-causing substance.

CARDIOVASCULAR: Relating to the heart and blood vessels.

CATHARTIC: A laxative, or drug which is used to treat constipation.

CENTRAL NERVOUS SYSTEM: The brain and the spinal cord.

CHOLESTEROL: A substance contained in animal fats. Eating large quantities of foods with animal fat (including dairy products) raises the level of cholesterol in the blood. High blood cholesterol levels are associated with a greater risk of having heart attacks.

CHRONIC ILLNESS: An illness of long duration.

CIRCADIAN RHYTHM: The "internal clock" by which each person functions. This clock has a regular cycle of sleeping and waking; when it is disrupted, insomnia may result.

COMA: A state of unconsciousness from which an individual cannot be aroused.

COMMON COLD: A viral infection of the nose and throat. Symptoms may include sneezing, runny nose, sore throat, cough and body aches.

CONGESTION: Fullness or blockage due to an accumulation of fluid in the tissue.

CONGESTIVE HEART FAILURE: A medical condition in which the heart does not pump blood adequately, fluid accumulates in the lungs and/or the legs, and the body tissues may not receive adequate blood.

CONTRACEPTIVE: A drug or device that prevents pregnancy.

CONTROLLED STUDY: A scientific study in which one group of people is given a drug, another group of people which is similar to the first group is given a sugar pill or placebo and differences between the two groups are measured. If the two groups are similar and the study is well-designed, differences that occur after drug treatment are likely to be a result of drug treatment.

CONSTIPATION: A decrease in the number of bowel movements, or difficulty in passing hard stools.

CONVULSION: A violent involuntary contraction of the muscles.

CORONARY ARTERY DISEASE: Blockage of the vessels which supply blood to the heart. This can cause angina (heart pain) or heart attacks.

CORROSIVE: An agent that eats away at something or produces deterioration.

CORTICOSTEROID: A hormone produced by the adrenal gland (or a synthetic equivalent). Its effects include changing the body's balance of water and salt and acting as an anti-inflammatory agent.

COUGH CENTER: The area in the brain which controls the coughing reflex.

COUNTER-IRRITANT: A substance applied to a body surface which produces a sensation that distracts the body from sensing pain, itching or burning.

DANDER: The tiny scales from feathers and animal hair that may provoke an allergic reaction.

DEBILITATED: Very weak.

DEBRIDING AGENT: A chemical that removes dead or infected skin.

DEFECATION: "Having a bowel movement": the removal of feces from the body through the anus.

DEFECATORY REFLEX: The reflex which controls defecation.

DEHYDRATION: Loss of water from the body without adequate replacement of the lost water. Dehydration may result from, (among other things), diarrhea, vomiting, fever or exercise.

DELIRIUM: A mental state characterized by confusion, hallucinations, restlessness and incoherence.

DEMULCENT: A substance used to soothe an irritated or inflamed surface.

DEPRESSANT: A drug, such as a barbiturate, antihistamine or alcohol, that slows down the central nervous system. It may reduce clear mental functioning and cause drowsiness.

DEPRESSION: A mental state which may be characterized by sadness, feelings of worthlessness, inability to concentrate, loss of appetite, trouble sleeping, daytime drowsiness and other symptoms.

DIABETES: A disease in which the body cannot use or store carbohydrates properly, resulting in high levels of glucose ("sugar") in the blood. Diabetes is of two types:

   "Juvenile onset" diabetes: A form of diabetes which usually develops before age 30 and which must be treated with insulin.

   "Adult onset" diabetes: This usually occurs in adults who are overweight and is best treated by diet, though some victims may need insulin.

DIAGNOSE: To recognize a disease.

DIGESTIVE TRACT: The long hollow tube which takes in, digests and absorbs food and rids the body of indigestible food waste. It includes the mouth, esophagus, stomach, intestines, rectum and anus.

DISTENSION: Swelling or enlargement of a part of the body.

DIURETIC: A drug that eliminaties fluids from the body by increasing the volume of urine.

DIVERTICULAR DISEASE: Inflammation or other complications of diverticulae (abnormal sacs protruding from the lining of the intestines).

DRUG METABOLITES: Substances which are produced when a drug is broken down by the body.

DUODENUM: The upper portion of the small intestine.

DYSMENORRHEA: Pain during menstrual periods, including cramps and backache.

ECZEMA: A skin ailment characterized by dry, red, itchy, flaking skin.

EFFERVESCING: Bubbly or carbonated.

EMETIC: A drug that induces vomiting.

ENEMA: Liquid that is injected into the anus, usually used to bring on a bowel movement.

ENTERIC-COATED DRUG: A drug coated to prevent its absorption in the stomach.

ENZYME: A chemical which acts on other substances, to speed a chemical reaction in the body. Enzymes in the intestines help to break down food.

ENTEROBIASIS (Pinworms): A medical condition in which small worms live in the intestinal tract and crawl out of the anus at night to lay eggs. The main symptom of the condition is intense anal itching.

ESOPHAGUS: The portion of the digestive tract that lies between the mouth and the stomach.

EUSTACHIAN TUBE: A tube that connects the throat and the middle ear, which helps to maintain middle ear pressure.

EXPECTORANT: A drug used to thin mucus in the airways, so that the mucus may be coughed up more easily.

FAD DIET: A diet which promises a quick, drastic reduction in weight, but may deprive the body of necessary protein and vitamins.

FAT: A substance found in food. Fat is contained in lard, egg yolks, meat, butter and other dairy foods, and vegetable oil. Usually (but not always), animal fats are saturated fats, while vegetable oils are unsaturated fats. Fat which is used for energy contains significantly more calories than the same weight of carbohydrate or protein.

FERROUS SULFATE: A type of iron supplement tablet.

FDA: The Food and Drug Administration; the U. S. government agency which regulates prescription and over the counter drugs.

FDA PANEL: A panel of medical experts appointed by the FDA to review over the counter drugs for safety and effectiveness.

FIBER (Dietary): The part of whole grains, cereals, raw vegetables, raw and dried fruit, and beans that is not digested by the body and becomes a part of stool. (See also HIGH FIBER DIET.)

FIXED-RATIO COMBINATION DRUG: A medicine that contains two or more ingredients, each in a fixed amount. This means that you cannot take more or less of one ingredient without also changing how much of the other ingredient you take.

FLATUS: Gas which is passed by the rectum.

FLU (Influenza): A specific viral infection characterized by fever, achiness and upper respiratory symptoms (such as earache or sore throat) or gastrointestinal symptoms (nausea, vomiting or diarrhea).

GASTRITIS: Inflammation of the stomach wall, which may cause bleeding from the stomach.

GASTRO-ESOPHAGEAL REFLUX: Acid indigestion, heartburn or sour stomach. A condition in which the contents of the stomach rise up into the esophagus (the top portion of the digestive tract), often producing a burning sensation.

GASTRO-INTESTINAL: Relating to the stomach and intestines.

GASTROSCOPY: A procedure in which a tube is swallowed allowing the doctor to examine the inside of the stomach.

GENERIC: A non-brand name, version of a drug that is not protected by a trademark. For example, acetaminophen is the generic name for the only active ingredient in Tylenol. When used in this book, the term "generic" includes "house brand" versions of drugs — drugs sold under a drugstore or supermarket's own label — because these are also usually much less expensive than brand name versions of the same drug.

GLAND: A group of cells that produce chemicals that are used by other parts of the body.

GLAUCOMA: A disease in which there is too much pressure in the eye. Glaucoma can cause impaired vision and blindness.

GOUT: A form of arthritis caused by uric acid crystals deposited in the fluid surrounding the joints.

GUT: Intestines.

HALLUCINATION: Seeing, hearing or feeling something that isn't real.

HEALTH CARE PROFESSIONAL: When used in the book, the term refers to someone who is trained to diagnose disease and determine whether there is a need for medical treatment. Examples include physicians, physicians' assistants and nurse practitioners.

HEMORRHAGE: Heavy bleeding.

HEMORRHOIDS: Enlarged blood vessels in the anorectal area that may cause pain, itching and burning. Internal hemorrhoids occur in the rectum; external hemorrhoids occur in the anus.

HERNIA: The protusion of all or part of an organ through a weak area in the body wall.

HIGH FIBER DIET: A diet rich in foods such as whole grain breads and cereals, raw vegetables, raw and dried fruits, beans and bran.

HORMONE: A chemical messenger carried by the blood from a gland to other parts of the body. Examples are insulin, growth hormone, thyroxine (a hormone produced by the thyroid gland) and sex hormones.

HOUSE BRAND: A generic form of a drug (often sold by a drug store or supermarket under its own label) that is usually much less expensive than brand name versions of the same drug. (See GENERIC.)

HYDROCORTISONE: A hormone produced in the adrenal gland (or a synthetic equivalent). Its effects include reducing inflammation. (See CORTICOSTEROID.)

HYPERCHOLESTEROLEMIA: A condition in which there is too much cholesterol (a fat-like substance) in the blood. (See CHOLESTEROL.) People with this condition have a greater chance of having heart attacks.

HYPERLIPIDEMIA: A condition in which there is too much fat in the blood.

HYPEROSMOTIC: A type of substance which attracts water to itself. Such substances are sometimes used as drugs to treat constipation.

HYPERTENSION: High blood pressure.

HYPERVENTILATION: A condition resulting from rapid, deep breathing, characterized by dizziness and lightheadedness and sometimes by numb or cramped fingers or chest pain.

IDEAL BODY WEIGHT: The appropriate weight for an individual of a certain height and build.

IMMUNE SYSTEM: The body's defenses, which fight off viruses, bacteria and other foreign substances which invade the body.

INDICATION: A recommended use of a drug.

INFECTIOUS ARTHRITIS: Infection of one or more joints. This type of arthritis is usually accompanied by fever.

INFLAMMATION: The body's response to infection or injury, usually characterized by pain, redness, heat and swelling.

INFLUENZA (Flu): A specific viral illness characterized by fever, achiness and upper respiratory symptoms (such as runny nose, earache or sore throat) or gastrointestinal symptoms (nausea, vomiting, diarrhea).

INHALANT: A medicine that is breathed in through the nose or mouth.

INSOMNIA: A disorder in which an individual feels that he or she is unable to sleep or has difficulty falling or remaining asleep.

INTESTINAL DISTRESS: The feeling of bloating, distension cramps and fullness which may occur from 30 minutes to several hours after eating a meal.

INTESTINAL OBSTRUCTION: A blockage in the flow of food contents through the intestines.

INTESTINE: The portion of the digestive tract that lies between the stomach and rectum; it digests and absorbs food and liquid.

INTRARECTAL: In the rectum.

IPPUAD: "Immediate Post Prandial Upper Abdominal Distress": Bloating, cramps, fullness and stomach discomfort experienced immediately after eating a meal.

IRRATIONAL COMBINATION: A medicine that has one or more ingredients which are not appropriate for the intended purpose of the drug, or two ingredients that act in the same way, when only one is needed.

JOINT: A connection of two bones which allows movement in at least one of the bones. Examples are the knee, elbow, finger, hip and ankle.

KERATOLYTIC: A substance which produces shedding of the surface layers of the skin.

LAXATIVE DEPENDENCY: A condition which develops from over-use of laxatives. The victim cannot defecate without using a laxative.

LEAN BODY MASS: All the body weight except fat (the weight of bone, muscle, etc).

LOWER ESOPHAGEAL SPHINCTER: The muscle which controls the passage of food from the esophagus to the stomach.

LUBRICANT: An agent which provides moisture or wetness.

LYMPH NODES: Body structures which act to combat infection in the body.

MENINGITIS: An inflammation of the meninges (the membranes which surround the brain).

MENSTRUAL: Related to menstruation, or monthly periods.

METABOLISM: The process by which food and stored fat are converted into energy. People with a higher metabolic rate burn food and fat more quickly than people with a lower metabolic rate.

MICROORGANISM: A tiny living thing, such as a virus, bacterium, yeast or mold.

MIGRAINE HEADACHE: A recurring headache (often on one side of the head) caused by temporary changes in the width of blood vessels in the head. Symptoms may include nausea, vomiting and sensitivity to bright light.

MONONUCLEOSIS: "Mono": an infectious disease caused by a virus, often charaterized by a sore throat, swollen glands, unexplained exhaustion, and liver or spleen abnormalities.

MORNING SICKNESS: Early-morning nausea and vomiting which occurs during pregnancy.

MOTION SICKNESS: Nausea and/or vomiting caused by car, boat or air travel.

MUCOLYTIC: A drug which breaks up mucus.

MUCOUS MEMBRANE: The thin, soft layers of cells that line the respiratory tract (including the inside of the mouth and nose), the throat, and the digestive and reproductive tracts.

MUSCLE RELAXANT: A drug that relaxes muscles.

MYOCARDIAL INFARCTION: "Heart attack": An abrupt reduction in the blood flow to the heart muscle, causing damage to the heart.

NARCOLEPSY: A disorder in which an individual has frequent attacks of uncontrollable sleepiness or sleeping during the day.

NARCOTIC: An addicting drug that is used to relieve pain or produce sleep. Examples are codeine, meperidine (Demerol), morphine and propoxyphene (Darvon).

NASAL: Relating to the nose.

NASAL DECONGESTANT: A drug that unclogs a stuffed nose, usually by causing the blood vessels in the nose to narrow and reducing the swelling of the mucous membrane in the nose.

NATIONAL ACADEMY OF SCIENCES: A U.S. government scientific research group.

NERVE IMPULSE: A message carried by nerves.

NERVOUS SYSTEM: The brain, spinal cord and nerves throughout the body.

NEURAL: Relating to the nerves.

NEURAL MISMATCH: The preception of conflicting sensory experiences. This is one theory used to explain motion sickness: the body sees that it is moving in one direction, but feels that it is moving in another.

NONPRODUCTIVE COUGH: A dry cough that produces no sputum.

NUTRIENTS: Substances found in food that are necessary for growth and normal functioning, including protein, carbohydrates, fats, vitamins and minerals.

OBESITY: Being overweight or having too much body fat, also defined as weighing more than 10 to 20 pounds over ideal weight.

ORAL: Relating to the mouth.

ORTHOPEDIC DEVICE: A device such as a crutch or brace which is used to preserve functioning of the back, neck, arms or legs.

OSTEOARTHRITIS: A form of arthritis caused by "wear and tear." It often affects weight-bearing joints of the body such as the hips and knees.

OTIC: Relating to the ear.

OVER-INDULGENCE: Excessive eating and/or drinking.

OVER THE COUNTER (OTC) DRUG: A drug that is sold without a prescription.

PEDICULICIDE: A drug that kills lice.

PEPTIC ULCER: An erosion of the wall of the stomach or the duodenum (the top portion of the small intestine).

PERI-ANAL: Around the anus.

PHYSICAL THERAPY: Treatment which uses exercise, massage, electrical stimulation, water and heat too improve body functioning after disease or injury.

PLACEBO: A pill, liquid or capsule that contains no active drugs. In medical research, placebos are used to test whether a particular drug treatment works better than no treatment at all. The *placebo effect* occurs frequently when people taking placebos or medicine experience relief of symptoms, not because of the effectiveness of the drug, but because they expect to feel better after using medicine.

PNEUMONIA: An infection of the lung.

PREMENSTRUAL TENSION: Symptoms which can occur the week before a menstral period, including tiredness, bloating, breast tenderness and irritability.

PRODUCTIVE COUGH: A cough that produces sputum.

PROLAPSE: Sagging or protusion of an organ or body tissue.

PROTECTANT: A substance which is applied over an irritated area to provide a protective coating and prevent further irritation.

PROTEIN: A substance found in food. Meat, eggs, fish, dairy products, seeds and beans are all foods high in protein. Proteins are made up of amino acids, which the body uses to build and repair cells.

PRURITIS ANI: Anal itching, often caused by hemorrhoids, enterobiasis (pinworms), body secretions, tight clothing or allergy.

PULMONARY: Relating to the lungs.

REBOUND EFFECT: An effect which may occur after stopping drug treatment, in which the symptom for which the drug was used returns and may even be more severe than before drug treatment began.

RECTAL: Relating to the rectum.

REFLEX: An automatic action of a muscle in response to nerve stimulation.

RESPIRATORY TRACT: The nose, lungs and air passages.

REYE'S SYNDROME: A rare, often fatal illness that occurs in children who have chicken pox or flu, characterized by severe vomiting and changes in consciousness such as lethargy or coma. It is almost always preceded by use of aspirin to treat the flu or chicken pox.

RHEUMATIC FEVER: A disease that can occur mostly in children and young adults after exposure to the bacteria that cause strep throat. Its symptoms include sudden fever, joint pain, and inflammation of the joints; It can lead to heart and kidney damage.

RHEUMATOID ARTHRITIS: A form of arthritis (joint inflammation) caused by a disturbance in the body's immune system.

SALINE: Containing salt.

SEDATIVE: A drug that produces a calming, tranquilizing effect.

SEEPAGE: The leaking of liquid from an inflamed or infected area.

SELF-LIMITING DISEASE: A medical problem that goes away after a few days and does not require medical attention.

SELF-MEDICATION: The use of medication without the recommendation of a health care professional.

SELF-TREATMENT: Treatment of a medical problem which may or may not involve the use of drugs.

SENSITIZATION: The stimulation of the body's immune system in response to specific substance, so that the body will have an allergic reaction when it comes into contact with that substance again.

SIMPLE SUGARS: Substances that the body produces by breaking down complex sugars and starches, and uses to provide energy. Glucose (dextrose) and sucrose (table sugar) are simple sugars.

SITZ BATH: A bath taken in warm water (about 110°F) to cleanse and heal inflamed or infected tissue in the genital or rectal area.

SKINFOLD THICKNESS: The thickness of a fold of skin (usually on the back of the upper arm), used as one measure of body fat.

SLEEP APNEA: A condition in which breathing stops for a time during sleep. It is often characterized by heavy snoring.

SODIUM: An element found in table salt (sodium chloride). Sodium is one of the components of blood and other body fluids.

SOPORIFIC: Sleep-inducing.

SPASM: A sudden contraction of a muscle which can cause pain and restricts movement.

SPUTUM: Mucus or phlegm which is coughed up.

STARCH BLOCKER: A product sold for weight reduction which claims to (but does not) block the body's absorption of starch (carbohydrate.).

STIMULANT: A chemical which stimulates the central nervous system, making it difficult to relax or fall asleep.

STREP THROAT: A bacterial infection, which may cause sore throat, swollen glands in the neck, fever and/or pus in the back of the throat. This infection must be diagnosed by a throat culture and treated with antibiotics because otherwise it may lead to rheumatic fever.

STROKE: A condition in which a blood clot blocks a vessel which supplies blood to the brain, or a blood vessel breaks, causing bleeding into the brain. A stroke causes temporary or permanent loss of physical or mental function.

SUPPOSITORY: A solid medicine which is inserted into an orifice of the body such as the vagina or anus.

SURFACE TENSION: The coherence of a surface which helps keep it intact.

THROAT CULTURE: A test for strep throat performed by a health care professional in which a swab is placed on the back of the throat. If the cells collected on the swab grow streptococcal bacteria over the next few days, the individual has strep throat.

THROMBOSIS: A blood clot.

TISSUE: A group of cells that performs a specific function.

TOPICAL MEDICATION: A medication applied to the specific area of the body which requires treatment, or a medication applied to the skin.

TOXIC: Poisonous or harmful.

TRANQUILIZER: A drug used to counteract the symptoms of anxiety. (See SEDATIVE.)

TRAVELER'S DIARRHEA: Diarrhea that may occur when traveling, especially in countries where water is contaminated.

TRAUMA: Wound or injury.

TREMOR: Involuntary trembling or quivering.

UPPER RESPIRATORY TRACT: The nose, throat and upper airways.

URIC ACID CRYSTALS: Crystals made of uric acid, which may form in joints and cause gout.

VASCULAR CONDITION: A disease of the blood vessels, including myocardial infarction (heart attack), hypertension (high blood pressure) and stroke.

VASOCONSTRICTOR: A drug that temporarily narrows the blood vessels and reduces the amount of blood that can flow through them.

VIRUS: A tiny living thing that can grow only within living cells. Viruses cause many different infections.

VITAMIN: A substance found in foods which does not provide energy, but is needed by the body in minute amounts for normal functioning.

VITAMIN C: A vitamin contained in citrus fruits and many vegetables. People who do not get enough vitamin C can develop scurvy.

VITAMIN K: A vitamin that helps the blood to clot. It is found especially in dark green leafy vegetables.

WOUND-HEALING AGENT: Drugs used to speed up the process of wound healing and tissue repair.

HOW THIS BOOK WAS COMPILED

Food and Drug Administration Evaluations

The FDA evaluations of the drugs and ingredients in the *Brand Name Index to OTC Drugs* and in the chapters on *Common Problems* are largely based on reports and notices published in the *Federal Register,* as part of the ongoing OTC Drug Review. (See *History of the OTC Review,* p. 300.) Reports of the FDA advisory panels account for most of the evaluations, though in a few cases the agency has published more recent monograph decisions in the *Federal Register* which differ from the panel's report. In some cases, results of New Drug Applications were also considered in these evaluations.

The *Ingredients Index* is based solely on an FDA list published in 1980 and/or *Federal Register* notices published since that time and up until December 31, 1982.

Health Research Group Evaluations

In addition to the FDA evaluations discussed above, scientific evidence submitted by manufacturers and correspondence between the agency and the manufacturer were obtained and reviewed by the Health Research Group in many cases. In this way we were able to judge the adequacy of evidence not published elsewhere and judge the apparent outcome of the FDA's as yet unpublished decisions. These and other documents were obtained through the Freedom of Information Act and were supplemented by other documents and information obtained from numerous FDA employees.

When our evaluation of a drug (either in the *Brand Name Index* or the chapters on *Common Problems*) differs from the evaluation of the FDA, our disagreement is based on the scientific evidence concerning safety or effectiveness, or on our evaluation of the value of a drug to the consumer.

When our problem with a drug is one of safety or effectiveness, our decision is based on information from medical publications such as the reliable, non-profit *Medical Letter,* and other reputable scientific journals and books. Additionally, we evaluated unpublished studies when necessary. Our final evaluation of a particular drug is also based upon consultations with specialists in that specific field, in many instances.

When our problem with a drug is one of value, our decision is based on the availability of other, equally good or better treatments that are readily available at less cost to the consumer.

Over the Counter Drug Products

The main sources for information on brand name drug products and their labeling and ingredients were the 1982 editions of the

Physician's Desk Reference for Nonprescription Drugs and the American Pharmaceutical Association's *Handbook of Non-prescription Drugs*. These volumes were supplemented in some cases by checking products currently available in Washington, D.C. area drugstores.

Price Comparisons

Price comparisions provided in this volume are based primarily on price to the consumer as seen in Washington, D.C. area drugstores and supermarkets during January and February, 1983. Additional sources of price information include *Drug Topics Red Book 1983* and *Facts and Comparisons*.

HISTORY OF THE OTC REVIEW

The Food, Drug and Cosmetic Act ("FDC Act") divides drugs into two categories. The first category is prescription drugs, which may be dispensed only with a doctor's prescription. In general, prescription drugs must be approved as safe and effective by the Food and Drug Administration prior to sale.

The second category is over the counter ("OTC") drugs, which are sold to consumers without a prescription. In general, OTC drugs do not require prior approval from the FDA. Instead, they are sold on the basis of their manufacturers' conclusions that they are safe and effective.

Prior to 1962, the FDC Act required manfacturers to show only that their products were generally recognized as safe. However, in 1962 Congress amended the Act to require general recognition of effectiveness as well. While this new requirement applies only to so-called "post-1962 drugs," it is now applicable to virtually all over the counter drugs. This is because most pre-1962 OTC drugs still on the market either have been reformulated or their uses have changed since 1962.

In 1966, the FDA appointed the National Academy of Sciences-National Research Council (NAS-NRC) to review the efficacy of a sample of OTC drugs which were broadly representative of the whole range of the products then on the market. In its 1969 report, the NAS-NRC concluded that only 25% of those drugs were effective even for one use.

Nevertheless, the agency waited three years to take any action. In 1972, it commenced the Over the Counter Drug Review ("OTC Review") to study the ingredients in the 100,000 to 500,000 brands of OTC drugs which it estimated were on the market. The goal of the review is to make final determinations on the efficacy of the OTC drugs on the market, so that ineffective drugs can be removed, as required by the 1962 Amendments. The FDA has made a commitment not to enforce the efficacy requirement of the statute against manufacturers of any OTC drugs until the completion of the OTC Review, which the FDA originally estimated would require 3 to 5 years.

The FDA adopted a highly complex system of conducting the OTC Review, with several procedural steps and many built-in delays. It first appointed 17 advisory panels to review the test data for each of 26 categories of OTC drugs. After their deliberations, receiving testimony and comments from the drug industry, each panel submits to the FDA one or more reports describing the uses and conditions under which OTC drug products reviewed are generally recognized as safe and effective. The FDA then reviews each panel report and publishes it, with revisions, in the Federal Register as a "proposed monograph" to give the drug industry a second opportunity to submit comments. After reviewing the comments, the FDA publishes a "tentative final monograph," and provides the manufacturers a third opportunity to comment. After this stage, the FDA reviews the comments and then publishes a "final monograph," which establishes the conditions under which particular ingredients are generally recognized as safe and effective.

FDA regulations require that the ingredients studied be classified in one of three categories: Category I, for drugs which are generally recognized as safe and effective, and therefore may be sold without FDA approval; Category II, for drugs which are not generally recognized as safe and effective and therefore may not be sold; and Category III, for drugs for which "the available data are insufficient" to classify them in Category I or Category II.

The 1977, the Health Research Group sued the FDA to challenge the regulation which allowed the continued marketing of Category III drugs. HRG's argument, which Judge Sirica of the U.S. District Court for the District of Columbia accepted, was that it was illegal for manufacturer to sell Category III drugs since Category III meant that the agency had made a final determination that the evidence to support the sale of those drugs was insufficient to establish their safety and efficacy, as required by the statute. Judge Sirica agreed and issued a court order invalidating the Category III regulation. However, the FDA took more than two years to amend its regulations to conform to the Court's decision, and even then adopted a regulation which the Health Research Group believes is also illegal. Under the new regulation, the FDA allows manufacturers to continue to test drugs that have not been proven safe and effective during the middle of the administrative process, and the FDA then postpones issuing its final decision about whether the drug is safe and effective. During the new testing phase, the drugs remain on the market.

The OTC Review has taken far more than the 3 to 5 years

301

originally projected by the FDA. The Review has lasted 10 years already, and there is no end in sight. The FDA does not even seem troubled by the fact that the scientific panels found that 69% of the ingredients reviewed lack the evidence of safety and effectiveness required by the law to support their sale for the uses for which they are intended. Moreover, in a recent interview with the Government Accounting Office, the Director and Deputy Director of the OTC Review estimated that the Review would not be completed until the year 2000.

During all this time, the FDA has refused to bring any enforcement actions against ineffective drugs, and it has brought only a handful of actions against drugs which its panels have found to be unsafe. Thus, the main beneficiary of the agency's policy has been and continues to be the drug industry, which can continue to market unsafe and ineffective OTC drugs until final monographs are issued, with virtually no risk of prosecution by the FDA. In some cases, the drug companies have reformulated their products to eliminate the unsafe or ineffective ingredients. But in many other cases, discussed throughout this book, the compainies have retained unsafe and ineffective ingredients, since those ingredients are often the sole basis for distinguishing among different brands of products.

In 1981, attorneys for Public Citizen Litigation Group filed a lawsuit against the FDA to challenge the new Category III regulation and to obtain a court order requiring the agency to expedite the OTC Review. The district court rejected their arguments, and the consumers have appealed that decision to the U.S. Court of Appeals for the District of Columbia Circuit.

However, even if Public Citizen Litigation Group succeeds in obtaining a court order requiring the FDA to speed up the OTC Review, many years will have passed before the agency begins enforcing the requirement that Congress adopted more than 20 years ago that drugs be safe and effective. Therefore, it is all the more important for consumers to learn as much as they can about over the counter drug ingredients so they can protect themselves from those which are unsafe and ineffective.